Pain Science · Yoga · Life

HANDSPRING
PUBLISHING
Edinburgh

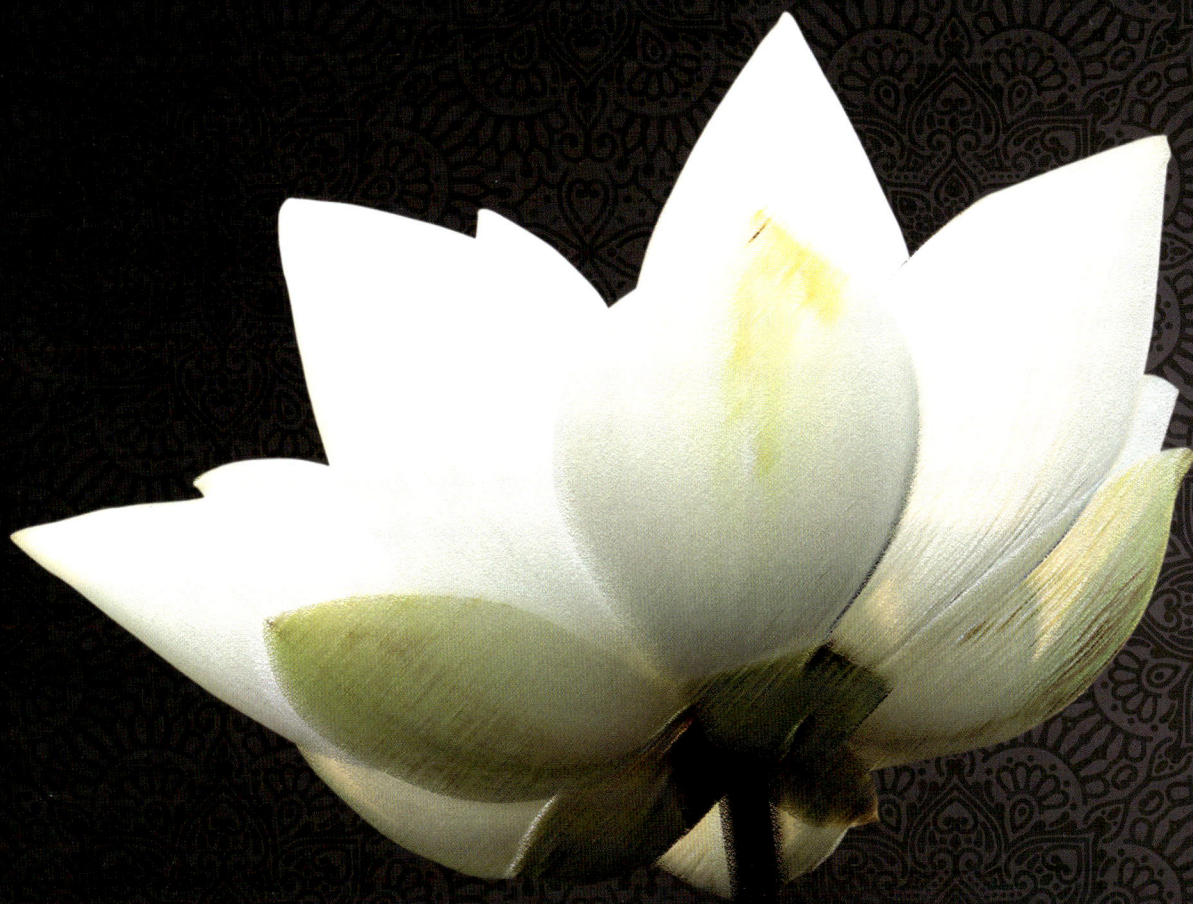

Pain Science · Yoga · Life

Bridging neuroscience and yoga for pain care

Niamh Moloney · Marnie Hartman

Forewords Tiffany Cruikshank · Gwendolen Jull

HANDSPRING PUBLISHING LIMITED
The Old Manse, Fountainhall,
Pencaitland, East Lothian
EH34 5EY, Scotland
Tel: +44 1875 341 859
Website: www.handspringpublishing.com

First published 2020 in the United Kingdom by Handspring Publishing

ISBN 978-1-912085-58-3
ISBN (Kindle eBook) 978-1-912085-62-0

British Library Cataloguing in Publication Data
A catalogue record for this book is available from the British Library

Library of Congress Cataloguing in Publication Data
A catalog record for this book is available from the Library of Congress

Notice
Neither the Publisher nor the Authors assume any responsibility for any loss or injury and/or damage to
persons or property arising out of or relating to any use of the material contained in this book. It is the
responsibility of the treating practitioner, relying on independent expertise and knowledge of the patient,
to determine the best treatment and method of application for the patient.

All reasonable efforts have been made to obtain copyright clearance for illustrations in the book for which
the authors or publishers do not own the rights. If you believe that one of your illustrations has been used
without such clearance please contact the publishers and we will ensure that appropriate credit is given in
the next reprint.

Commissioning Editor Sarena Wolfaard
Project Manager Morven Dean
Copy Editor Susan Stuart
Designer Bruce Hogarth
Indexer Aptara, India
Typesetter DSM Soft, India
Printer Melita, Malta

The
Publisher's
policy is to use
paper manufactured
from sustainable forests

CONTENTS

DEDICATION

To all who have crossed the bridge from pain and suffering back to life. Your resilience has taught us that moving beyond pain is possible. You have inspired us to develop deeper roots for teaching and facilitating others to embark on this journey.

FOREWORD *by Tiffany Cruikshank*

Pain is one of the most common reasons why people go to the doctor and turn to the practice of yoga. Especially important in a time when opioid addiction has reached into every community in the world, yoga offers us a precious drug-free alternative or adjunct that does more than just relieve pain. Yoga helps us build strength and mobility while also triggering innate biochemical mechanisms that can heal, soothe and break the pain feedback loop to strengthen our physical, mental and emotional resilience.

I have known Marnie for many years: first as a student, now as a trusted peer and colleague in the Yoga Medicine® community. All of us in this community feel it is our privilege to be part of our clients' care team. Thus, as teachers, when we engage in pain care, we must take seriously our responsibility to understand pain and to connect with people suffering from persistent pain. We must do this using science and research alongside the traditional yoga practices and simple themes of connection, loving kindness and acceptance. In *Pain Science Yoga Life,* Marnie and Niamh offer a powerful guide to holding both spaces at the same time, to give us the confidence that the results we see on the mat are also being demonstrated and supported in the current medical literature.

In the past several years, traditional practices that have been in existence for millennia have started to be validated by emerging research in neuroscience and neuroplasticity: how the nervous system continues to change its function to adapt to our circumstances throughout our lifespan. Research is now starting to support what we in the yoga world have always believed, on a bone-deep level: yoga *is* medicine.

What the science has given us is a great deal of detailed information and data about how the nervous system responds to yoga, thus offering us deep insights into the specific individual practices that can influence our pain. It has moved us from solely considering tissue health and pathology, to embracing and protecting structures, to a place where we appreciate broader factors that influence how our nervous system functions. In the last couple of decades, mainstream healthcare has increasingly been supporting and embracing the importance of lifestyle, positive psychology, emotional wellbeing, accurate and balanced information and perspectives on pain – all factors deeply embedded in yoga philosophy and practice.

In *Pain Science Yoga Life*, Marnie and Niamh fuse together this cutting-edge research on the science of pain and explore the practices that can be utilized in pain care. The structure of the book is unique in that Marnie and Niamh provide the direct connection between the medical research and its exploration on the mat, closing the loop and bringing the science back to daily life. *Pain Science Yoga Life* offers readers a strong, easy-to-grasp understanding of dense medical literature, seated in a keen awareness that both knowledge and compassion are important qualities in a caregiver working with people in pain. They recognize that knowledge, yoga and clinical pain care, used together or separately, are not supposed to stop at the mat or the clinic door. Marnie and Niamh eloquently guide us in combining all modalities together to help our clients build resilience and to move beyond pain, both on the mat and in their lives.

As caregivers we are always driven and guided by the Hippocratic Oath: first do no harm. In the delivery of any healthcare or teaching, even though our intentions may be sound, we all have the capacity to heal but also to harm. Yoga teaching is no different. Recognizing some of the areas where we might inadvertently contribute to pain, *Pain Science Yoga Life* provides guidance on how to watch out for these pitfalls, taking care in the use of our words and practices, as well as working within our scope of practice, so that we mindfully craft care that will not only do no harm but also help guide the healing process.

Ultimately, Marnie and Niamh help us to recognize that working with our patients deepens our own practice. We learn to see pain as part of our life experience and our humanness. Seeing pain from this perspective helps us realize that pain is not a problem to fix, escape from or get rid of – pain is a portal into our own inner lives, a lens through which we can grow our self-compassion, a way of connecting to the suffering inherent in all life, and an opportunity to grow. In *Pain Science Yoga Life*, Marnie and Niamh help us to tap into this deep inner well, to better help ourselves and our clients change our relationship with pain, thus altering our pain experiences, for life.

Tiffany Cruikshank LAc, MAOM, E-RYT
Founder of Yoga Medicine®
May 2020

Followers of the WHO Global Burden of Disease study are well aware of the personal and societal burden of chronic musculoskeletal pain disorders. Many people with chronic pain seek assistance to try to alleviate or manage their pain, to improve their quality of life. Assistance is sought from a variety of practitioners and considerable time and money is often invested in this venture. Thus interventions need to be accountable in terms of their evidence base and effectiveness.

Pain Science Yoga Life is a text which presents a novel integration of contemporary pain science into the philosophy and practice of yoga. If you are a clinician managing persons with chronic musculoskeletal pain or a yoga teacher having to adjust teachings and techniques to suit and assist people with chronic pain, then I suggest that this book is a must-read. The text is written by two physiotherapists who, between them, have a wealth of knowledge and expertise in pain research and clinical practice across both physiotherapy and yoga. This has produced a work with a unique cross-pollination of knowledge and practice which will add value to both yoga and physiotherapy practices in pain care.

The pain experience, especially in its chronic form, is complex. The authors have created a Pain Mandala in the form of a lotus flower. In eastern culture, the lotus is the symbolic representation of enlightenment. In this spirit, the Pain Mandala certainly enlightens the reader by clearly conceptualizing the multidimensionality of the human experience of pain. It is the road map for this text and helps the reader from the outset to appreciate the many factors that can influence an individual's health and wellbeing and their pain experience.

What I most definitely valued in the text was that the information presented was informative and well balanced, reflecting current research and knowledge in pain neuroscience and in the framework in which a person's pain experience is considered in contemporary practice. Physical, pathological and psychosocial contributors to the pain experience are all considered, together with their potential inter-relationships and moderating effects in the acute, subacute and chronic pain states. The text has been beautifully crafted and most chapters are presented in an engaging way under three headings: Headspace, Out of the Head and Onto the Mat, and Off the Mat and Into Life. Thus readers are provided with the current science and research base, which is then very adeptly translated into practice and daily activities. Many examples are provided, which applies the knowledge in practice. The individual nature of a person's pain experience has been emphasized throughout, which is so important to appreciate when developing physical and psychologically informed programs.

I read this text with only a very basic knowledge of yoga and its physical, mental and spiritual practices. Yet, as I soon learned and as this text has demonstrated, there are many synergies between yoga and the science and practice informing more traditional pain management approaches. For example, the current evidence base for the health benefits and hypoalgesic effects of exercise in pain management support the use of yoga asanas, and the benefits of Dhyana and Dharana are paralleled in many of the conventional cognitive behavior therapy approaches. I firmly believe that interventions for pain (or any other condition) must be accountable in terms of their evidence base. The evidence base for yoga currently, like many other interventions, is looking positive but not strong when put under the scrutiny of a systematic review. However, as illustrated in this text, many yoga practices can be regarded as research-informed, and the evidence base for yoga needs to be tested in future well-designed clinical trials that ask specific and relevant questions.

The authors aimed to explain the human experience of pain and to illustrate the contribution yoga may offer to change and positively assist an individual's pain experience. I think they have achieved this in a very readable book that is packed with both information and numerous clinical examples and applications. I commend this book, without reserve, to yoga teachers and practitioners using insights of yoga in the management of the patient in pain.

Gwendolen Jull AO, MPhty, PhD, FACP
Emeritus Professor in Physiotherapy
School of Health and Rehabilitation Science
The University of Queensland
Australia
May 2020

ACKNOWLEDGMENTS

Our heartfelt recognition and appreciation to the following, who reviewed various chapters of the book, scrutinized the content and offered insightful suggestions:

Dr Samantha Bunzli PhD, University of Melbourne, Australia

Dr Jean Byrne PhD, The Yoga Space, West Perth, Australia

Dr Kathryn Mills PhD, Macquarie University, Sydney, Australia

Narendar Nalajala, Consultant Physiotherapist, Ashford & St Peter's Hospitals NHS Foundation Trust, Ashford, UK

Edel O'Hagan MSc, Neuroscience Research Australia & Prince of Wales Clinical School, University of New South Wales, Australia

Dr Martin Rabey PhD, THRIVE Physiotherapy, Guernsey, UK

Dr Rob Schutze PhD, Curtin University, Perth, Australia

Associate Professor Jessica Van Oosterwijck PhD, Ghent University, Belgium

Professor Benedict Wand PhD, University of Notre Dame Australia, Fremantle, Australia

Also, warm regards to Anne Coates, BSc, PgD, THRIVE Physiotherapy, Guernsey, UK, and Rachel Saitzyk, BFA, CMT, Haines, Alaska, USA for their help with drafting illustrations, particularly the mandalas. And to John Hagen, Haines, Alaska, USA for photography.

Niamh's Acknowledgments

My deep fascination with pain has been influenced by many great minds. In somewhat of a chronological order my thanks go to: Claire O'Donnell, Lecturer, University College Dublin, for some early acknowledgments that pain was complex well before this was widely recognized in the field of physiotherapy. Ruth Magee, without whom I would never have considered staying in physiotherapy – you demonstrated a compassionate, knowledgeable and insightful approach to physiotherapy. David FitzGerald, for encouraging me to read and study as much as I could and for modeling that for me so well. Without doubt, my deepest gratitude extends to the late Max Zusman, who taught Pain Physiology during my Masters program at Curtin University, Perth. He was insightful, learned and practical, and taught us to really think about the effects of movement-based treatment in a physiological and behavioral way. To the late Bob Elvey, for being an inspirational clinician and teacher, for really making me think about what I was doing in clinical practice. To Peter O'Sullivan, for so much inspiration as a true 'clinician–researcher'. To David Butler and Lorimer Moseley: you've inspired me from a distance for many years through your writing, research and very witty repartee – thank you for making pain science so accessible and for helping me and many other teachers and clinicians translate pain science to the people we see every day and help them make sense of their pain. To Catherine Doody and Toby Hall, for your guidance during the formative years of my PhD, as I learned how to research and explore the world of pain science in more detail. And last but by no means least, to Marnie Hartman – what an incredible journey it's been. You've deepened my roots, built bridges and softened the edges and impacts, in this book, on this journey and into my life – thank you.

To the many, many inspiring yoga teachers I've had over the years who have shared nuggets of wisdom and facilitated me putting that into practice. You have served me in more ways than you can imagine and enabled me to serve others – thank you.

Heartfelt thanks to my friends and family for all your support over the writing of this book. Particular thanks to Kay Rabey and Ilze Jansone Briggs.

To my beautiful daughter Freya Seoda – you came into my life halfway through this project and have been busy ever since showing me how to live a more mindful, creative and open-hearted life. You are beautiful and joyful – a true treasure.

Finally, to my partner in life, parenting, clinical practice, research and teaching, Martin Rabey: you are more to me than you could ever imagine. You are a beautiful, loving companion, an inspirational clinician, and are wiser and more insightful that you ever give yourself credit for. Thank you for all of your support, emotionally and practically, from taking care of Freya when I needed to research and write, to proofreading those endless drafts – you inspire me every day to be a fuller me.

Marnie's Acknowledgments

It seems remiss if I start with anyone else but Niamh Moloney – you are a great teacher. Through all the highs and lows with the heavy weight of research, you remained true to your mission – all pain information shared must have a strong foundation in evidence. Thank you for leading (sometimes dragging) me down this path. And to Martin Rabey: you are so much more than our 'twaddle meter'.

My warmest gratitude goes to all the teachers, mentors, patients, friends and family who have walked in my life. It is they who paved the way for me to be the teacher, clinician and human I am today. Most of you know who you are and the special place you hold in my life and heart. I'd like to bow to a specific few whose seemingly endless faith, support and leadership either directly or indirectly gave me all I needed to participate in, and complete, the writing of this book. In no particular order, I bow in gratitude to each of you: Lorimer Moseley, Adriaan Louw, Jim Clover, Ashleigh Reed, Russ Lyman, Phillip Saunders, Beth MacCready, Andrew Cardella, Janine Allen, the Bombers, Russell Kennedy, my family, and as a whole: the community of Haines, Alaska. I'll close with a special note of appreciation for Kris Miller – thank you, dear one, for your patience.

ABOUT THE AUTHORS

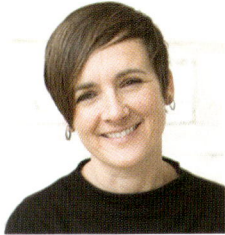

Niamh Moloney (PhD, MManipTh, BPhysio, SMISCP) is a Specialist Musculoskeletal Physiotherapist, Yoga Teacher and Pain Researcher. She practices in Guernsey, in the Channel Islands, but also holds an Honorary Fellow position with Macquarie University, Sydney, where she was previously a Senior Lecturer. A passionate advocate of evidence-based practice, she has over 50 peer-reviewed publications from her pain-related research. Her increasing appreciation of how yoga philosophy and practices can help address some of the complex aspects of pain and its care has led her to integrate yoga into her clinical practice and has ultimately inspired the writing of this book. She runs pain education and yoga courses for people with persistent pain, and teaches widely to healthcare professionals.

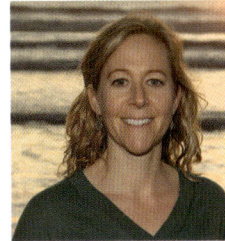

Marnie Hartman (DPT, CSCS, RYT) is a Doctor of Physical Therapy, a Certified Strength and Conditioning Specialist and Registered Yoga Teacher. Her drive for compassionate, authentic interactions and connection to the good in all humans and the wild led her to a simple life and challenging practice in the bush community of Haines, Alaska. It was here that she first developed an interest in learning how to care for those in persistent pain. She quickly realized the supportive container yoga held for people engaging in pain care. She has incorporated pain science education and yoga as part of her clinical care and teaching for nearly a decade. Marnie owns and operates a private physical therapy and yoga practice, and has been an instructor for the International Spine and Pain Institute, and an Education Contributor for Yoga Medicine.

You can connect with Niamh and Marnie through their website painscienceyogalife.com.

*We all come into this world with the need for **connection, protection** and a sense of **freedom**.*

Esther Perel

INTRODUCTION

Pain is a primary *protection* response; it is normal and necessary. Yoga offers us an opportunity to *connect* first to ourselves, and then to the world around us. When we yoke the two of these together (protection and connection) we may gain *freedom* from persistent pain. Welcome to *Pain Science Yoga Life*, a passage through the science of pain, blended with the art and science of yoga to help bridge the gap that exists between a person in pain and their ability to move beyond suffering and back to life. It also aims to bridge the gap between clinicians and yoga teachers. It was the identification of these two gaps that first sparked the composition of this book.

When we, Niamh and Marnie, met in 2010 at the Neuro Orthopaedic Institute (NOI) pain conference, it was clear from the start that we were kindred spirits. We reunited again at NOI's second conference in 2012. It was there that the conversation about using yoga for pain care began. As our studies and clinical experiences deepened, the connection between yoga and pain became more and more apparent to us; however, these gaps seemed so vast it was difficult to determine the best way to start constructing a bridge. Should it be a research project? Hmm...ideas were floated, but what about what is available now? So, we decided to take a little inspiration from others, particularly our teachers and mentors: why not marry what we know or can learn from the currently available research with our clinical experience and experience as yoga practitioners and teachers and put it in a book? Maybe we can inspire a few clinicians and teachers to test our question – *Can yoga offer a helpful bridge to those who are stuck on the suffering side of pain to cross back into life?* You didn't know you were signing up for such a challenge and joining our tribe when you opened this book, did you? That's OK because we have faith in you. You wouldn't have picked up this book and started reading the introduction if you weren't up for such a challenge. So, let's get into it.

Who this book is for – the tribe members

1. The yoga teacher who has a special interest in working with individuals who are struggling with pain.

2. The clinician who is curious about the art and science of yoga and how it might be used in pain care.

3. Anyone interested. No previous training or education is required to process the information presented. All you need is an open mind and sense of curiosity.

Mindset for the tribe

Be curious, be kind, be open, be ready to learn, accept challenges to pre-existing knowledge, and lastly be ready to practice for yourself, before teaching or caring for others.

Helpful Knowledge: Pain Science Overview

Pain *is* critical for survival; however, pain can also cause suffering and impact our ability to participate in a full life. Until relatively recently, pain was considered a good indicator of tissue damage or disease. This perspective has shifted and continues to evolve. While the state of the tissues is important, other contributions to pain, ranging from general health to mood, social engagement and environment, all influence the experience of pain and are key targets for moving beyond pain. People will have their own perspectives on pain, due to their culture, history, profession and knowledge base.

The experience of pain varies. It ranges from a degree of unpleasantness to terrible suffering and disability. While we all experience pain, the sad fact is that millions of people, approximately 20% of the global population, suffer from persistent pain.[1] UK statistics indicate higher rates of 35–51%.[2] Pain-related disability associated with conditions like persistent back pain now ranks as the leading cause of disability globally.[3] Persistent pain can have far-reaching effects for the individual on personal suffering, shifting the sense of self, relationships, living a life with a sense of value, financial stability, ability to work and provide for self and family, and on and on. Fundamentally, each individual is on their own unique pain journey – each person in pain has their own unique past, story, diagnosis, and contributing factors to their pain and suffering. The impact of pain on people's lives demands that we continue to improve how we understand and treat pain. As yoga is the study of self and living with awareness, and encompasses philosophies and tools to facilitate this and to promote self-regulation, it may provide a vehicle to improve wellbeing and move beyond pain.

What to Expect and How to Approach this Book

While this book is written to be read in sequence, we appreciate that readers might find themselves drawn to different topics and may wish to read individual chapters. However, the first three chapters of this book lay down foundational information that is threaded through the rest of the chapters, so we recommend you read these three chapters as well

as the case study of 'Phillip' first before delving further.

Chapter 1 will build a foundation on the neurobiology of pain – what happens in your body when you have a pain experience. We will explore a little history and how we have come to understand pain, and introduce models of pain to help deepen your understanding. You will be introduced to what we call the *Pain Mandala*. We developed this model to capture a multidimensional picture of the pain experience and mechanisms that appear to drive it. We haven't covered every dimension possible, nor every mechanism, but we hope it's enough to get you thinking broadly. In Chapters 2 and 3, we describe yoga and mindfulness principles that we weave into the context of pain care. There are many aspects of yoga we have not covered; however, we hope to set a scene to demonstrate bridges between yoga and pain care. We encourage you to include your own yoga and/or pain care knowledge to build even more bridges.

Through the remaining chapters, we take several elements important to pain and describe each in more detail. We have addressed key elements we frequently see when using yoga as part of pain care. The topics covered range from physical aspects of pain, psychological aspects, sleep and how we perceive our body. We will relate each chapter area back to the Pain Mandala and explore how each element fits within the broader pain landscape. (And, although we use the first person singular when writing about specific experiences, the 'I' refers to either of us.)

There are other aspects that may be relevant for a person in pain which we have not covered, e.g. trauma, diet and nutrition, specific pathologies and many others. Our decisions to include or exclude should not be interpreted as some sort of hierarchy but as a reflection of our own scope of practice in writing this book.

Chapters 4–9 are divided into three sections: 1) Headspace; 2) Out of the Head and Onto the Mat; and 3) Off the Mat and Into Life.

Headspace

The biology of pain as we know it will be explored, along with evidence available for yoga and mindfulness traditions or philosophies. This does not come without its limitations. For example, yoga is increasingly being studied from an empirical perspective, but much of this scientific research is at an early stage. Therefore, many times we highlight that not enough is known from an evidence-based perspective at this point. This does not mean that we should completely discount the possibilities of yoga's effects, but sometimes we simply cannot confidently advocate for certain interventions, right now. This may change. We also regularly lean on evidence from the fields of pain science, physical therapies and growing data on mindfulness and meditation practices to explain some of the possible effects of yoga. It is important to acknowledge that when we extrapolate these results to imply their potential benefits, we often do not actually know yet whether we will see the same responses using yoga as the intervention – we are simply pointing out similarities and considering the potential that may exist for these effects from yoga. There are two specific factors that are almost impossible to really study using research. The first is the connection or direct interaction that occurs between the clinician or teacher and the person in pain and how this influences pain and recovery. The second is that yoga is a practice to be fostered over a lifetime – studying the effects of short courses of yoga is important, but may not show us what is possible if we commit to regular, sustained and evolving practice. With these considerations in mind, we encourage an open approach as we step out onto the bridge between yoga and science.

Fundamentally, yoga teaches us to study our self; through this study we learn to be vulnerable and authentic. As professionals and caregivers, when we are able to be curious and vulnerable, we are able to set the stage for those seeking pain care to do the same. Thus, you will be asked to practice, which brings us to the next two sections of each chapter.

Out of the Head and Onto the Mat; Off the Mat and Into Life

The second and third sections of each chapter are for your practice: in these we will be putting the knowledge shared from 'Headspace' into a specific yoga practice (onto the mat) and then into daily life. They are directed to the reader as the practitioner: as a clinician or teacher, you may be tempted to skip this practice and simply share it with your patient or client. We strongly encourage you to first try each practice to experience it for yourself from your own perspective. With your mind clear of those you provide care for, be your own subject. There is something to be gained in each exercise, regardless of the amount or duration of pain one has experienced. If you are a person in persistent pain you may find it best to take on these practices with the assistance of a teacher or clinician, and know that shifts may happen slowly and only with consistent attention. Physical, mental or emotional responses may come up during the practice that may benefit from further explanation and guided exploration.

Without taking on the actual practice, this book will only offer the reader knowledge. Knowledge without practice loses its worth: it is what you do with the knowledge gained that can change your perspective and the way you choose to live, and this can greatly impact the care we give and receive.

These practices are based on information gained from evidence-based research, yoga training, clinical practice with patients, practice with yoga students and personal yoga practices. Individually they have not been specifically studied and therefore may not be fully supported by empirical evidence. Consider using them, teaching them and prescribing them as a practice of getting to know the self. The more you practice, the more you will know and understand your own needs at any given moment. Encouraging those around you to do the same can only benefit the therapeutic exchange.

A Note About Armoring

We use the term 'armoring' to demonstrate the potential of being on the defensive – physically, emotionally or in thought. Like pain, armoring can be a protective response, sometimes helpful and sometimes not. There may be times along the way where you will want to disregard what you are reading. When you sense this armoring, choose to take a pause and breathe. We might notice what arises for us when our thoughts and beliefs are challenged, or a different perspective is

offered. Do we hold onto our previous ideas or beliefs with vigor? Can we allow our perspective to shift with integrity, knowing that what we have learned may hold some truth, and that other valuable perspectives exist? Can we make space for another viewpoint or accept that all of this may change again in the future? This might be a struggle for some but we believe this struggle is worth the investment of time and energy. The people we work with may also demonstrate the tendency to armor, question and reject, as a reaction to education regarding pain, or attempts at using mindfulness or yoga as part of their care plan. When we play with leaning in and changing our own reactions, we may improve our ability to identify and assist others to do this as well.

Thank you for reading *Pain Science Yoga Life*.

References

1. Goldberg, D.S. and S.J. McGee. Pain as a Global Public Health Priority. BMC Public Health, 2011. 11: 770.

2. Fayaz, A., P. Croft, R.M. Langford, et al. Prevalence of Chronic Pain in the UK: A Systematic Review and Meta-Analysis of Population Studies. BMJ Open, 2016. 6(6): e010364.

3. GBD 2016 Disease and Injury Incidence and Prevalence Collaborators. A Global, Regional, and National Incidence, Prevalence, and Years Lived with Disability for 328 Diseases and Injuries for 195 Countries, 1990-2016: A Systematic Analysis for the Global Burden of Disease Study 2016. Lancet, 2017. 390(10100): 1211–59.

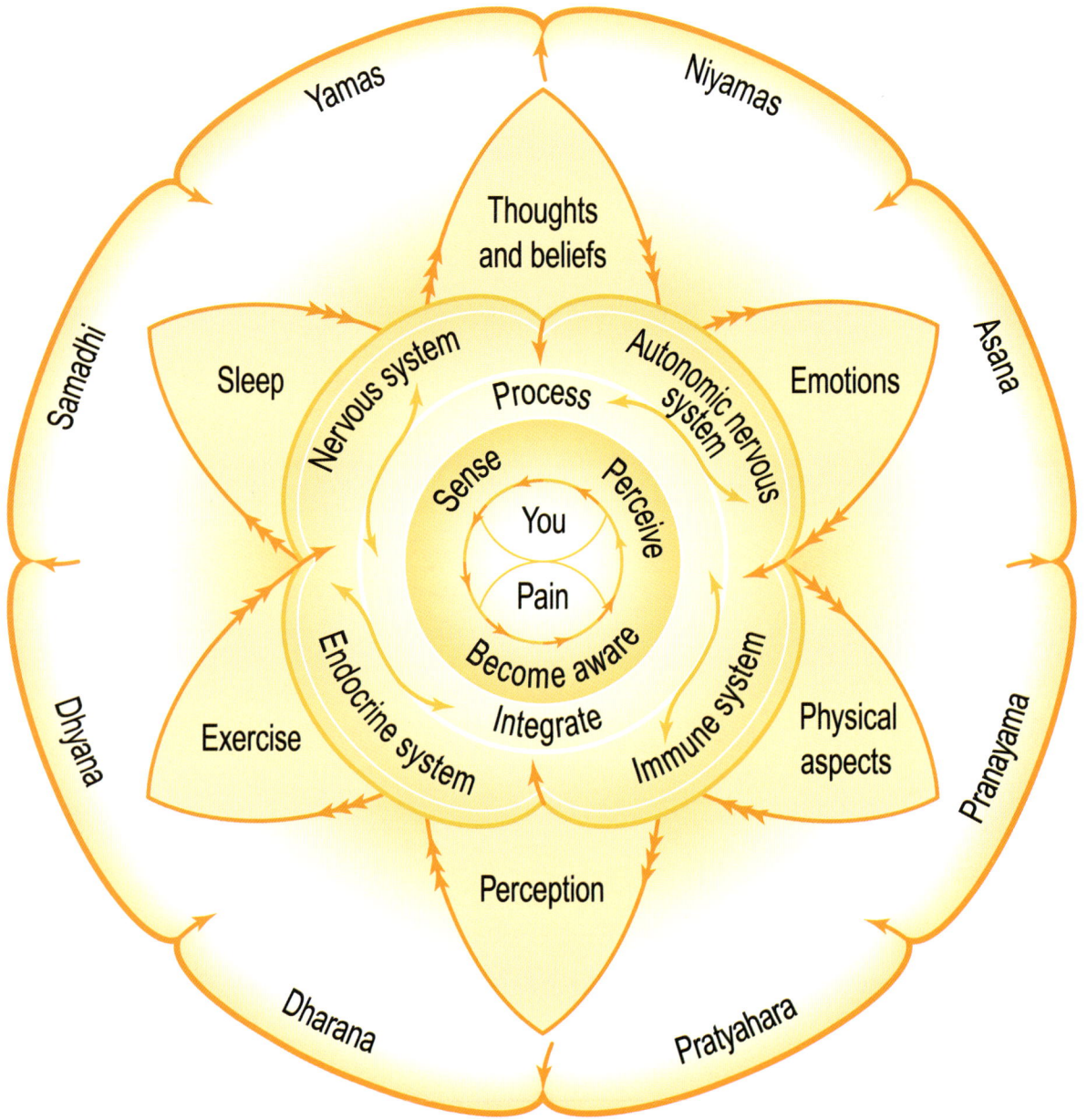

1

When your roots run deep there is no reason to fear the wind.

African proverb

Perception of Threat and Protection by Pain

Pain is a key protective mechanism, critical for our survival. However, our understanding of pain has evolved considerably over the years. We now appreciate that rather than being a sole measure of tissue damage, pain has many contributions – from how we think, to the culture we live in. How is this possible? In this chapter we explore the roots of neuroscience to explain how inputs from many dimensions of life and health underpin our pain experiences.

The currently accepted definition of pain is that: "Pain is an unpleasant sensory and emotional experience associated with actual or potential tissue damage, or described in terms of such damage."[1] So, rather than just being a measure of tissue damage, pain is a protective response produced by our brain and nervous system, whenever we, or our tissues, are under threat, or perceive ourselves (consciously or unconsciously) to be under threat.[1,2] This is important to bear in mind as we continue this journey into pain and its care because any credible sign that we are under threat can generate a pain response.[3] These 'cues for protection' or 'inputs' can relate to tissue problems, as commonly considered. However, 'inputs' aren't limited to the tissues; they can also arise from our thoughts, mood, sleep, body perception, physical activity and environment. We will continue to use the terms 'cues for protection' or 'inputs' to describe these contributions.

While the formal definition of pain reflects the present understanding of pain science and is applicable to all pain experiences, minor or major, ask a person disabled by persistent pain if they think that 'pain is an unpleasant sensory and emotional experience' and they may feel short-changed, given the impact of pain on their lives.

As we continue, we aim to honor the science underpinning the current understanding of pain, while including the scope of the human experience that pain and its associated suffering bring. As we will explain, traditional models of pain are limited in their ability to address pain fully: hence understanding the complexity of pain from a more holistic viewpoint and using multidimensional and broader approaches to pain care are increasingly advocated.

The Traditional Model of Pain

Let's start the journey toward a modern understanding of pain by looking at some historical perspectives that have led to our current knowledge. The traditional understanding of pain is embedded in what's called the *Biomedical Model* of pain. This model suggests a discoverable disease process or pathological source of pain can be identified, and that once identified, can be treated, leading to resolution of pain.[4] This might include inflammation, arthritis, muscle tears, disc problems, or other diseases of the tissues or organs: in other words, tissue inputs. This idea that the source of pain is directly related to tissue changes emanates from a model of pain proposed by René Descartes in 1664.[5] Descartes proposed that when tissues were damaged, a nerve signal was sent from the tissues to a pain center in the brain. This ultimately meant that: 1) pain emanated from the tissues; and 2) pain was registered in a specific center in the brain. This is a linear approach to understanding pain and, because it maintains a primary focus on 'finding and fixing' a tissue source, it can limit options for pain care. There is of course a lot of merit in examining the tissues to explain pain. For example, if someone presents to a clinician with back pain, it is reasonable to screen for signs that the pain indicates something serious, or is linked with specific pathology that might warrant further screening with scans or blood tests, or, indeed, surgery. However, back pain associated with serious causes occurs less than 1% of the time, and specific pathology that requires surgery occurs in less than 10% of cases.[6,7]

A next step in clinical practice for the remaining 90% of cases is to look at how the pain is behaving. Traditionally, this has meant looking for a 'mechanical pattern' associated with back pain, i.e. pain that might be attributable to physical stressors and how the muscles, joints and nerves of the spine are responding. While there is nothing wrong with this, the problem is that for many people this is where the examination ends, with failure to recognize broader contributions to pain by both the individual and the clinician. Studies that investigate the extent to which pathology explains pain demonstrate that the contribution from pathology is actually more limited than was once considered, and that pain is more complex.[8-11] Without a broader understanding of the person, and how the pain experience works, explanations for back pain in the 90% of people with 'non-specific back pain' will fall short. Explaining pathological or mechanical terms or using vague terms of reassurance like 'There's nothing serious wrong' simply won't cover the whole of what is happening and thus will likely leave people frustrated and suffering.

While Descartes's theory was revolutionary at the time, it is fair to say that the science of pain has moved on dramatically. Here are a few ways in which the biomedical model of pain fails to serve many people:

- It relies on finding a 'source' of pain and fixing it. Studies show this isn't always possible, and our confidence in attributing pain to identified pathology is waning, given that so-called 'pathology' is common among people *without* pain.

- It separates the mind from the body and focuses solely on physical contributions. Failing to recognize wider contributions means that important factors (e.g. sleep, mood, stress, relationships, environment) are often ignored, potentially leading to poorer outcomes.

- When a clear pathological or biological source cannot be identified, persistent pain can become stigmatized as 'all in the head' or associated with drug-seeking.

- It can lead to unnecessary investigations and consultations.

- It often perpetuates 'passive' treatments aimed at addressing tissue sources, and facilitates more rest than is healthy.

- It often perpetuates beliefs that the body is weak and easy to damage, and must be protected, and often does not support beliefs that the body is strong, resilient and capable of healing.

Changing Tides in Understanding Pain

In the late 19th and early 20th centuries, the theory that there is a specific pathway for pain prevailed. Some researchers such as von Frey and Goldscheider (cited by Melzack and Wall[12]) noted that certain nerve fibers reacted to particular sensations, and that some nerve fibers preferentially responded to noxious stimulation, i.e. intense, potentially harmful inputs. These fibers originally became known as pain fibers, and some argued that this was evidence that specific pain pathways existed. This reinforced the biomedical model of pain.

However, the tide was about to turn. During World War II an anesthetist, Henry Knowles Beecher, made some startling observations. Comparing his role serving in the war to his previous job as Chief of Anesthesia at Massachusetts General Hospital, he noted a decreased need for morphine among soldiers awaiting evacuation.[13] The soldiers certainly had equally severe injuries as the patients he had previously treated, so this was a first clue that context was important for pain: perhaps awaiting evacuation was less of a 'threat' and therefore there was less need to 'protect'? This was one of the earliest records of *psychological contributions to pain* and Beecher went on to champion research into placebo effects in pain.

Placebo research continued to grow post World War II, and placebo-controlled trials are now the gold standard for many forms of medical research. Placebo-controlled research highlights that people often demonstrate positive responses to 'inert' interventions, simply because they think they have been treated. This shows the power of psychological contributions to pain and pain relief. When we think we have been treated, cognitive and emotional cues for protection may lessen and therefore the brain no longer needs to produce pain to protect us.

Another major milestone in the evolution of our understanding of pain came from Ronald Melzack and Patrick Wall. They proposed the *Gate Control Theory of Pain* in 1965.[12] To understand what they showed, we need to briefly introduce the concept of nociception. Nociception, from the Latin *nocere*, to harm or hurt, translates in this context as 'danger detection'. Nociceptors are nerve endings that respond to noxious (potentially harmful) cues like intense pressure, extreme temperatures or changes in chemistry, and which then generate a signal. These were essentially what earlier researchers had called pain fibers. Nociceptive signals are the warning signals these nerves transmit. Based on a series of experiments, Melzack and Wall demonstrated that the intensity of nociceptive (warning) signals from the tissues could be 'turned down' at the spinal cord. They showed that if sensory fibers responding to touch and vibration were stimulated at the same time as nociceptors, this could inhibit the nociception. They likened this to a gate that could be opened or closed, i.e. facilitating or

blocking these warning signals being projected to the brain.

Therapies like electrical stimulation (e.g. TENS units) and spinal cord stimulators were developed as a result, and we began to understand the mechanisms underlying traditional therapies like massage and manual therapy. This challenged the idea that pain directly originated from the tissues, in that Melzack and Wall's research highlighted that warning signals could be adjusted along their pathways, and that sensory inputs interact with one another. So, the sensations a person experiences weren't only a result of 'tissue inputs'. While the evidence was yet to evolve, Melzack and Wall also proposed that descending influences from the brain existed that could open or close the gate, e.g. psychological influences. This aligned with Beecher's findings and the placebo research that was emerging at the time.

> Nociception: perception of harm or danger detection.[2]
>
> Noci: 'harm' from the Latin *nocere*, to harm; ception: from the word perception.

Moving into the latter part of the 20th century, the *Biopsychosocial Model* became more widely advocated throughout health care. This proposed that illness be considered from the perspective of having biological, psychological and social contributions, all culminating in the impacts and suffering associated with the illness or disease[14] (Figure 1.1). This was subsequently applied to pain.[15] Gatchel[16] later outlined *how* biological, psychological and social interactions could lead to processes that could drive ill-health. Peripheral inputs from tissue injury and inflammation were considered to interact with hormonal, immune and stress systems, as well as mood, thoughts and beliefs. Feedback loops between these systems are increasingly recognized, influenced by social contexts and environmental factors.

Chapter 1

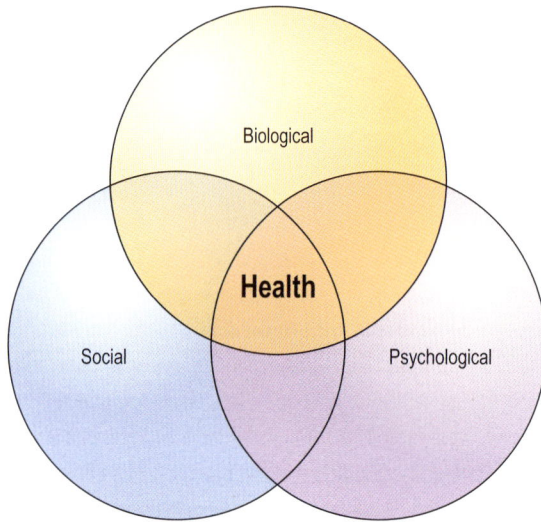

Figure 1.1

The Biopsychosocial Model of health. This diagram illustrates the interconnection of biological, psychological and social aspects that contribute to our health.

As recognition of complex interactions of bodily systems with psychology, emotions and social contexts increased, a number of important models for understanding pain emerged. The *Neuromatrix Model* was proposed by Ronald Melzack in 1999,[17] which elaborated on biopsychosocial interactions and proposed that the body-self neuromatrix (a conscious awareness of the self) activates perceptual, homeostatic and behavioral responses following injury, pathology or chronic stress. Around the same time Louis Gifford proposed the *Mature Organism Model* (more on p.20)[18]: that the mature organism (human) has to scrutinize and make sense of many inputs (e.g. from tissues, thoughts and beliefs) and produce many outputs (e.g. muscle tension, immune and hormonal responses), including pain when under threat. Specifically, we have to 'sample' our environment, 'scrutinize' it and then produce appropriate responses for our survival. Both models highlight the circular nature of inputs

and responses, as they start to interact and the effects accumulate.

Ultimately, a more contemporary understanding of pain considers multiple health and social contributions and numerous physiological processes and interactions. Key to this is that pain is a protective response produced by our brain and nervous system, whenever we are under threat or perceive ourselves to be under threat.[1,2] This perception of threat might arise from various inputs – from tissues, thoughts and beliefs, mood, our society, etc. Further, pain responses occur in tandem with responses from other biological systems and these interact. In doing so, the 'whole response' will often be greater than the sum of the parts. As one of my patients said as he reflected that his back pain was less related to spinal pathology and more about stress, lack of sleep and a sensitive nervous system: "What you're saying is that the problem is in the software in my case, and not just the hardware." Maybe this is a nice analogy – our body tissues/structures are the hardware but our physiology is the software. They both contribute to the 'output' or experience of pain.

While these contemporary models of pain are increasingly advocated, there are large barriers to implementation. Commonly held beliefs about pain (what we think we have always known) are often more aligned with a biomedical model ('find it and fix it') of pain than a biopsychosocial model. To improve pain care, it is imperative that the wider population, clinicians and teachers recognize a broader approach to understanding and working with pain. So, let's deepen the roots of our pain knowledge and dive into the nervous system to learn more about how pain emerges.

Pain Processing

In this section we'll explain: 1) how inputs from tissues can generate warning signals; 2) how events in our nervous system can cause these signals to be turned up or down; 3) how interactions within the brain drive our pain experience; and 4) briefly how the brain and nervous system interact with our immune and hormonal systems to shape pain and related physiological responses.

A Brief Look at Pain Science in Life

Picture this: you're out walking a trail and you roll your ankle. It hurts! You can see your ankle is swelling and when you try to put weight on it, it's really painful. Clearly, you've sprained your ankle and the injury has caused some inflammation. So, you assume that the pain you're experiencing is coming from your ankle. Here's the thing: pain itself can't biologically *come from* your ankle. It is more a product of your nervous system, and as a lived experience is complex, even with this simple acute injury.

When you roll your ankle, nociception occurs: nociceptors detect the intense pressure and are activated, sending warning signals from your ankle to your spinal cord and on to your brain to warn that your ankle has been stretched and that there is a potential threat to your ankle tissues. The important thing is, this isn't pain at this point; nociception is simply a warning that there is some *potential* threat in the body.[2,19,20] Warning signs are just that, a warning. Despite what Descartes and early pain researchers thought, pain receptors don't exist! These warning signals are relayed through your spinal cord and from there projected to the brain. In the spinal cord, they can be modulated – turned up or down before they are sent on their way to the brain. In the brain, a cascade of communication occurs as it integrates these warning signals from your tissues with knowledge about the situation you are in, your prior experiences, memories, thoughts, concerns. Your clever brain then orchestrates a response. This can result in pain, hopping around, rubbing your ankle, limping back to your car, and if you think it's bad enough, seeking medical help. Let's keep this example in mind as we look at the science underpinning this.

The Nervous System and Nociception

Let's start by looking at the structure and function of our nervous system, starting with our peripheral nerves (Figure 1.2).

Receptors: In our skin and tissues we have receptors and free nerve endings that respond to various stimuli: changes in temperature, tissue chemistry and pressure.[21] Remember, pain receptors don't exist. When our receptors detect a change in temperature, pressure (force, changes in movement, tension) or tissue chemistry (e.g. inflammation), they can stimulate nerve fibers by opening channels on the nerve (called ion channels), which generates a signal, called an action potential.[21] This signal is then transmitted through neurons to the spinal cord and can be projected to the brain. When there is intense (noxious) pressure, extreme cold or heat, or noxious changes in tissue chemistry, warning signals can occur: nociception. Not all stimuli result in action potentials, though, as the stimulus needs to be sufficiently intense. Our receptors are being stimulated continually but only some of this stimulation results in nerve signals.

Nerve fibers: Sensory nerves that relay signals to the spinal cord are divided into four main types:

1. Aα (A alpha): relay information about joint or muscle position and are known as proprioceptive fibers.

2. Aβ (A beta): relay information about touch, light pressure or vibration.

3. Aδ (A delta): relay information about temperature and noxious pressure. Noxious pressure means pressure that is intense and potentially harmful and the resultant signal can be considered a warning signal.

4. C: relay signals about any noxious (potentially harmful) input.[21]

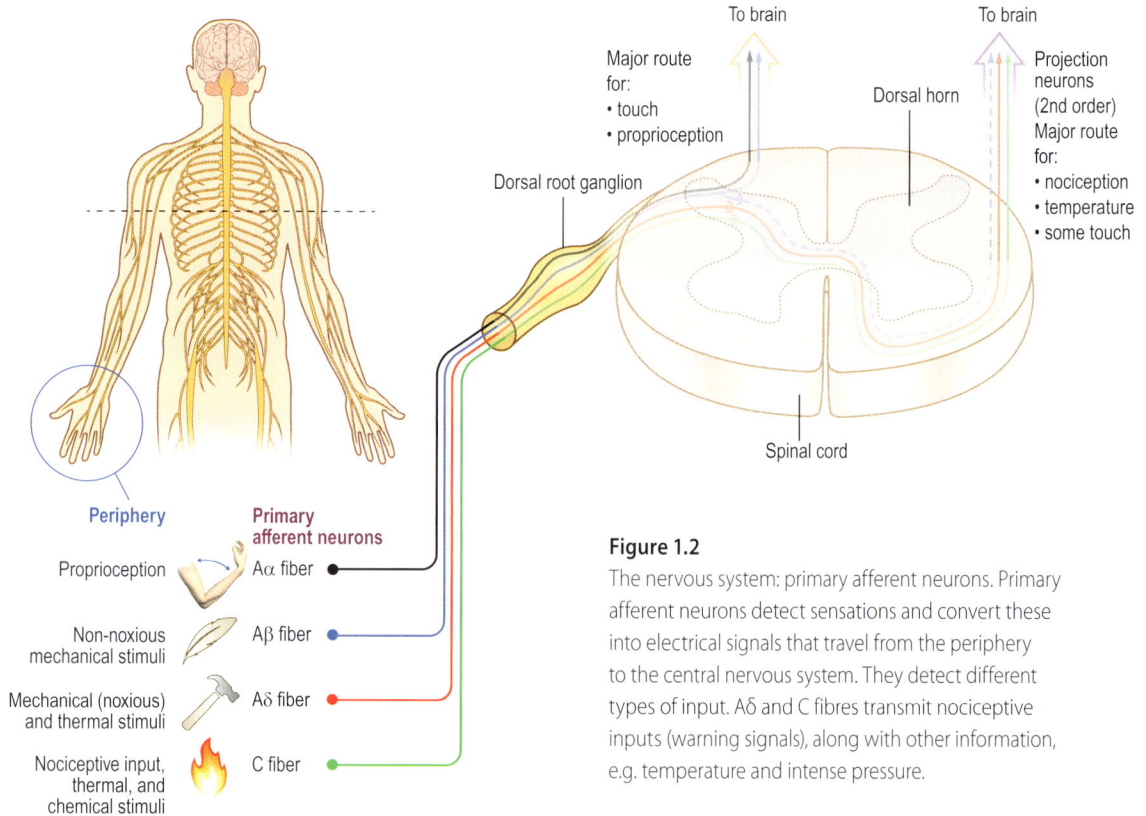

Figure 1.2

The nervous system: primary afferent neurons. Primary afferent neurons detect sensations and convert these into electrical signals that travel from the periphery to the central nervous system. They detect different types of input. Aδ and C fibres transmit nociceptive inputs (warning signals), along with other information, e.g. temperature and intense pressure.

None of these nerves actually transmits 'pain', but Aδ and C fibers are called nociceptive fibers because they preferentially transmit 'warning' signals.[20]

Spinal Cord and Brain

As nociceptive signals are relayed through the nervous system to the brain, they synapse (communicate) with 'projection' neurons in the spinal cord[20] (Figure 1.3). These neurons then relay or 'project' information to the brain. Let's look at the basic structure of the synapse – where one neuron communicates with another (Figure 1.4). Synapses in the spinal cord are gaps between incoming neurons and projection neurons. When incoming signals reach the terminal of the neuron, they cause the release of neurotransmitters (chemical messengers), which diffuse across the synapse. On the receiving end of the projection neurons are ion channels which, when activated by the right neurotransmitters, open and allow a signal to be projected onwards within the nervous system. At these synapses, inhibitory interneurons also exist. These release neurotransmitters that calm the synapse down after some activity (signaling and transmission described above) has occurred.[22,23] Think of your synapse like a gathering at your home. The neurotransmitters are your guests, the ion channels are the doors into your home and the inhibitory interneurons are your sensible friends who turn the music down. When our nervous system is working well, there is a nice balance between excitation and inhibition at synapses. The gathering doesn't get out of control.

From the spinal cord, sensory information can be projected to the brain.[24] To ensure our survival and protection, sensory information must be interpreted by the brain and responses generated when needed.

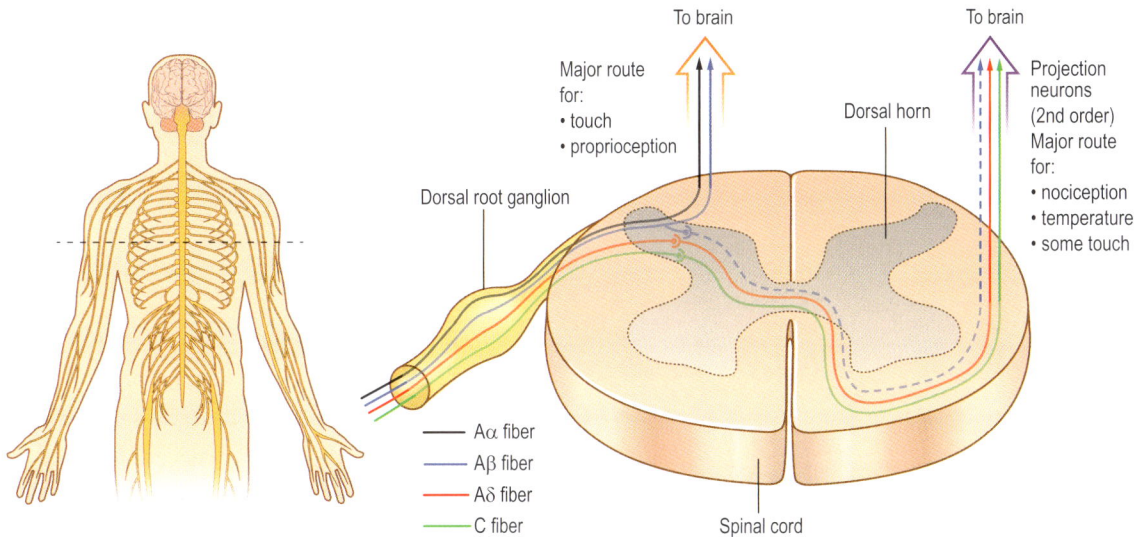

To brain

To brain

Major route
for:
• touch
• proprioception

Projection
neurons
(2nd order)
Major route
for:
• nociception
• temperature
• some touch

Dorsal horn

Dorsal root ganglion

—— Aα fiber
—— Aβ fiber
—— Aδ fiber
—— C fiber

Spinal cord

Figure 1.3

The nervous system: dorsal root ganglion and projection neurons. Information from the periphery is relayed to the brain via the dorsal root ganglion, part of our spinal cord. Here, information about nociception, temperature and intense pressure (along with some touch) crosses the midline and 'synapses' with projection neurons (also called second-order neurons). They carry the information to the brain. Information about touch and proprioception is carried further into the central nervous system before synapsing with its second-order neurons.

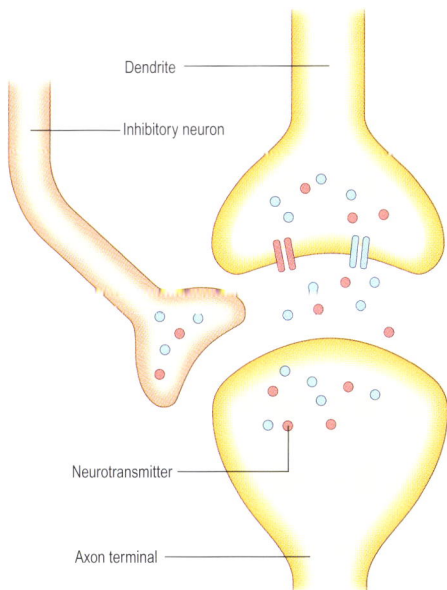

Dendrite

Inhibitory neuron

Neurotransmitter

Axon terminal

Figure 1.4

The nervous system: synapse. This synapse demonstrates how nerves communicate with one another. At the axon terminal, neurotransmitters are released which open ion channels on neighboring neurons. This communication can be modulated by inhibitory neurons via the release of more neurotransmitters that have a calming effect on the synapse.

11

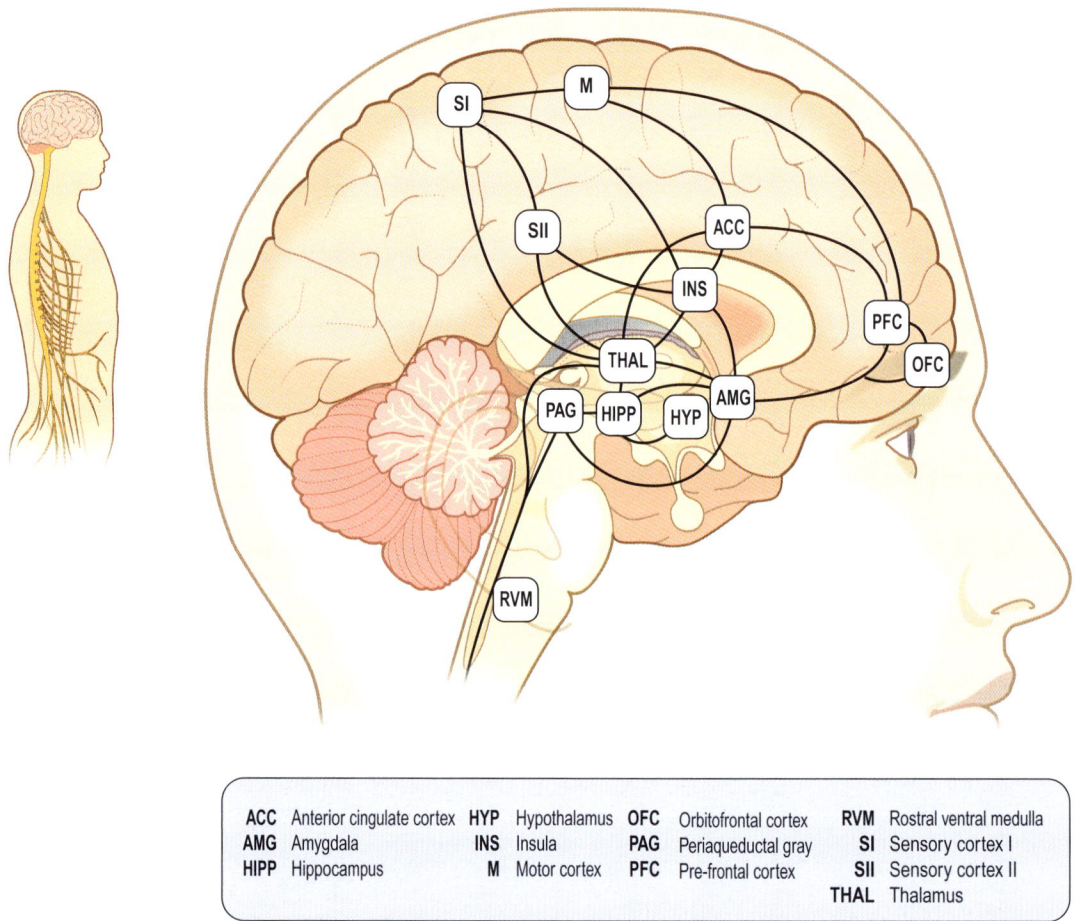

ACC	Anterior cingulate cortex	**HYP** Hypothalamus	**OFC** Orbitofrontal cortex	**RVM**	Rostral ventral medulla
AMG	Amygdala	**INS** Insula	**PAG** Periaqueductal gray	**SI**	Sensory cortex I
HIPP	Hippocampus	**M** Motor cortex	**PFC** Pre-frontal cortex	**SII**	Sensory cortex II
				THAL	Thalamus

Figure 1.5

The nervous system: brain and brain stem. The above areas indicate regions of the brain known to be activated during a pain experience. These include regions responsible for sensation, motor planning and execution, as well as emotions, memories and cognition. All of these areas come together to process whether potential threat exists and can produce pain as an output.

The relay of warning signals to the brain, and subsequent activation of multiple brain areas, allow us to respond appropriately at a physiological level, as well as at cognitive and emotional levels. Functional MRI (fMRI) scans of the brain can map activity in different parts of the brain in real time. During pain experiments or pain experiences, fMRI scans demonstrate activation of and connectivity between many different brain areas during a pain experience.[25] Figure 1.5 outlines those areas of the brain known to be activated during pain.[26–29]

The relay of information to our sensory cortices (somatosensory cortex I and II – SI and SII) allows us to localize where the signals are coming from. Activation of the limbic system or 'emotional brain' causes us to react (mostly unconsciously) to protect ourselves.[30] In detecting potential danger (when we rolled our ankle), we behave in protective ways like hopping, taking the weight off our leg or rubbing the ankle when we have a sprain. These initial actions are all largely driven by the limbic system,[30] but of course they involve movement and hence our motor cortex too. Activation of the limbic system causes us to feel emotions around the experience – it adds emotional context to the sensory information.[31-33] Now we might feel anxious or worried. This response can drive physiological stress responses, which can also be helpful for our survival.[34,35] Memories are created, and this involves the hippocampus.[36] Creation of memories of the event or experience is again designed to protect us in the future – it's why we don't put our hand on a hot pan twice! The fact that the limbic system is activated by incoming nociceptive signals is one reason why, when we have pain, we don't just feel a sensation in a bodily part but we experience unpleasantness, react in physically protective ways and feel worried or anxious. This relates to the 'emotional experience' part of our definition of pain. *These are normal, biological responses.*

The cognitive areas of the brain are recruited too. Areas like the pre-frontal cortex (PFC), orbitofrontal cortex and anterior cingulate cortex (ACC) start to integrate information about the significance and impact of this suspected injury: your brain is making sense of what has happened.[30,37] Your brain is drawing on information from your past: have you sprained an ankle before and what were the consequences? And it's drawing conclusions about the consequences of you spraining your ankle. The ankle sprain happened on a remote trail. How will you get back to your car? Is something broken? Do you need medical help?

Your brain's job right now is to decide how much threat you are facing. If the brain decides that the various 'cues for protection' mean you or your tissues could be harmed, you will likely experience pain as part of your body's natural protective response. If the brain, for whatever reason, concludes that you are not

under threat or indeed if something else is going on that's more important, then you will experience less pain or no pain.[2] For example, if at the time of your ankle sprain, you received a call saying your partner had been in an accident and had been taken to hospital, it's very likely you wouldn't experience much pain at all, as it's more important for you to get to the hospital. Saying that 'the brain decides' often makes it sound like this happens under our conscious control but, at least initially, much of this occurs automatically.[30] Indeed, cues for protection manifest in different ways, and often we're not aware of this on a conscious level (e.g. a deep memory of past pain). Nevertheless, while many of our responses occur at a subconscious level, bringing awareness to these reactions can allow us to start to understand them, and can offer avenues for change when we choose different responses.

> Take home message: The pain that we experience is the result of various inputs. Triggers can sometimes (but not always) be warning signals (nociception) from the tissues, but pain is a response from processing and integration within the nervous system and brain.

Neuroplasticity and Modulation of Nociception

There are a number of mechanisms important for understanding how pain is fine-tuned and produced as an experience. Modulation of nociception refers to amplification or inhibition of nociceptive signals within the nervous system: in other words, turning up or turning down the intensity of warning signals. Sometimes this is called pain modulation, but as pain is the eventual experience after all of this modulation and processing, it's probably more correct to call this modulation of nociception. Here we describe two main processes that drive this: 1) peripheral and central sensitization; and 2) descending modulation of nociception – the role of the brain.

These processes reflect how the nervous system adapts and changes in response to the demands that are placed on it. This is called *neuroplasticity,* and works in the following way: when neurons are regularly activated together, they increase their strength of connection – synapses strengthen.[38,39] More neurotransmitters are released and more receptors are laid down to accommodate this, which makes it easier to relay signals between neurons. As this process repeats, genetic coding occurs, allowing the synapse to 'remember' this activity, and making it easier to activate signaling in the future.[39] Remember learning to play a sport or a musical instrument? The reason you improved with practice was down to neuroplasticity: neurons became more efficient at activating and networking. Some of these patterns of firing become so deeply embedded in your nervous system's memory that even if you haven't played that instrument or sport in years, you still remember the skills. On the other hand, without continued practice, you lose some of your skill and what was once automatic becomes less coordinated.

You may have heard of the phrase 'neurons that fire together, wire together'. When neurons from different regions of your brain regularly act together, the connections can become automatic.[17] It becomes more difficult to activate one brain area involved in the task without activating another – the network strengthens. Think about playing a musical instrument: you need to coordinate movement with hearing, and reading the music. This is difficult at first but becomes much easier as your brain improves the necessary connections, and eventually it becomes well trained and automatic. Neuroplasticity and coordinated networks are key to learning, but they become very important in understanding pain and its persistence too.

Peripheral and Central Sensitization

Peripheral Sensitization

Sensitization means a reduction in how much stimulus a nerve needs in order to be activated.[1,40] The neuroplastic changes highlighted above mean that nerves can become more sensitive – more responsive, firing more easily. When this happens at nerve endings in our tissues it is called peripheral sensitization. For example, with inflammation, sensory nerve endings become more sensitive, lowering their threshold for firing. As outlined above, they do this by generating more ion channels, and these ion channels can stay open for longer. Now it takes less stimulation to generate a nerve signal (action potential). This peripheral sensitization is a normal response to injury and inflammation. It explains why, after you sprained your ankle, the area was sensitive to touch. Touch doesn't normally generate a pain response, but with peripheral sensitization, touch and gentle movements can feel painful. This sensitization also means that noxious stimuli (e.g. firm pressure on your ankle's ligaments) can produce greater responses. While peripheral sensitization is protective and normal, it can sometimes become a problem, and mean your body's warning system is very active. In some situations, such as arthritis, this peripheral sensitization can be problematic.

> Peripheral sensitization: increased excitability of neurons in the *peripheral* nervous system, making it easier for them to fire.

Central Sensitization

Central sensitization means a reduction in the threshold for neurons within the spinal cord and brain to transmit signals.[1,40] It takes less stimulus for warning signals to be transmitted within your central nervous system (CNS). This occurs because of neuroplastic changes in the CNS and has two main effects: it's easier for incoming signals from the tissues to be relayed to the brain, and these signals can be amplified – 'turned up'. As with the neuroplastic changes outlined above, sensitization occurs because more neurotransmitters are released and more ion channels are expressed and stay open for longer than normal (Figure 1.6).[20,41,42] (It also results from reduced

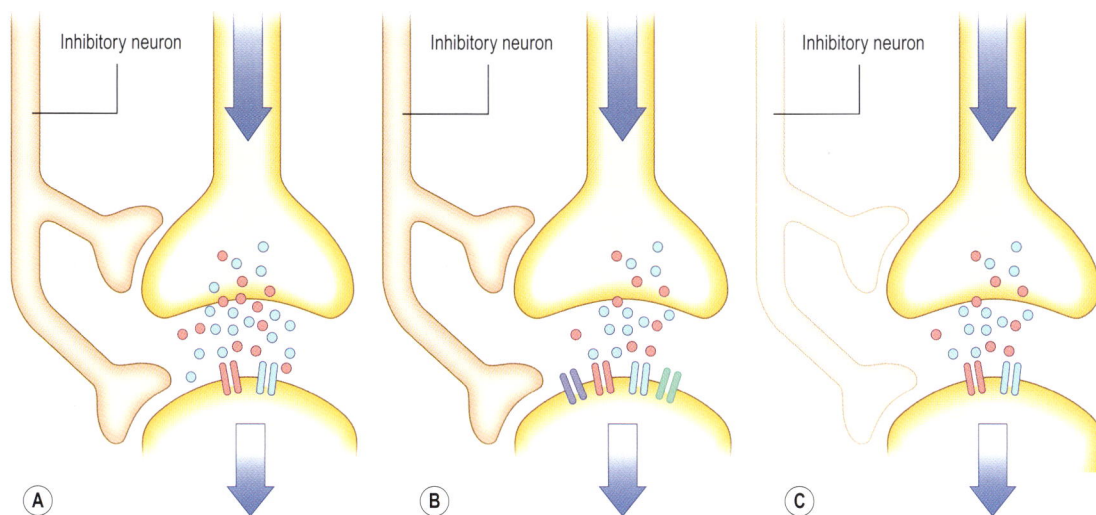

Figure 1.6

Synaptic changes with neuroplasticity: sensitization. Sensitization results from three main processes at synapses in the central nervous system: **(A)** increased expression of neurotransmitters, **(B)** increased expression of ion channels, and **(C)** loss of inhibition.

inhibition, but more about that in a moment.) If we think about that social gathering again: more people (more neurotransmitters) show up and there are more doors open into your home, which are held on a latch keeping them open (more ion channels expressed and they stay open). The result is that there is more activity and the noise goes up at your gathering – the nervous system has become more efficient at sending signals: in this case, warning signals.

> Central sensitization: increased excitability of neurons in the *central* nervous system, making it easier for them to fire.

Modulation of Nociception at the Spinal Cord Can Turn Down Signals

We mentioned our nervous system's natural control mechanisms earlier: inhibitory interneurons release neurotransmitters or chemicals that calm synapses down

after activity has occurred.[41] These chemicals may be familiar: they include endorphins (our natural opioids), serotonin, GABA (gamma-aminobutyric acid), adrenaline and noradrenaline (also known as epinephrine and norepinephrine), and more.[41] Returning to the gathering analogy, these are your sensible friends who help control the noise – turning the music down.

Remember Melzack and Wall's gate-control theory from earlier in this chapter? Gate-control experiments showed that competing stimuli like touch or vibration could activate these inhibitory interneurons and therefore effectively block nociceptive signals from being projected to the brain. In other words, the gate between the spinal cord and the brain closes so that fewer warning signals reach the brain. In this way, it makes sense to rub your sprained ankle as a way of blocking some of these warning signals. This inhibitory system is also influenced by activity in the brain, as Melzack and Wall had proposed.

When there is loss of inhibition, the synapse can stay activated so that it takes a less intense signal to activate it next time. It is easier for the synapse to be activated, to stay active, and for signals to be transmitted through the nervous system. So, previously the gathering was being controlled, but now your sensible friends get fed up and leave. It doesn't take much from your boisterous friends to get things kicked off again: this gathering is on its way to becoming a full-blown party. In pain this is important: the nervous system has adapted, allowing warning signals to be sent, received and processed more easily. The nervous system has become really effective at what it has been practicing: protection.

It's important to bear in mind that these neuroplastic changes happen to all of us to some degree when we have an injury or pain. In the case of the ankle sprain, peripheral and central sensitization may be more pronounced if the ankle sprain was more severe. However, the longer pain persists or is recurrent, the more likely it is that this sensitization causes 'over-protection' and becomes an important input for pain. It can amplify the 'cues for protection' by changing information about the state of the tissues. While this 'turning up' means that warning signals can be amplified, it also means that, in some cases, normally harmless stimuli result in pain. This is because these normally harmless stimuli can now access a warning system in the spinal cord and essentially project mixed messages (e.g. danger instead of touch) to the brain. These processes may result in people describing how pain is spreading, or how harmless things like touch or gentle movements are painful, even very painful.

Take home message: Our clever nervous system adapts its structure and function to respond to demand. In pain, this can result in peripheral and central sensitization and loss of inhibition, turning up the volume on pain and sensitivity.

Neuroplasticity and the Brain

The brain has many jobs in pain: to interpret how much danger the person/person's tissues are in, register where in their body sensations are arising from, interpret the impacts of pain, recall what happened in the past, decide to pay attention to these sensations or not, make decisions on what to do next, and generate a host of physical, emotional and cognitive responses. This involves many areas of the brain (see Figure 1.5).

Results from brain imaging studies have highlighted that the neurons in our brains are very plastic and become more active and efficient at signaling in certain conditions, e.g. if we are afraid or stressed, or if we have pain for a long time.[43] The processes are the same as those we've already outlined. People with persistent pain also demonstrate increased signaling in the limbic system (emotional brain).[44,45] The result is that for the same input from our tissues, we can experience enhanced pain because of greater brain activity. This is called a 'pronociceptive' state. In other words, anxious thoughts, and being stressed and worried can enhance our pain. Further, greater brain activity can mean that nociception from tissues isn't needed to produce pain: pain can be produced without any significant tissue input.

On the other hand, the brain can have 'anti-nociceptive' effects. The brain can drive the release of neurotransmitters that calm activity within the brain: for example, the neurotransmitter GABA, released from the medial PFC, can calm activity in the amygdala.[32,46] The calming effects of meditation are thought to act in part on this pathway and this may be one reason why meditation can help with pain.[47-49] The brain also exerts descending or 'top-down' effects on nociception. Let's look at that next.

Descending Modulation of Nociception: the Brain's Pharmacy

Have you ever had a cut or bruise that you don't remember getting? Clearly, there was some tissue input and no doubt warning signals were sent from the tissues to the spinal cord and brain, but why didn't you feel anything? I've recently taken up off-shore rowing and I've noticed plenty of bruises the day after I row that I wasn't aware of at the time. Getting the boat in and out of the water is challenging as we try to hold the boat still against the swell, lift it to get the wheels under and secure it to get out of the water. I'm completely focused on the tasks at hand.

I'm obviously incurring a couple of knocks along the way but why don't I feel anything at the time?

The anti-nociception or inhibition we described above is largely driven by the brain. Let's think of this as the pharmacy in your brain (Figure 1.7).[2] Downstream from the cortex lies the brain stem, and within it are areas called the periaqueductal gray (PAG) and rostral ventromedial medulla (RVM). For some time now

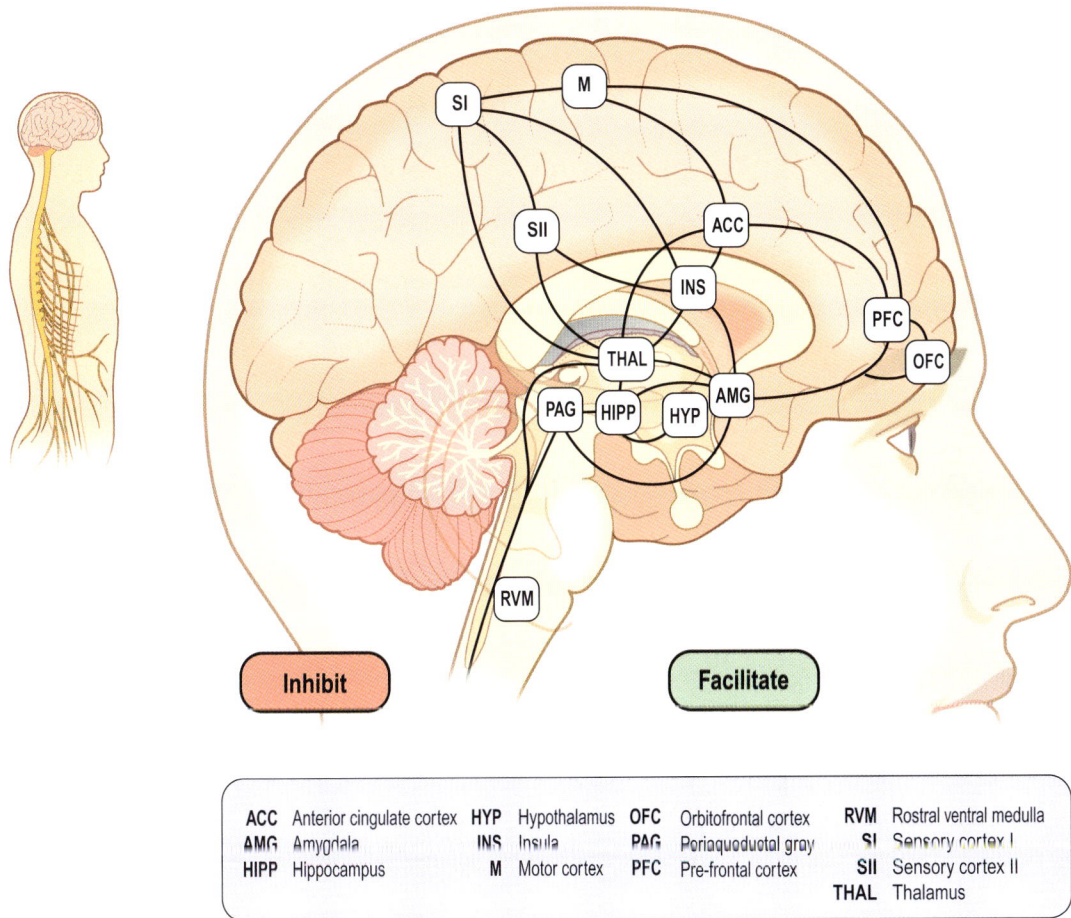

ACC	Anterior cingulate cortex	HYP	Hypothalamus	OFC	Orbitofrontal cortex	RVM	Rostral ventral medulla
AMG	Amygdala	INS	Insula	PAG	Periaqueductal gray	SI	Sensory cortex I
HIPP	Hippocampus	M	Motor cortex	PFC	Pre-frontal cortex	SII	Sensory cortex II
						THAL	Thalamus

Figure 1.7

The nervous system: the 'brain's pharmacy' and descending modulation of nociception. The PAG/RVM can inhibit or facilitate nociception, turning the dial up or down on nociception. When neurotransmitters that inhibit nociception are released, nociceptive signals are turned down: result = less pain. When neurotransmitters that facilitate nociception are released, nociceptive signals are turned up: result = more pain.

we've known that the PAG and RVM are key players in controlling how much pain relief (or not) we receive in the presence of nociception.[41] The 'brain's pharmacy' releases natural painkillers to inhibit or reduce nociceptive signalling.[41,50] This is called 'anti-nociception' and can result in pain reduction. The brain's pharmacy does this frequently in response to inflammation, injury or even threat of injury. It might not feel like it when you've had an injury but the brain's pharmacy will be active, working to keep your pain manageable. These natural painkillers primarily target the nociceptive pathways of the spinal cord,[41] i.e. descending inhibition from the brain stem to the spinal cord. Thus, they form an important part of the 'pain gate mechanism' in the spinal cord, controlling or blocking further nociceptive signals from the tissues and spinal cord from accessing the brain.

If we think about my bruises from rowing, perhaps my brain considers it more important to focus on the task at hand, so with my attention elsewhere, my brain pharmacy gives me a hit of pain-relieving chemicals to cause an anti-nociceptive effect.

> Anti-nociception: a state within the nervous system where nociceptive signaling is reduced. *Warning signals are turned down.*
>
> Pro-nociception: state within the nervous system where nociceptive signaling is enhanced. *Warning signals are turned up.*

The Pharmacy Out of Kilter

Now here's the thing: the brain's pharmacy can also fail to release natural painkillers or indeed it can release neurotransmitters that enhance nociceptive signaling – 'pro-nociception'. Because of the chemical release by the brain stem, the spinal cord pathways may be rendered very sensitive or reactive, taking much less input from the body's tissues to send warning signals to the brain. It's a vicious circle. Like all pharmacies, the brain's pharmacy receives instructions about what to release and when to release it. At least some of these prescriptions come from the emotional and cognitive brain areas.[30] While

a very complex process, there is growing evidence that when areas of the brain like the amygdala (part of the limbic system) are highly active, they signal to the PAG and RVM to stop releasing inhibitory neurotransmitters (painkillers) to reduce nociception, and instead release chemicals that actually enhance nociception, and thus the pain experience.[30] This would occur in situations where people are anxious or stressed, or expect pain.[50–52] If people are worried about doing further damage, are concerned that something has been missed, or habitually expect pain with certain movements, they are likely to feel more pain. Even the presence of persistent anxiety or stress that is unrelated to pain causes the brain's pharmacy to become *less effective* at releasing painkillers.[30] This is common for many people with chronic pain.[44,53,54] On the other hand, better mood, reduced anxiety and better knowledge about pain can reduce pain unpleasantness and intensity, partially due to descending modulation.[55,56]

Drivers of Nervous System Sensitization

There are many factors that can drive peripheral and central sensitization and influence descending modulation of nociception. Some that we'll explore throughout this book include:

- Sustained or intense peripheral inputs: e.g. repeated joint inflammation in arthritis or sustained muscle tension with back pain.

- Thought processes: e.g. thinking the worst about pain, feeling helpless or worrying about doing more damage.

- Our mood: feeling depressed, anxious or stressed.

- Altered perception.

- Sleep disturbance.

- Low physical activity and poorer general health.

Using Pain Science Models to Make Sense of Pain

To help us understand how 'cues for protection' or inputs from multiple health and social dimensions integrate to create and perpetuate pain and associated suffering, let's consider the conceptual models mentioned a little earlier: the Neuromatrix and Mature Organism Models. We describe these models here to help explain the integration of the dimensions important to the pain experience. We have incorporated these concepts into a Pain Mandala (Fig. 1.10), a schematic that we will refer to throughout this book. You will get a full introduction to the pain mandala in a bit (see p. 21); first, let's continue looking at some traditional pain models in more detail.

Neuromatrix Model

The Orchestra of the Brain

The Neuromatrix Model was proposed as a conceptual model to help us understand pain and its responses, but arguably could be applied more broadly to our perception of our self and all of our experiences. It highlights interactions within the brain and connectivity with bodily inputs and responses.[17] The concept is that our conscious awareness of the self – the body-self neuromatrix – is influenced by integrated brain activity. This activates responses: perceptual, physiological (homeostatic) and behavioral, which are important following injury, pathology or chronic stress. For example, responses include the stress response, inflammation, psychological responses such as how we feel or think, and behavioral responses that drive how we move and act. Importantly, each response can in turn become an input to the system, as highlighted by the loops depicted in Figure 1.8: a cycle of inputs influencing outputs, and in turn, outputs or responses becoming inputs. While this model was initially reported to explain pain and its associated responses, it's noteworthy that similar patterns may be relevant for

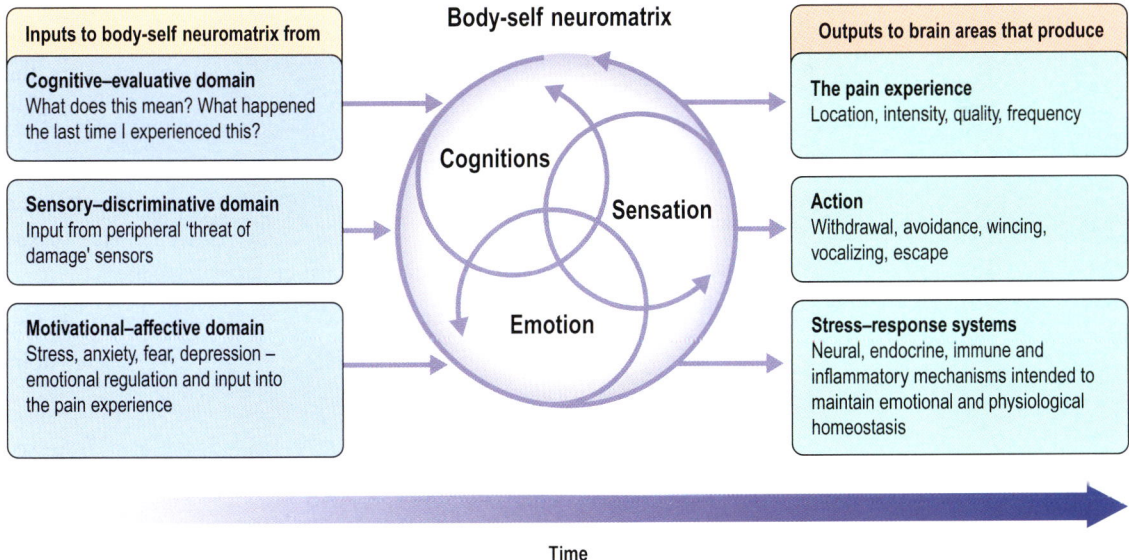

Figure 1.8

The Body-Self Neuromatrix Model for explaining how pain emerges. (Reprinted with permission from Melzack R. Pain and the Neuromatrix in the Brain. Journal of Dental Education, 2001. 65(12): 1378–82.) This model depicts how inputs (perception of threat) from multiple systems are processed within the brain to determine an appropriate output. To aid protection, one response is pain; others could include stress responses and movement adaptations.

our awareness of the self in various experiences, e.g. fear, or love, or simply how we sense our body (body perception or body awareness).

The model proposed that our responses or 'outputs' were driven largely by connections of neuronal activity in the brain: a neuromatrix. Many different areas of the brain become active to produce a pain response, and while there are key areas activated in most pain experiences, for each of us it will be slightly different. This basic neuromatrix is like a template based on genetics and learned experiences. It was proposed that the neuromatrix could be triggered by incoming sensory information from the body, but that the responses involved much greater activation and interaction of brain areas, i.e. the neuromatrix. As experiences repeat, the signaling across the neuromatrix starts to strengthen and become more automatic (neuroplasticity). Butler and Moseley nicely describe this as the 'Orchestra in the Brain'.[2] Just like a musical orchestra relies on all of its components for optimal performance, it takes many parts of the brain to coordinate their activity to produce a pain response. Sometimes, the orchestra plays harmoniously together but sometimes some instruments dominate. In pain there are typical areas that will be activated but they will vary subtly for different people: there will be different inputs triggering the whole neuromatrix to produce a response. In one person's pain experience, stress or anxiety may dominate, while for another, negative thoughts and hence over-activity of areas like the ACC may prevail. Or for another still, it will be inputs from muscle tension. Returning to the orchestra analogy, like preludes that might be led by the violin or piano, pain preludes could be 'cues for protection' from the tissues, stress, poor sleep, or an environmental cue like driving near a crash site. The evidence supporting this theory has grown exponentially in recent decades while the clinical relevance of the concept continues to hold.

Mature Organism Model

The Mature Organism Model[18] (Figure 1.9), as outlined by Louis Gifford, proposed that the mature organism (the person) has to make sense of or process many inputs and produce many outputs for survival, and this can be related to pain experiences, much of which may occur without conscious awareness. *Inputs* might include nociception or other signals from tissues (inflammation/muscle tension), our thoughts and beliefs, our worries, as well as contextual factors like the environment we live in and societal norms, e.g. how we should manage pain and injury. These inputs are potential 'cues for protection'. *Outputs* include bodily responses like pain, muscle tension, nervous system sensitivity, immune and hormonal system responses such as how much cortisol to produce, and indeed, thoughts and beliefs we develop as a result of all of these processes.

Like the loops in the Neuromatrix Model, 'inputs' are also 'outputs', e.g. muscle tension can activate warning signals (*input*), but in turn, to protect us, our body produces more muscle tension (*output*). As the nervous system becomes more sensitized, there may be more *input* from our nervous system. With greater nervous system activation comes increased activity in our sympathetic nervous system in preparation for 'fight or flight' (*output*). When we have pain we automatically become concerned about the problem (*input*), and take action to protect ourselves (*output*), but more concerned thoughts (*output*) can also result from pain (*output*). When presented in this framework, the inability to clearly identify a beginning or an end, or a cause and effect, at first might seem confusing and overwhelming. However, by appreciating the cyclical nature of inputs/outputs and all the in-betweens that occur, we can consider addressing the suffering of pain in a variety of ways, without getting caught up with the need to always identify a 'cause' or to fix a problem.

This is not unlike the *Polyvagal Theory* that suggests, for our survival, we are vigilant against risk: safety, danger and life threat. Our risk evaluation involves assessment or scrutiny of various peripheral

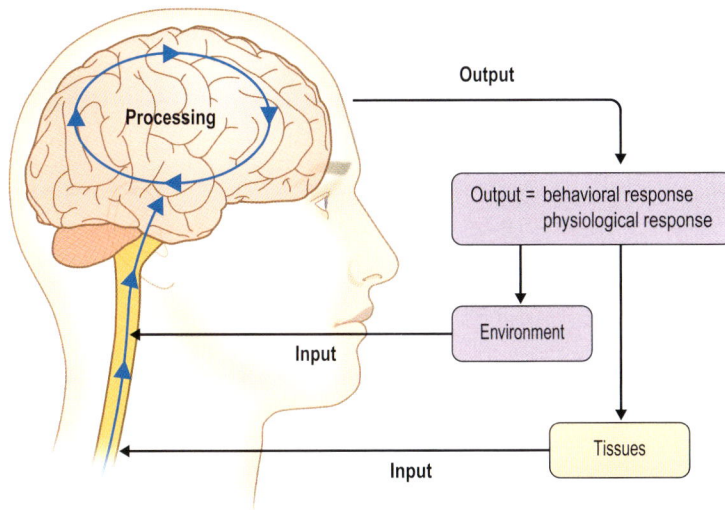

Figure 1.9

The Mature Organism Model for explaining bodily survival and how pain emerges. (Reprinted with permission from Louw A., et al. Pain Neuroscience Education 2018. Adapted from Gifford L.S., 1998. Pain, the Tissues and the Nervous System: a Conceptual Model. Physiotherapy 84(1):27–36.) This model also depicts how inputs (perception of threat) from multiple systems come into the brain for process and scrutiny to determine the best output as a response. For our protection, one response produced may be pain but others include altered behaviors and physiological responses. It is also clear here how some of these outputs, such as behavioral responses, can loop back as inputs.

inputs from the body, prior to conscious involvement of higher brain areas. Threat versus safety is weighed and measured against the things we may have already experienced as a means to offer a response, all prior to our awareness.[57,58] Taken together, these models may help connect the dots between the thinking mind (cognitive perception), body perception and body responses designed for protection and survival.

Can you see the common ground between these frameworks for understanding pain? All of them ask us to consider how multiple systems – our physical, emotional and thinking selves – interact. All of them include a cognitive–emotional element that scrutinizes, or tries to make sense of, what's going on. Is there reason to believe we are under threat? If the conscious or unconscious conclusion is that we are under threat, then physical and physiological responses will be produced, as well as thoughts and feelings regarding the scenario of perceived threat. These responses then feed back into the loops of inputs. Therefore, inputs can be a first-line stimulus (e.g. nociception) or the input could be an output of protection (e.g. muscle tension or a belief of threat); this then becomes an additional input and the circle continues and grows in layers and depth, not unlike the image of a mandala.

The Pain Mandala

Mandala, meaning circle in Sanskrit, is a diagram used traditionally to broadly symbolize the multi-dimensional aspects of life as a whole, from the relationships within our minds and bodies to the interconnection with others and the infinite nature of the universe. We use the Pain Mandala (Figure 1.10) to illustrate how integration of multiple inputs from

21

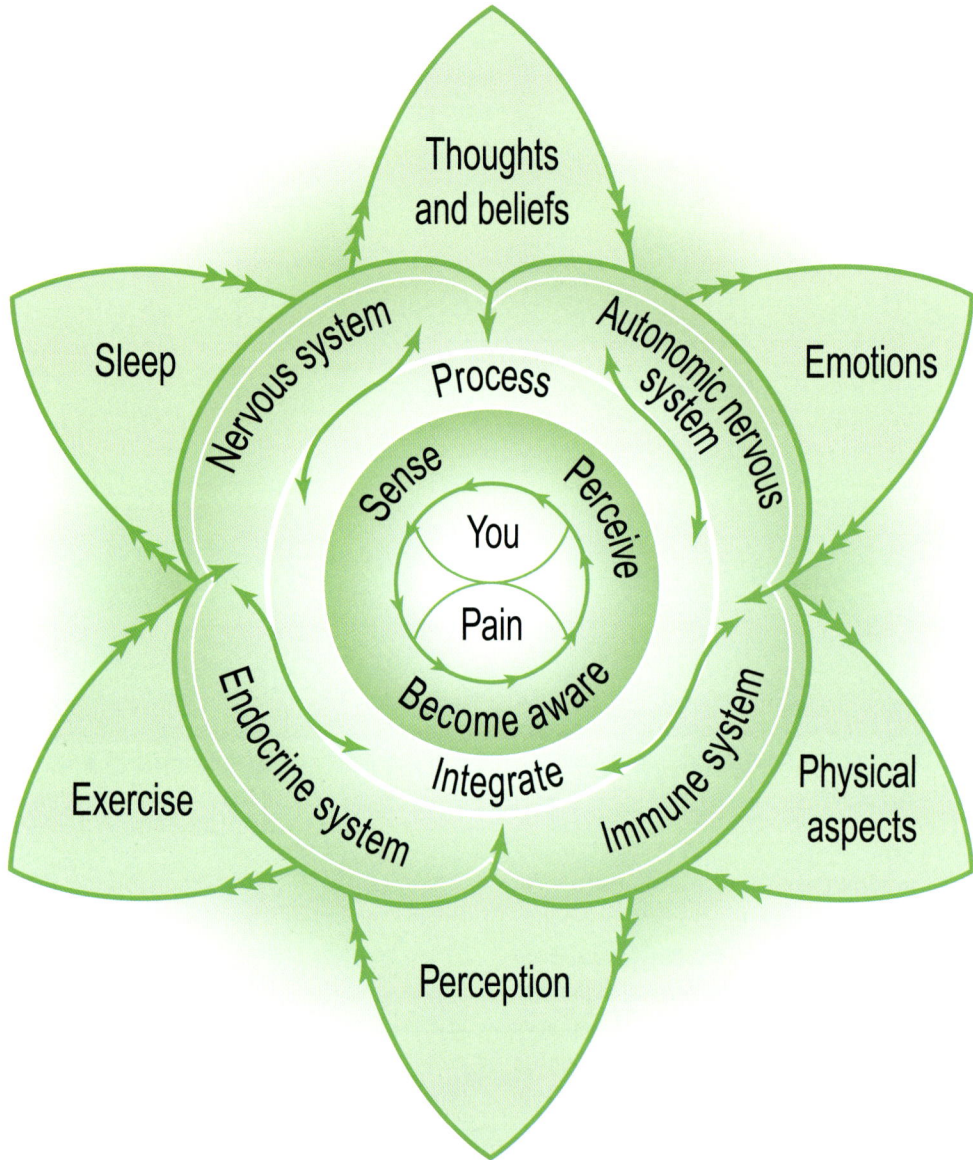

Figure 1.10

The Pain Mandala. This mandala depicts aspects of the human experience of pain covered in *Pain Science Yoga Life*. The petals represent 'inputs' to the pain experience. The next layer demonstrates systems that are influenced by these 'inputs'. Listed here are: the somatosensory nervous system (listed as nervous system), the autonomic nervous system, the endocrine (hormonal) system and the immune system. The inner circles represent how this information is processed and integrated to culminate in our awareness, our perception, and our sense of an experience. This processing, integration and creation of awareness primarily happens within the central nervous system. The mandala as a whole represents the circular nature of the pain experience; each aspect can interact with others. At the heart is you: you are you, with and without pain.

Note: Other inputs, dimensions and body systems than those noted here can contribute to pain.

different dimensions converges to explain how pain emerges. We will use it as a prompt to deepen awareness of the integration of dimensions with each aspect described in Chapters 4–9. This mandala has a lotus as the visual focus. At the heart of the flower live 'pain' and 'you'. 'You' to represent the inner you; you that is individual, unique and constant in each of us. 'Pain' because it is the key experience we are exploring. The next layer is circular, representing how this information is processed and integrated into our awareness, perception, and sense of an experience. The outer layer refers to some of the body's systems that are influenced by the 'inputs'. Those listed here are key systems that we will continue to reference: the somatosensory nervous system (listed as nervous system), the autonomic nervous system, the endocrine (hormonal) system and the immune system. The arrows represent how all inputs, outputs, systems and processes influence each other and the overall perception and experience of pain. The petals of the lotus flower relate to the key health dimensions covered in this book. These petals represent some of the key 'inputs' into the body's systems that feed the pain experience; each could also be an output or response driven from the body's systems. The person remains constant at the core of all of these 'inputs', 'systems' and 'processes'. You are always you, even when pain is in your life. The mandala will expand to include the Eight Limbs of yoga (more in Chapter 2; see Figure 2.2). This will demonstrate the bridge yoga offers, to provide strategies that may interact with the mechanisms involved in pain, to shift the pain experience.

Yoga and Pain

In Chapters 2 and 3, the philosophy of yoga and a few mindfulness principles will be outlined and considered in the context of pain care. With the emergence of this holistic view of pain, it becomes easier to see how a broader approach to pain care, involving self-regulation with compassion and mindful living, may provide an optimal modality to move beyond pain and back to a meaningful life. Within the Buddhist-inspired principle of '*and this too*', we are encouraged to hold space for all lived experiences, good and bad, without getting lost in a spiral of judgment and emotion. This is particularly relevant for pain, where we encourage the ability to hold space for diagnoses, consequences and different contributions to pain, without losing a sense of ourselves or compounding our suffering further with reactions. This makes sense not only philosophically but also (neuro)scientifically when we see how pain is modulated, and the various inputs and outputs interact within a pain experience.

Summary

Pain, an important lived experience, is the brain and nervous system's attempt to produce a helpful response to protect us that is based on many contributions (inputs). These might be thought of as 'cues for protection' and range from a variety of inputs from physical aspects and general health, to what we think, our attention and focus, memories and our emotional states. Some of the cues come from our previous experiences, pre-existing expectations, or information we've picked up throughout our lives that reflect the norms and expectations of our society. Indeed, we may be quite oblivious to the source and relevance of some inputs that contribute to the template of our perceptions and our pain. Sometimes our pain responses indicate our nervous system has become over-protective, and we experience pain even with minimal or no stimulation. By understanding pain's complexity, we can start to appreciate the need for holistic pain assessment of each individual and, in turn, holistic models of pain care. Pain care should never be solely in the hands of clinicians or teachers – optimally, it is the individual in pain who takes the lead role – but we as clinicians and teachers can provide guidance and help people acquire the necessary knowledge and skills needed to do so.

References

1. International Task Force on Taxonomy. Part III: Pain Terms, A Current List with Definitions and Notes on Usage, in: Classification of Chronic Pain, H. Merskey and N. Bogduk, Editors. 1994, Seattle: IASP Press. pp. 209–14.

2. Butler, D.S. and G.L. Moseley. Explain Pain. 2003, Adelaide: Noigroup Publications.

3. Moseley, G.L. and D.S. Butler. The Explain Pain Handbook: Protectometer. 2015, Adelaide: Noigroup Publications.

4. Quintner, J.L., M.L. Cohen, D. Buchanan, et al. Pain Medicine and Its Models: Helping or Hindering? Pain Medicine, 2008. 9(7): 824–34.

5. Descartes, R. Treatise of Man. 1664 (republished 2003), Amherst, NY: Prometheus Books.

6. Henschke, N., C.G. Maher, K.M. Refshauge, et al. Prevalence of and Screening for Serious Spinal Pathology in Patients Presenting to Primary Care Settings with Acute Low Back Pain. Arthritis and Rheumatology, 2009. 60(10): 3072–80.

7. Maher, C., M. Underwood, and R. Buchbinder. Non-Specific Low Back Pain. Lancet, 2017. 389(10070): 736–47.

8. Brinjikji, W., P.H. Luetmer, B. Comstock, et al. Systematic Literature Review of Imaging Features of Spinal Degeneration in Asymptomatic Populations. American Journal of Neuroradiology, 2015. 36(4): 811–16.

9. Minagawa, H., N. Yamamoto, H. Abe, et al. Prevalence of Symptomatic and Asymptomatic Rotator Cuff Tears in the General Population: From Mass-Screening in One Village. Journal of Orthopaedics, 2013. 10(1): 8–12.

10. Schwartzberg, R., B.L. Reuss, B.G. Burkhart, et al. High Prevalence of Superior Labral Tears Diagnosed by MRI in Middle-Aged Patients with Asymptomatic Shoulders. Orthopaedic Journal of Sports Medicine, 2016. 4(1): 2325967115623212.

11. Teunis, T., B. Lubberts, B.T. Reilly, and D. Ring. A Systematic Review and Pooled Analysis of the Prevalence of Rotator Cuff Disease with Increasing Age. Journal of Shoulder and Elbow Surgery, 2014. 23(12): 1913–21.

12. Melzack, R. and P.D. Wall. Pain Mechanisms: A New Theory. Science, 1965. 150(3699): 971–9.

13. Beecher, H.K. Pain in Men Wounded in Battle. Annals of Surgery, 1946. 123(1): 96–105.

14. Engel, G.L. The Need for a New Medical Model: A Challenge for Biomedicine. Science, 1977. 196(4286): 129–36.

15. Loeser, J.D. Perspectives on Pain, in: Clinical Pharmacology & Therapeutics, P. Turner, C. Padgham, and A. Hedges, Editors. 1980, London: Palgrave Macmillan.

16. Gatchel, R.J. Comorbidity of Chronic Pain and Mental Health Disorders: The Biopsychosocial Perspective. American Psychologist, 2004. 59(8): 795–805.

17. Melzack, R. From the Gate to the Neuromatrix. Pain, 1999. Suppl 6: S121–6.

18. Gifford, L. Pain, the Tissues and the Nervous System: A Conceptual Model. Physiotherapy, 1998. 84(1): 27–36.

19. Butler, D.S. The Sensitive Nervous System. 2000, Adelaide: Noigroup Publications.

20. Woolf, C.J. and Q. Ma. Nociceptors: Noxious Stimulus Detectors. Neuron, 2007. 55(3): 353–64.

21. Kingsley, R.E. Concise Text of Neuroscience. 2nd ed. 2000, Baltimore: Lippincott, Williams & Wilkins.

22. Woolf, C. Pain: Moving from Symptom Control Toward Mechanism-Specific Pharmacologic Management. Annals of Internal Medicine, 2004. 140: 441–51.

23. Woolf, C.J. Dissecting Out Mechanisms Responsible for Peripheral Neuropathic Pain:

Implications for Diagnosis and Therapy. Life Sciences, 2004. 74: 2605–10.

24. Willis, W.D. and K.N. Westlund. Neuroanatomy of the Pain System and of the Pathways that Modulate Pain. Journal of Clinical Neurophysiology, 1997. 14(1): 2–31.

25. Jutzeler, C.R., A. Curt, and J.L. Kramer. Relationship between Chronic Pain and Brain Reorganization after Deafferentation: A Systematic Review of Functional MRI Findings. NeuroImage: Clinical, 2015. 9: 599–606.

26. Knudsen, L., G.L. Petersen, K.N. Norskov, et al. Review of Neuroimaging Studies Related to Pain Modulation. Scandinavian Journal of Pain, 2018. 2(3): 108–20.

27. Monroe, T.B., J.C. Gore, S.P. Bruehl, et al. Sex Differences in Psychophysical and Neurophysiological Responses to Pain in Older Adults: A Cross-Sectional Study. Biology of Sex Differences, 2015. 6: 25.

28. Schweinhardt, P. and M.C. Bushnell. Neuroimaging of Pain: Insights into Normal and Pathological Pain Mechanisms. Neuroscience Letters, 2012. 520(2): 129–30.

29. Tracey, I. and M.C. Bushnell. How Neuroimaging Studies Have Challenged Us to Rethink: Is Chronic Pain a Disease? Journal of Pain, 2009. 10(11): 1113–20.

30. Lumley, M.A., J.L. Cohen, G.S. Borszcz, et al. Pain and Emotion: A Biopsychosocial Review of Recent Research. Journal of Clinical Psychology, 2011. 67(9): 942–68.

31. Neugebauer, V. Amygdala Pain Mechanisms. Handbooks of Experimental Pharmacology, 2015. 227: 261–84.

32. Thompson, J.M. and V. Neugebauer. Amygdala Plasticity and Pain. Pain Research and Management, 2017. 2017: 8296501.

33. Thompson, J.M. and V. Neugebauer. Cortico-Limbic Pain Mechanisms. Neuroscience Letters, 2019. 702: 15–23.

34. Dampney, R.A. Central Mechanisms Regulating Coordinated Cardiovascular and Respiratory Function During Stress and Arousal. American Journal of Physiology: Regulatory, Integrative and Comparative Physiology, 2015. 309(5): R429–43.

35. Herman, J.P., J.M. McKlveen, S. Ghosal, et al. Regulation of the Hypothalamic-Pituitary-Adrenocortical Stress Response. Comprehensive Physiology, 2016. 6(2): 603–21.

36. Vachon-Presseau, E., M. Roy, M.O. Martel, et al. The Stress Model of Chronic Pain: Evidence from Basal Cortisol and Hippocampal Structure and Function in Humans. Brain, 2013. 136(Pt 3): 815–27.

37. Wiech, K., C.S. Lin, K.H. Brodersen, et al. Anterior Insula Integrates Information About Salience into Perceptual Decisions About Pain. Journal of Neuroscience, 2010. 30(48): 16324–31.

38. Squire, L., D. Berg, F.E. Bloom, et al. Learning and Memory: Basic Mechanisms, in: Fundamental Neuroscience, L. Squire, D. Berg, F.E. Bloom, et al. Editors. 2013, Waltham, MA: Academic Press. pp. 1009–27.

39. Sandkuhler, J. Models and Mechanisms of Hyperalgesia and Allodynia. Physiology Reviews, 2009. 89(2): 707–58.

40. International Association for the Study of Pain, IASP Terminology. 2019; Available from: http://www.iasp-pain.org.

41. Ossipov, M.H., K. Morimura, and F. Porreca. Descending Pain Modulation and Chronification of Pain. Current Opinions in Supportive and Palliative Care, 2014. 8(2): 143–51.

42. Woolf, C.J. Central Sensitization: Implications for the Diagnosis and Treatment of Pain. Pain, 2011. 15(3): S2–15.

43. De Felice, M. and M.H. Ossipov. Cortical and Subcortical Modulation of Pain. Pain Management, 2016. 6(2): 111–20.

44. Kupers, R., N. Witting, and T.S. Jensen. Brain-Imaging Studies of Experimental and Clinical Forms of Allodynia and Hyperalgesia, in: Hyperalgesia: Molecular Mechanisms and Clinical Implications, K. Brune and H. Handwerker, Editors. 2004, Seattle: IASP Press.

45. Jiang, Y., D. Oathes, J. Hush, et al. Perturbed Connectivity of the Amygdala and Its Subregions with the Central Executive and Default Mode Networks in Chronic Pain. Pain, 2016. 157(9): 1970–8.

46. Likhtik, E., J.M. Stujenske, M.A. Topiwala, et al. Prefrontal Entrainment of Amygdala Activity Signals Safety in Learned Fear and Innate Anxiety. Nature Neuroscience, 2014. 17(1): 106–13.

47. Menezes, C.B., N.R. Dalpiaz, L.G. Kiesow, et al. Yoga and Emotion Regulation: A Review of Primary Psychological Outcomes and Their Physiological Correlates. Psychology & Neuroscience, 2015. 8(1): 82–101.

48. Taren, A.A., P.J. Gianaros, C.M. Greco, et al. Mindfulness Meditation Training Alters Stress-Related Amygdala Resting State Functional Connectivity: A Randomized Controlled Trial. Social Cognitive and Affective Neuroscience, 2015. 10(12): 1758–68.

49. Taren, A.A., P.J. Gianaros, C.M. Greco, et al. Mindfulness Meditation Training and Executive Control Network Resting State Functional Connectivity: A Randomized Controlled Trial. Psychosomatic Medicine, 2017. 79(6): 674–83.

50. Zhuo, M. Descending Facilitation. Molecular Pain, 2017. 13: 1744806917699212.

51. Lockwood, S.M., K. Bannister, and A.H. Dickenson. An Investigation into the Noradrenergic and Serotonergic Contributions of Diffuse Noxious Inhibitory Controls in a Monoiodoacetate Model of Osteoarthritis. Journal of Neurophysiology, 2019. 121(1): 96–104.

52. Nation, K.M., M. De Felice, P.I. Hernandez, et al. Lateralized Kappa Opioid Receptor Signaling from the Amygdala Central Nucleus Promotes Stress-Induced Functional Pain. Pain, 2018. 159(5): 919–28.

53. Fingleton, C., K.M. Smart, and C.M. Doody. Exercise-Induced Hypoalgesia in People with Knee Osteoarthritis with Normal and Abnormal Conditioned Pain Modulation. Clinical Journal of Pain, 2017. 33(5): 395–404.

54. Rabey, M., C. Poon, J. Wray, et al. Pro-Nociceptive and Anti-Nociceptive Effects of a Conditioned Pain Modulation Protocol in Participants with Chronic Low Back Pain and Healthy Control Subjects. Manual Therapy, 2015. 20(6): 763–8.

55. Villemure, C. and M.C. Bushnell. Mood Influences Supraspinal Pain Processing Separately from Attention. Journal of Neuroscience, 2009. 29(3): 705–15.

56. Lee, H., J.H. McAuley, M. Hubscher, et al. Does Changing Pain-Related Knowledge Reduce Pain and Improve Function through Changes in Catastrophizing? Pain, 2016. 157(4): 922–30.

57. Sullivan, M.B., M. Erb, L. Schmalzl, et al. Yoga Therapy and Polyvagal Theory: The Convergence of Traditional Wisdom and Contemporary Neuroscience for Self-Regulation and Resilience. Frontiers in Human Neuroscience, 2018. 12: 67.

58. Kolacz, J. and S.W. Porges. Chronic Diffuse Pain and Functional Gastrointestinal Disorders after Traumatic Stress: Pathophysiology through a Polyvagal Perspective. Frontiers in Medicine (Lausanne), 2018. 5: 145.

Out beyond the ideas of wrongdoing and rightdoing there is a field. I'll meet you there.

Rumi

Yoga: An Introduction

The word yoga can elicit a number of reactions from the general public, including: 'I am not flexible enough to do yoga' or 'I already have a faith system.' These responses represent a misunderstanding of what yoga is and what the practice involves. Yoga is the study of self and living with awareness. It encompasses philosophies and tools to facilitate this, to promote self-regulation, and hence to improve wellbeing. The yoga philosophy presented here and throughout the following chapters, as we weave the concepts of yoga with pain science, is a product of the combination of our individual yoga teacher training, clinical experience, self-study and contemplations. While reading, we encourage you to keep in mind the primary purpose of this book, which is to utilize yoga to facilitate a change in one's relationship with pain. We recognize that yoga as it is presented may feel over-simplified for some or difficult to fully digest for others. It may be helpful to proceed with the mindset of 'take what you need and leave the rest.'

Yoga misconceptions:

- It is not a religion.
- It is not a fixed series of exercises for flexibility or handstands.
- It is not a trendy lifestyle of clothing, foods and social media posts.

Yoga does encompass:

- A spiritual connection and practice with the many layers of ourselves and the world we live in.
- Exercises or postures known as *asanas* that promote strength, proprioception, flexibility and mindfulness or awareness.

- Positive thinking and mindfulness with meditation practices.
- Awareness of, and activities to promote understanding of, our own perceptions of body, emotions and the self.
- Awareness of, and activities for, breathing known as *pranayama*.
- Awareness of how we nourish ourselves through food, society, nature, thought, etc.
- Promotion of rest and relaxation.
- Positive social and environmental living, harnessing wisely from these entities, taking no more than we need and learning to give back as well.

At its core, yoga is the study of self and living with awareness. In Sanskrit, yoga's root language, the word yoga comes from the root word, *yuj*, meaning to yoke, to unite or bring together. This can be thought of simply as connecting the body, mind and spirit. For our purposes spirit can be thought of as the way our inner self connects with the outer world. At a more in-depth level, this union is the ability to detach from dualistic thinking. Non-dualism allows the bringing together, yoking, of all things. Comprehension of dualism is challenging; we will look more closely at it in just a moment.

A Look at the Self – One Potential Viewpoint

People spend years attempting to understand and define 'the self'. To keep it simple and for the purpose of pain, we will consider the self as one entity with two distinct layers. The *superficial self* is the physical body, including the senses, the brain and the psychological mind. The mind here is all of your thoughts, beliefs and opinions. This is the self that we tend to identify strongly with, the one that we put up against others for comparison. This is the ego-driven self. The second or deeper layer of self can be thought of as the *true self*. The true self is not driven by ego or comparison. It is the consistent center of you, the one that doesn't change based on the outer environment. When yoga is thought of as the study of self, it is this deeper layer of self that one is seeking to connect with and understand. With practice we can learn to live our lives more connected to and rooted in this deeper, more consistent self. It is from here that we can process the vicissitudes of life with greater equanimity.

An Introduction to Dualism

Dualism is a philosophical concept that is centuries old. Simply stated, it is the idea that for most experiences or entities a division into categories can occur.[1] We, as humans, tend to view the world through the lens of expectations, judgments and comparisons. For example, good versus evil, you versus me, mind versus body. Dualism is a recognition of differences. It is rooted in comparison and often in the idea of better or worse, good or bad, success or failure, power or submission. If we live primarily from the superficial layer of self it is difficult *not* to live with a dualistic outlook. This comparative outlook can be prevalent in pain states and may be a root of unnecessary suffering. Pain is perceived as a negative experience or negative state, a state to be rid of. A non-dualistic outlook on pain would suggest that pain is not good or bad, it just is: a normal sensory or emotional experience and a part of all human life.

Non-dualism is the recognition that all living things are made equal and are precious: everything made from nature (humans, animals, plants, etc.) is made of particles and elements, and is connected as one aspect of a bigger whole. It is the recognition that life's experiences will be varied, including pleasure and pain, neither being more or less important than the other. This view can be incredibly challenging to grasp because it is not exactly tangible. However, once

accepted, even on a conceptual level, it can be healing for many human struggles and promote a place of loving kindness for ourselves and others. Think of this: a water molecule at the top of a wave looks at its neighbor and says: 'Why would you think you are less worthy than the entire ocean? You are in fact the same, just in a different form' (Figure 2.1). Can you see that we humans are all the same, just in different forms? The connectivity and likeness don't stop at humans. When we find this ability to recognize connection rather than separateness, we can begin to step away from unhealthy attachments to our own sufferings, comparisons and perceived short-comings. This perception or 'awakened/enlightened' mindset is not easy and will only come with observation and practice.

When we think about persistent pain, we often think of it as a negative, as a disability. These thoughts come from comparison: 'I used to be able to…', 'Because of my pain I can no longer…', but what if we choose to

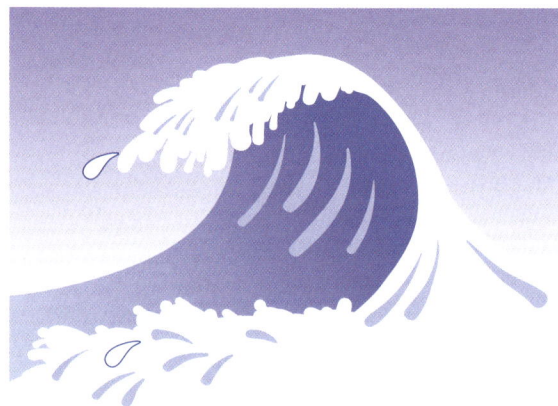

Figure 2.1
This figure depicts the concept of non-dualism. As humans and part of the natural world we are all simply molecules in different forms. One human to another is no different than these two water molecules: here one molecule is in wave form while the other is part of the spray, different but the same.

see pain and its effects as one part of a whole? Take Russell, for example. He is an Alaskan smoke-jumper: he hurls himself out of helicopters to fight forest fires and ensure the safety of humans and wildlife. At age 34 he began to struggle with recurrent back pain. To him, this pain could easily have become a disability, and a threat to his sense of self-worth: 'If I can't jump with the crew, what good am I?' If he attached his sense of self to this vocation, he would undoubtedly suffer with catastrophic thinking patterns which would most likely drive his pain and sensitivity further (see Chapter 4 for more details on this process). However, by recognizing that smoke-jumping is something he *does* and not who he *is*, he was able to see this scenario as an opportunity to simply continue to learn and grow and add to his life skill set. Now 37, Russell has returned to university to pursue a career in teaching literature. He gets to be a smoke-jumper with back pain and a literature student, and still he is Russell – a human, a part of nature, not better, not worse. Because he has learned to relate to the world from his true self, he can smoothly transition into this additional role without comparing it or getting lost in dualistic thinking and suffering.

The Eight Limbs of Yoga

Historically, yoga was taught only verbally and by direct instruction from sage to student. This was said to keep the knowledge pure and prevent excessive intellectual contemplation. Sometime around 400 CE, Sage Patanjali wrote the Yoga Sutras, which have become known as the first comprehensive system of yoga, also known as the Eight-Fold Path or Eight Limbs.[2,3] The Eight Limbs – 1. *Yamas*, 2. *Niyamas*, 3. *Asana*, 4. *Pranayama*, 5. *Pratyahara*, 6. *Dharana*, 7. *Dhyana*, 8. *Samadhi* – help to establish a formula for practice. Each limb could be considered a window for observation with curiosity of the various features of ourselves. Each serves as a means to learn who we are and how we tend to connect with what surrounds us.

There are many other tools in yoga traditions. If you already have a yoga foundation or practice that delves into other traditions, please don't think you need to abandon that in any way. If we blend traditional practices with pain science, we may see yoga as a toolbox for self-regulation and self-care (Figure 2.2): first becoming aware of the integration of inputs and outputs associated with pain, and then starting to regulate these processes. With consistent practice the ability to use tools such as self-regulation becomes more natural and efficient.[4]

1. Yamas

The first limb represents self-restraint, moral discipline or vows, and incorporates five subsets:

- *Ahimsa*: non-violence.
- *Satya*: truthfulness.
- *Asteya*: non-stealing.
- *Brahmacharya*: positive use of energy (*prana*).
- *Aparigraha*: non-greed, non-attachment, non-grasping.

It is easy to see how these can be practiced as outward expressions and vows of moral actions toward others. However, in yoga these are also emphasized as behaviors toward ourselves. To practice non-violence (ahimsa) with others we must first find self-compassion and loving kindness inwardly. Harboring feelings of guilt and shame are two of the most violent acts we endure. We must also hold ourselves accountable for our own truths (satya). If I have feelings of anger or jealousy, I can choose not to act out these feelings but I have to admit to myself that they are there. Denying or ignoring such emotional states is an act of lying to the self.

In the context of asteya and aparigraha, it is said if we take more than we need we are indeed stealing and acting out of greed, be it with food, material objects or

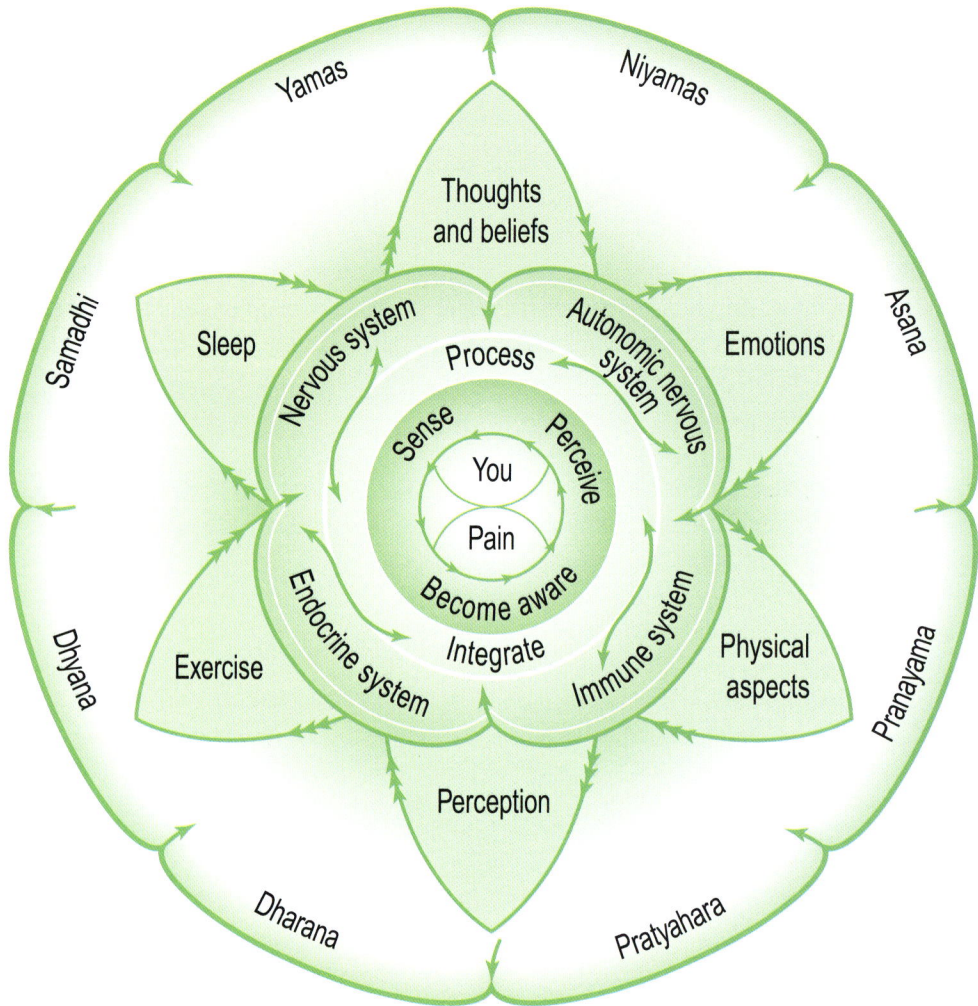

Figure 2.2
Pain and Yoga Mandala. This mandala depicts aspects of the human experience of pain covered in *Pain Science Yoga Life*. The petals represent 'inputs' to the pain experience. The next layer demonstrates systems that are influenced by these 'inputs'. Listed here are: the somatosensory nervous system (listed as nervous system), the autonomic nervous system, the endocrine (hormonal) system and the immune system. The inner circles represent how this information is processed and integrated to culminate in our awareness, our perception, and our sense of an experience. This processing, integration and creation of awareness primarily happens within the central nervous system. The mandala as a whole represents the circular nature of the pain experience; each aspect can interact with others. At the heart is you: you are you, with and without pain.
The Eight Limbs of yoga surround the lotus to offer a depiction of how yoga philosophy and practices may aid in changing inputs and outputs that feed the pain experience. Yoga may also deepen the relationship you have with your inner self and potentially soften the impacts of pain.
Note: Other inputs, dimensions and body systems than those noted here can contribute to pain.

emotional/intellectual justifications. These practices suggest that being mindful of our true needs ensures we don't take more than we need and we balance the act of taking with the act of giving back. Activities we participate in can either feed our energy or deplete it (brahmacharya). The five positive aspects listed above are all a means of nurturing and boosting ourselves physically, emotionally and psychologically. In yoga, giving back to the self may be referred to as increasing one's prana or lifeforce.

Yamas and Pain

Ahimsa: non-violence

Many of us have a metaphorical tendency to beat ourselves up, especially when we are in pain. This can be a result of negative thought patterns, for example: 'I am broken/I can't/my bad back…' This can also manifest in the actions we take, participating in too much or too little activity. Even though violence can be a bit of an extreme word, these negative thoughts and actions toward our physical body can be an act of harm for ourselves. If we learn to shift to a more compassionate thought process and learn a balance of physical participation, we may feel a shift in pain.

Satya: truthfulness

It is quite common to hear things like: 'Everything hurts, I can't do anything, my pain is horrible, my shoulder is ripped to shreds, it's all because of the stupid driver who hit me.' All of these things might feel real. Are they actually true? We will look specifically at a practice of 'real but not true' in the next chapter. While learning to be fully honest with ourselves can be difficult and uncomfortable, truthful examination allows us to see the entire scenario for what it really is. This practice may give insight into the areas we have the ability to control and shift us toward the direction we need for healing and recovery. A patient recently stated he has had 18 years of back pain. He said he can no longer do his work as a composer: "I just can't work

at all," he firmly stated. However, with further questioning he revealed he spends four hours per day for at least five days per week in his studio, composing – working. He hasn't been fully truthful to himself; this simple misrepresentation of the truth might lead to a belief, an input, that adds to his pain experience.

Asteya: non-stealing

If we think of non-stealing, for pain this might be over-utilizing medical or health care or asking more from our friends and family than we are giving back to them. Stealing sounds intentional and malicious but it may be an unintentional lack of awareness and realization. Are we taking more than we are giving? Expecting someone else to heal us or fix something? Are we contributing equally to our health care, doing as much as we can to improve the situation? There are times in life that we need others to take care of us, but even during these times it is important to take only what is actually needed and to continue to offer what we can to give back to those around us, as well as ourselves.

Brahmacharya: positive use of energy (prana)

This means keeping our thoughts and actions around pain in a positive perspective. This could be as simple as focusing on what we can still do instead of what we can't. Let us look at again at the composer. How much time in the studio does he spend ruminating about what he can no longer do, and how his studio time is much less than he would like it to be? This is not a productive use of his time or physical tolerance. He may actually be more productive if he can shift into the optimistic and grateful outlook – he then has four hours to accomplish his desired tasks. This is written as if it is a simple shift to put in place. Of course, it is more complex. Emotional lability about what has been lost will happen and is important to process. But grieving the loss during times of attempting productivity becomes unproductive for both emotional processing and, in this case, composing.

Aparigraha: non-greed, non-attachment, non-grasping, non-possessiveness

In yoga this goes beyond the idea of wanting money, power or food. This limb also reflects the side of human nature that can lean toward grasping and clinging. In a persistent pain scenario, aparigraha may be practiced through the ability to maintain realistic expectations. If walking for 10 minutes is difficult, then having a goal of returning to mountaineering in the next month may be greedy, or grasping at a past demonstration of physical ability. A goal to improve walking tolerance to allow a 30-minute stroll in the woods may be more realistic and obtainable. This isn't to say mountaineering will never be possible, but learning to accept smaller yet meaningful achievements might actually aid a fuller recovery. This may also mean accepting the scenario at hand, feeling the discomfort or pain, learning how to cope with it and regulate it without trying to escape it or simply get rid of it.

2. Niyamas

This second limb encompasses self-observances or self-study, and also has five subsets:

- *Saucha*: cleanliness.
- *Santosha*: contentment.
- *Tapas*: discipline, self-will.
- *Svadhyaya*: self-reflection and spiritual studies.
- *Isvarapranidaha*: surrender to a system of faith or higher power.

In this limb, the greatest aim is to create a flexible mind, releasing the tendency toward rigid thoughts and beliefs. Again, these can be looked at as outward acts with an inner shift of perspectives.

Saucha: cleanliness

This includes cleansing the mind and emotions of attachment. For the purpose of pain, this might be thought of as a means of cleaning out unhelpful and automatic reactions of our minds or movement patterns. Have you ever noticed how sights and sounds can cause our posture to shift? For instance, every Wednesday in the summer, a giant cruise ship full of curious passengers arrives in my small community in Alaska. On Wednesday mornings, pedaling around the corner to my office, my eyes land on the large structure docked in my view. Automatically, I can feel my body 'armor'. My chest will puff a little, my shoulders rise up toward my ears. I begin to avoid eye contact with tourists and edge toward being unapproachable. I know the day will be filled with interruptions, and slowed internet and cellular services. Because of past experiences, my physical posture is affected, based on the visual cue of a cruise ship. Practicing saucha might mean letting go of my patterned reactions and allowing the day to unfold however it may.

Santosha: true contentment

This is an intention to accept and understand that all is impermanent and nothing in the outer world will supply us with joy or acceptance; we have to find these for ourselves from within.

Tapas: discipline, self-will

Tapas does not mean Spanish appetizers, rather it is said to be the internal fire that drives us or motivates us. It is said that within our tapas is where we find the strength to change our behaviors, emotions and perspectives and to endure when things become uncomfortable. Tapas is also how we promote the output of energy or physical strength and endurance. This could be seen as the driving force behind self-regulation.

Svadhyaya: self-reflection

This acts as a catalyst for change. Making space for awareness is the first step toward a shift in regulation and responses. It is encouraged to be practiced as an observation of patterns with kindness and compassion. What would change if we began to treat our own mind and emotions like a small child? We each have the ability to make a friend or a slave out of ourselves. Positive encouragement toward desired changes rather than self-resistance can create a greater balance toward healing for the whole system.

Isvarapranidaha

This is the recognition or belief in a higher being or power; it can be inclusive of all faith systems.

Niyamas and Pain

Saucha: cleanliness

With respect to pain, this practice could be thought of as a means to starting and ending each day 'fresh and clean'. Pain, especially as it persists, is unpredictable and often unreliable. This in itself can be very frustrating. Waking each day and expecting it to go in the same way as the last may not be helpful, even if yesterday was a 'good day'. Each evening we can recognize the difficulties and the celebrations of the day, then set both aside equally so the next day can start anew without a comparison or expectation of what will be or what has come before.

Santosha: contentment

I asked my patient with an 18-year history of back pain whether he was OK. He answered that he wasn't. I reflected back to him:

"Are you currently in an active state of dying?" *"No."*

"Do you have shelter and food?" *"Yes."*

"Do you have a wife that loves and supports you?" *"Yes."*

"Are you OK?" *"Yes."*

It can be an important realization that contentment is a state of mind that is truly a choice. Even when things are not exactly as we want them to be, we can still choose to acknowledge we are, indeed, OK, content. If we consider that pain is a means of protection, driven in part by our emotions, beliefs, and examination of threat, what might happen to the intensity of protection if we simply shift a belief from 'I am not OK' to 'I am OK'?

Tapas: discipline, self-will

To take on an active state of recovery from one of persistent pain we must first find the will to persevere. It can be stunning how some people continue to seek answers to their personal painful experience. On one level we might call it over-utilization or 'doctor shopping' but on another they are persevering. While suffering, they are also continuing to search for someone who might have another perspective that provides a tangible way forward. When pain has been associated with an activity for a period of time, movement adaptations and reactions to pain may begin to become part of our normal way of being. Think about an injury that has led to a pattern of limping. Sometimes the limp is outside the awareness of the person and becomes difficult to change, even if the injury has healed. Another way to look at this is that it takes self-will, or tapas, to change ingrained training or patterns of thinking and even moving; these occur in our biological systems as a response to life and to pain. There are a number of biological processes involved in the multidimensional (initial and lasting) experience of pain. As you read on, you will see some of these in detail. You will also be exposed to evidence that shows us it is possible to change these responses. It is our tapas, the internal fire, that will allow us to be uncomfortable and be OK, to fall and stand back up, to face the hard facts of what we learn as we study ourselves and our experiences of pain or otherwise.

Svadhyaya: self-reflection and spiritual studies

This practice of self-reflection could be the anchor pin for incorporating yoga into pain care. It is here that we get to ask ourselves the potentially challenging questions. For example: How do I respond to threats? Are they true or perceived? What are my mental and emotional reactions to being physically uncomfortable? Are my pain triggers purely physical or are there social and emotional triggers too? When I'm in pain, do my internal reactions act as a helpful way to engage and protect myself or do these reactions create a barrier, preventing me from true connection to others?

Isvarapranidaha: surrender to a system of faith or higher power

Yoga does not dictate the exact nature of this faith system, but rather encourages recognition that we as humans are not in full control of our lives; surrendering to something bigger than ourselves can be helpful in all aspects of human suffering. The 'who' we surrender to is an individual choice. As care providers, we can simply support and recognize the benefit of a faith system that others may have and that this may aid their pain care.

3. Asana

Meaning a position that is comfortable and steady, asanas are the physical postures of yoga. Originally, these postures were intended to be performed prior to meditation to prepare the body to be comfortable for extended periods in a state of physical stillness and relaxation. Traditionally, meditation would be performed in a cross-legged seated position, and relaxation would take place in *savasana* (flat on the back, arms open to the side and palms facing upward). In Sanskrit, *sava* means corpse and *asana* means pose: therefore, *savasana* is corpse pose. When read in Sanskrit, posture names will finish with *-asana* at the end, and the prefix tends to describe the position. For example, *badaconasana* is bound angle pose.

In the context of yoga and pain care we consider any exercise or body position as an asana, if it is entered into with the right state of mind and connectivity to the breath. In yoga, through mindfulness and breath awareness, we attempt to view our body as a tool to find connection and awareness, be it the simple connection of the mind, body and breath, or the grander connection of all things. When we look at asanas as a therapeutic tool, the positions or movements might be an avenue to connect with our fears, conditioned reactions and movement patterns. The gained observations

can begin to challenge, change and allow us to recognize helpful and unhelpful reactions and patterns: physical, psychological and emotional. Through observation and awareness, we use asanas to help us move beyond our areas of resistance and struggle.

4. Pranayama

Prana means life force and *ayama* means extension. *Pranayama*, simply stated, is a breath practice. It is used as a tool to promote connection between the body, mind and spirit. Focus on the breath can act as a vehicle for mindfulness. Pranayama can be a practice in itself or in combination with meditation or asana. Breathing or respiration is a physiological function that occurs automatically (under the control of the autonomic nervous system) but can also be consciously regulated.[5] Emotionally difficult and physically painful scenarios can stimulate physiological responses that lead to a rapid heart rate and rapid, shallow breathing.[5,6] We may not be able to immediately or directly change the physical sensations involved nor directly slow our heart rate. We can, however, ease our breath and this, in turn, can alter the physiological responses and potentially soften the painful experience.[6] A very simple example is someone who fears going to the doctor to get an injection. If this person practices slowing and deepening their breath, they may immediately feel comforted, and better able to endure the needle-prick. Our breath can be powerful in times of stress and pain; it can add to the negative or help us to shift back to a more balanced place. Pranayama practices are outlined in Appendix 1: Meditation and Pranayama.

5. Pratyahara

This limb refers to dissociation of consciousness from the outside environment. *Pratya* means to withdraw or draw in, and *ahara* is taking in, referring to the things our senses continuously perceive, e.g. sight, sound, touch. It is in this limb that yoga realizes that all senses rely on the presence of the conscious mind. Our sense organs are responsible for picking up on elements but do not actually create the sensory experience as we know it. For example, our auditory receptors are responsible for receiving vibrations but it is our brain as a whole that makes sound into something that carries meaning for us. This is true even of pain. Through pratyahara we may also be able to identify with a true sense of interoception, the ability to feel and give meaning to what is going on inside the body. Yoga does not look at the dissociation of consciousness in this direct biological way, but through the practice of pratayahara we begin to recognize our senses for what they are: the perception of light, vibration, pressure, muscle tension, heart rate variability, etc. Instead of immediately attaching a meaning to them, we can choose to just be aware.

Through meditation or focused attention, we can begin to practice focusing the mind on desired tasks without getting distracted by inputs from the outside world or being overly alert to physical inputs from the body. This attention can directly help us moderate our responses to physically unpleasant sensations and in turn change our relationship with pain. This practice allows us the realization that we can choose our reactions regardless of what is happening in the external environment, and that we have the ability to focus and produce an internal environment that promotes less suffering and more contentment.

6. Dharana

Dha means holding or maintaining, and *ana* means other or something else. This is the ability to maintain focus, attention or concentration. Dharana and pratyahara are symbiotic. To gain full focused attention or concentration, one must withdraw from the senses that distract from the desired focus. Remember sitting for an exam in a room with an air-conditioning unit that is repetitively turning on and off? If you allowed your brain to let this sensory input be registered each time the unit switched on, your focus would have shifted far

from the exam in front of you. This ability to dampen the senses occurs only with focused concentration – dharana. Pranayama, *mudras* (symbolic hand gestures) or external objects such as candles can be used to assist in narrowing the focal point. We will offer some elements of dharana in the practice sections later. These could be introduced simply as choosing a specific object, a gentle movement or a breath to bring your attention to, while simultaneously choosing to let other sensory, potentially even painful, experiences occur without shifting focus. This is not meant to suggest that we ignore or deny that pain may be present. We are instead actively choosing to place our focus on a different element. If you are making a conscious choice of focused concentration, then you are practicing dharana.

7. Dhyana

This limb represents meditation, which can be thought of as an exercise of mindfulness. Mindfulness is the ability to be in the present moment in our daily life: not thinking about this ability or congratulating ourselves for it, but actually being in it. This state of presence doesn't happen easily without practice. So, meditation is a specific time in which we practice. It can be thought of as a silencing of self-resistance, pausing the tendency to ruminate about the past or grasp at the future. It is the practice of intentional focus or concentration, dharana, that allows us to achieve a meditative state and the ability to be mindful in our daily lives.

Have you ever notice how distracted we tend to be in life – how continuous the thought stream is? And how often it contains some sort of judgment, opinion or comparison? 'I should/I'm not as good/I will never/Why, why, why…?' This tendency creates a disconnection from ourselves and may facilitate an unhelpful state of vigilance. A constant stream of thoughts is normal for all of us. We can engage in those thoughts and turn them into full-blown stories that feel like realities. We can allow them to distract us and shift our awareness away from the present moment and what is really here. Or, we can choose to let the thoughts be present without giving them attention: this is mindfulness or a meditative state.

Meditation ultimately is time with yourself, to intentionally practice being mindful, with a promise to leave all self-judgments, stories and questions behind. During this time there is a goal to let go of the lens of society and stop the comparative and judgmental natures of our minds. Meditation is not a space of emptiness, void of all thoughts. Naturally and consistently, our thoughts come without choice or permission. No thought stands independent of another thought. This leaves us without space for true observation. What we add to a thought creates perspective, and perspective may lead to emotions or physical responses. These perspectives and emotions begin to carve our reality – our stories. When you have thoughts and intentionally choose not to add or engage in a 'conversation' or analysis with the thoughts, you are in a state of meditation.

In Chapters 4–9, meditation tools and techniques will be introduced. When first attempting these practices, it can be helpful to acknowledge that a meditative state or a state of mindfulness does not occur through the act of doing; it is the culmination of what happens as a result of the foundation of focus or intention. Mindfulness is not the act, it is the result; meditation is the practice. If you are sitting and thinking, 'I am meditating, I am meditating, I am meditating,' well, you aren't actually meditating; you are thinking about it. The state of mindfulness happens when you stop actively thinking and are able to be fully present with your chosen focus. Learning to sit without ruminating on our painful experiences ('Why me/Why has this happened?/If only/What does this mean for my future?'), we may naturally begin to let go of all that content and chatter and then true emotions (e.g. grief) around the experience can be felt.

When we have the ability to acknowledge and feel our genuine emotions, we gain the ability to move past them. We may then be able to identify and separate the emotional experience from the physically painful experience. We can then learn to address each for what it is and take actions to move ourselves into a more productive future. Without taking this purposeful pause, it can be difficult to even notice how much this brain chatter has been clouding our ability to recover – physically, emotionally and psychologically. The act of being aware or in a state of mindfulness is not something easily understood from reading alone; it takes experiential practice, and lots of it, to fully grasp.

8. Samadhi

Samadhi represents identification with pure consciousness, and this limb is broadly thought of as reaching a final stage of bliss or enlightenment. Using the other seven limbs to realign the relationships we have with our inner and outer environments, we have the potential of reaching this arena of realization. This is not about floating away on a cloud of joyful bliss. The Sanskrit roots tell us *sama* means same or equal, and *dhi* means to see. Therefore, this state of consciousness is reached when we can see equally the reality in front of us. A reality that releases the conditioning of judgment or patterned habits of comparison, likes and dislikes, good versus bad and the ability to release the need to attach to any specific aspect. This state of being becomes bliss or joy that is present regardless of what else is also here. In regard to pain, it might be the path of life beyond suffering.

Conclusion

Ultimately, yoga is the opportunity to study yourself – the true self. Yoga offers tools such as the Eight Limbs to facilitate this study and practice of self-regulation. Through the yoga practice we can gain the ability to recognize that we have a body to inhabit and use to physically interact with the external environment. We have a mind that we use to learn, process and retain knowledge and experience. We have emotions we can acknowledge and feel in order to connect with ourselves and others. But, these are not the limit of who we are. We are not solely our bodies, or our minds or our emotions. The better we know the constant state of self that runs beneath these superficial entities, the more resilient we can be when one or more of these areas begins to feel threatened.

You certainly don't have to learn or be able to pronounce the names of the Eight Limbs to understand or practice the concepts they hold. We hope that you can already see the holistic container yoga supplies for pain care and the bridge it may offer to get back to a full life. These practices are as important for us as clinicians and teachers as they are for those suffering from pain. The more willing we are to go deep into cleaning out our own cobwebs of struggle – physical, emotional or psychological – the more available we will be in facilitating the journey of others beyond pain.

References

1. Robinson, H. Dualism. Stanford Encyclopedia of Philosophy, 2016. Available from: https://plato.stanford.edu/entries/dualism/.

2. Saraswati, S.S. Asana Pranayama Mudra Bandha. 2013, Bihar, India: Yoga Publications Trust.

3. Iyengar, B.K.S. Light on Yoga. 1979, New York: Schocken Books.

4. Gard, T., J.J. Noggle, C.L. Park, et al. Potential Self-Regulatory Mechanisms of Yoga for Psychological Health. Frontiers in Human Neuroscience, 2014. 8: 770.

5. Zaccaro, A., A. Piarulli, M. Laurino, et al. How Breath-Control Can Change Your Life: A Systematic Review on Psycho-Physiological Correlates of Slow Breathing. Frontiers in Human Neuroscience, 2018. 12: 353.

6. Jafari, H., I. Courtois, O. Van den Bergh, et al. Pain and Respiration: A Systematic Review. Pain, 2017. 158(6): 995–1006.

Physician must convert or insert wisdom to medicine and medicine to wisdom.

Hippocrates

A Pause for Mindfulness

In Chapter 1 we laid a foundation for the biology of pain. We hope that you gained a glimpse of how far beyond the physical aspects pain stretches, and that you can see the complexity of this multidimensional experience. Before we continue to dive into other aspects, let's take a pause for a few less tangible spiritual and emotional characteristics.

As a clinician or teacher working with people in pain, it is important to recognize the individual in front of us. When we struggle with pain, it can be soothing to know it is in fact normal for all humans at some point in time to sense pain. However, the individual experience is unique: how it will impact life and the sense of self will never be exactly the same. Each person will come with a past history, diagnosis, imaging records, faith/spiritual foundation and cultural background. All of these elements will go into one's own personal pain experience and eventually the way each individual will view and relate to pain. Something I ask almost every student or patient I work with is, 'And what else is going on in your life?' It is imperative that we provide care for all the areas on which pain can impact: the physical, emotional and spiritual. By implementing a Buddhist-inspired mindfulness practice of *and this too*, we can potentially make space for gained knowledge and struggles without losing connection to ourselves and the direction we want to move in life. In this chapter we will explore *and this too* as well as other mindfulness practices.

Mindfulness is "moment to moment awareness".[1] The Buddhist view of mindfulness asks us to take this awareness one step further with a gentle self-inquiry in an observational sense of 'What's going on here?'

Mindfulness in this sense encourages awareness of the present and inclusion of all thoughts, sensations and emotions without judgment or interpretation. The goal of this focused attention and self-inquiry is to free us from our own suffering. It may teach us to release our patterns and allow us to experience the openness, warmth and essence of an aware heart and mind.[1-3] Let's explore a few practices to help develop awareness and the idea of inclusion.

Some of these practices may resonate with you right away. Some may cause you to armor and you may want to immediately reject the idea presented. If you haven't directly experienced significant physical pain forcing you to take pause in your life, maybe you can look at these perspectives through the lens of a significant struggle you have been through, perhaps emotionally, within an intimate relationship or in a professional setting. If, as a caregiver, you can learn to practice some of these shifts in your own life, you may be more apt at facilitating change in those you work with in pain care. As previously suggested, initially reading from a mindset of 'take what you need and leave the rest' may help to soften any defensive reactions that arise. You can always come back to it again, and again, as you are ready. When you begin to practice mindfulness, it gets easier to see the potential for shifts in perspective, and then engagement occurs from a new place. These practices help us to dive deeper into the investigation of knowing our true self. Through mindfulness, we may recognize that the way we view our scenarios can keep us stuck in suffering.

And This Too

We, as humans, tend to view the world through a lens of expectations, judgments and comparisons. Few of us are immune to dualistic thinking (see Chapter 2). We think things should be a certain way. When they are not that way, we view them as a problem. And then we either look for a solution to the problem or simply choose to exclude the problem altogether. In some cases, we may allow the problem to define us and change how we identify ourselves. We do this with our bodies, our beliefs and our interpersonal relationships. We each have a conception of what we think our bodies look like, what they feel like and how they perform for us. When we are faced with injury, pain or altered performance, it is easy to automatically view this sensation as a problem – a problem that we have to find the root cause of and solve. We go to clinicians and we have scans and tests to help us locate the issue. When we don't hear what we are hoping to hear, we pass judgment on the people we have sought help from, and we may lose faith and trust in others and ourselves.

Take, for example, my friend Kyle, a champion Australian rules footballer, who suffered a back injury (spondylolisthesis). This has resulted in persistent pain in his lumbar spine as well as intermittent numbness in his feet. He could choose to handle his injury from this 'problem' perspective: clinicians and teachers may tell him that he can't participate in sports any longer, or that he can't extend his back or lift heavy things. These 'can'ts' could then begin to make him question the way he identifies himself, since if he is no longer a top-level athlete, who is he, and what does he have to offer the world? He may lose his hopes and dreams, and it would be understandable if he subsequently fell into a state of depression as a result. He could adopt patterns of escapism, because who would want to be faced with thoughts and feelings like these? His escape could be to begin reaching for food or alcohol to give him some sort of immediate comfort. He might react with anger toward his family and friends, who don't understand why he is no longer the person he was before the injury. Or he could decide he is a top-level athlete and happens to have a spondylolisthesis – *and this too.*

Instead of pushing what appears to be a problem or negative experience away or trying to change things in order for them to be as we want them to be, what if we include them? Can we simply decide we will hold them for what they are and bring them as they are into our lives? 'I am _____, *and this too.*' Kyle's scenario now becomes a very different picture. He works with his clinicians and yoga teachers to learn how to move and support his spine. He decides to use this opportunity to retire from competitive participation in high-contact sport and begin to train harder for his other athletic passion, triathlons. His aspirations of participating in the grand final change to qualifying for Iron Man. He learns to breathe with the pain in his back instead of splinting against it. He learns to change his self-talk of pain and disability to discomfort and choice. These lessons bring an inner sense of self-compassion. This actually begins to carry over into his relationships with others because he can tap into this place of self-understanding and use it to be more compassionate with the people around him.

When we seek a problem and expect a solution in a scenario that isn't as easy as black and white or cause and effect, the result tends to be unnecessary suffering brought on by our own mindsets. If we can relax and be inclusive of all experiences, we may be able to walk the path without feeling like we are constantly falling over the roots of struggle encountered along the way. This is a Buddhist-inspired practice; however, it can be incorporated into any belief system.

Changing these patterns does not come easily or without effort. However, change is possible, and the potential for recovery from painful situations may make the effort worthwhile. The easiest way to begin to pull this inclusive mindset into your life is to first recognize problem-seeking tendencies. When your mind begins to shift to a problem viewpoint, pause and ask yourself: is this actually a problem, or can it just be included as something that is here and part of me for the moment?? It does not need to be defined, analyzed or changed.

A patient who underwent a total knee arthroplasty (replacement) walked into my practice one month after his operation with the statement: "The surgeon must have put this knee together wrong, it feels different from my other one I had replaced a year ago." Can you see how the belief that something is 'wrong' and the immediate tendency to want to blame someone could feed into a greater need for protection? As we learned, pain is the body's way of protecting, and therefore a sense of greater need for protection could also lead to greater pain. What if this patient, at least for the moment, decided to shift this 'problem' perspective to: 'This knee feels different from my other one.' Not better, not worse, just different. With this simple shift in perspective we reduce the need to protect and the need to fix. When we begin to include and hold things for what they are instead of what we want them to be, we may actually begin to become more resilient.

As clinicians and teachers, it is good to become gently aware of own negative biases and the tendency to seek a problem and provide a solution, either for ourselves or for the people we work with. When you start to look for it, you may be surprised at how pervasive it can be.

Learning to Practice

Out of the Head and Onto the Mat

- Take a comfortable seat.
- Consider placing one hand on your belly and one hand on your heart.
- Bring a current scenario to mind that you have been struggling with physically or emotionally.

- Take a few long, slow breaths and then see if you can start to change the way you think about or view the situation.
- Can you start to alter the problem into just a statement of fact? ('I feel sad,' 'My back is sore').
- Can you hold that statement without asking why it is present or how to fix it or change it?
- Hold that feeling with a sense of inclusion – embracing *and this too*. Keep sitting and breathing for a few minutes.

Off the Mat and Into Life

See what happens as you return back to your life. Each time that particular situation presents itself, take an observational scan of the thoughts that follow it. Notice the negative statements, the problem-seeking, the desire for a solution, the blame, etc. Choose to replace each of those thoughts with the neutral statement: 'I am sad.' 'My back is sore.' You can even choose to add *and this too* to the thought pattern, as a mantra for inclusion.

The following are a few other mindfulness practices that may be helpful in shedding this tendency of problem-seeking and learning to lean toward inclusion for all experiences, including pain. As Buddha said, we shall incline the mind: *what we think, we become.*

Real But Not True

Some Buddhist teachers have instructed the mantra 'Real but not true' as a means to open the line between the conscious processing areas (frontal lobe) of the brain and the more emotionally driven areas (limbic system).[2,4,5] Tsoknyi Rinpoche, a Tibetan Buddhist teacher who coined this phrase, says this connection is opened via kindness, empathy and reassurance.[2] You will learn a great deal more about these brain areas and the connections between them in Chapters 4 and 5. Take, for example, the fear of heights. The fear is real but peering off a cliff's edge does not equate to dying. You are afraid of dying: real. You are actually dying: not true. The feelings are real but they do not carry fact behind them; they are simply feelings. We can utilize this investigation tool in all realms of perceived suffering: physical, emotional and spiritual (interpersonal).

Let's look at a simplified example of a runner with knee pain. He has seen many clinicians. Scans and clinical tests have been performed. He has been assured his knee is not structurally compromised. Yet every time he runs, he suffers from pain in his knee. This has led him to stop running, mostly out of fear that he is damaging himself. The pain: real. Damage, disease, danger, need to protect: not true. As a runner he is most likely fairly well practiced at accepting physical discomfort from things like muscle fatigue and skin breakdown. Because he knows these sensations are not actually threatening to him, he does not fret about them and can continue running without a sense of suffering. He may choose to take some further action like applying a layer of Vaseline to his skin to prevent chafing but that's it. He is not looking for a bigger problem. If he can begin to gently shift the sensations around his knee to a similar viewpoint, then he may be able to take a simple treatment approach like balancing his running with some stretching, or addressing a slight mechanical dysfunction with some corrective exercises, but in the end he will mostly be able to return to running. Even if the physical discomfort does not dissipate immediately or completely, it does not turn into a sense of suffering or loss of sense of self-worth as a runner because no further problem or story is attached to it.

Learning to Practice

To further understand how this *real but not true* mindfulness practice can work in our own lives and those of the people we are working with, let's take it onto the mat.

Out of the Head and Onto the Mat

- Bring to mind a fairly simple reproducible pain you experience. Think about the other sensory stimuli that may come along with it: change in breathing, heart rate, movement, muscle tension, thought pattern, emotions, etc.

- Now, take a comfortable seat.

- Maybe close your eyes.

- Place one hand on your belly and one hand on your heart.

- Begin to deepen your breath.

- Let yourself slowly begin to imagine a movement, activity or position that can be painful. You might start to actually feel some pain.

- Let your awareness lean into the other sensory experiences: breathing, heart rate, movement, muscle tension, thought patterns, emotions, etc.

- Now, can you place your attention on softening the reactions around the painful experience? Keep the breath even, slow and full.

- Allow the heart rate to settle.

- Encourage the muscles to relax.

- Imagine the movements as fluid and efficient.

- Let your thoughts run but choose not to engage in them. If you notice fears and catastrophic thoughts begin to creep in, recognize them, acknowledge they are there – they are based on a real feeling – but begin to find the holes present in the truth behind them.

- With practice you may be able to temper the physical and emotional reactivity to the painful experience.

Off the Mat and Into Life

This mindfulness practice can be taken into an activity that produces pain for you or for someone you work with. You can simply repeat the cues given in the practice above during the troublesome activity. For example, the runner who experiences pain a few miles into running could choose to keep running, taking note of the other sensations and reactions that arise. He could choose to alter the thoughts and focus away from the painful stimuli and instead direct his attention toward other aspects. What has changed with the gait pattern? What muscles are holding tone that don't need to? How is his breathing? What thoughts arise? Are these negative, problem-seeking, blameful or comparative in nature? If he chooses to notice a few of these reactions, he can shift attention to an aspect that is controllable. He can choose to move his awareness toward steadying the breath or allowing the exhalation to be slightly longer than the inhalation whilst maintaining nostril breathing. This altered focus may actually begin to quieten the uncomfortable sensations and slow the negative thought spiral. Then he will be able to feel what is real and what is potentially being fed by reactions that aren't necessary or true.

First Dart, Second Dart

When we are faced with injury or threat, be it physical or emotional, the initial encounter is considered the *first dart* in Buddhism. The stuff we lay down on top of it are darts we throw at ourselves and are considered *second darts*, which tend to be the primary source of suffering. "If a person was struck by a dart, would it hurt?" asked the Buddha of a student. "Yes," replied the student. The Buddha then asked, "If the person was struck by a second dart, is it even more painful?" "Yes, it is," replied the student.[4] Chapter 1 began to demonstrate the biological processes behind increased nervous system sensitivity and that these processes are not all driven by tissue inputs; some of the drivers are emotions, thoughts or perceptions. This will be explored in greater detail in the following chapters.

The Buddha was not speaking in pain science terms, but see if you can start to draw the parallels between these lessons. The Buddha was referring to the stream of thoughts and stories we conjure up as a response to an initial insult. Self-created emotional wounds can happen often, and in everyday circumstances: for example, let's say I am waiting tables in a café, I slip on a banana peel and fall, causing a bruise to my hip. The bruise is a first dart and minor enough that I will heal within a couple of days. However, instead of seeing this event as an accident, I get angry at my co-worker for being negligent, and then my thoughts spiral into wondering whether he did it on purpose because he never really liked me anyway – maybe I thought I saw him snicker a little, just before asking if I was OK. On and on I spin: all these thoughts and fears are second darts. The bruise on my hip will heal long before all these emotional wounds that I just hurled around at myself. These second darts carry a potential of driving my emotional and physical pains.

To give an example from my own experience, I went through an emotionally loaded break-up a few years back. The thoughts that spun through my head, 'I am broken, abandoned, tossed aside, worthless, unlovable', began to create a place of internal struggle and made me feel like the victim of a harmful act. A decision my ex had made elicited a *first dart* reaction from me with feelings of sadness, grief and anger. But these are just feelings; they don't carry harm. When recognized as such they can be felt and processed. Allowing the actions of another person to determine my own value or worthiness is the *second dart* and is self-created. It is here in the head full of darts that an emotion of sadness turns into an experience of suffering.

In the book *Buddha's Brain,* it is described in this way: "As long as you live and love some of those darts will come your way."[6] First darts may feel hurtful but it is the *reactions* we add to them, second darts, that cause the suffering. I was sad. I felt betrayed. These emotions are real and carry a feeling of hurtfulness. But when recognized as simply uncomfortable rather than harmful they can settle and run their course, eventually softening. It was all the second darts I was throwing at myself that created a place of suffering. I was the one that attached my sense of worthiness and value to the actions of another. And I could make this suffering stop.

Returning to a more tissue-based example, let's look again at the runner with knee pain from earlier, who also has discomfort in his knee. When he pushes into the third mile of a run, he begins to feel the twinge of pain in his knee – *first dart*. He may then start to think 'My knee is all torn up, I will never run a marathon again' – *second darts*. To learn what can be done with these darts let's put it into a practice.

Learning to Practice
Out of the Head and Onto the Mat

- Take a comfortable seat.

- Place one hand on your belly and one hand on your heart.

- Start to find your breath.

- As you settle in, can you begin to think of an experience, physical or more emotionally driven, where you can clearly identify a first dart? Once you have that, then begin to look at the second darts you put into play. Try to label each one 'second dart'. Work through this as long as you need, to feel confident you are able to separate the initial event from the reactions you placed around it.

- Finish with a few long, slow, cleansing breaths and an intention to try to be more mindful of second darts in real time.

Off the Mat and Into Life

Emotional: The next time you find yourself in a scenario of feeling hurt by the actions of another, pause. Ask yourself what is the emotion – the first dart? Identify it. Give it time to be fully present, felt and realized. See what thoughts start to surface beneath it. Is this part of the actual experience? Or is it a second dart, the thing you are creating all on your own? Find the holes, lean in a little deeper to the root of the spinning thoughts or darts you are throwing at yourself. In a gentle way, begin to separate your sense of self from the action of the other, recognize the simple emotions instead. Let them be felt and expressed. Allow yourself to feel porous so the emotions can run through instead of attaching. This may sound easy, but it is not. It takes practice to pause and feel emotions. The very first step may be to simply take a long, slow, deep breath. This will allow the moment of pause to happen. Then try to clearly name the feeling: for example, I feel sad. Just feel that for a while. With time and practiced attention, the rest will begin to unfold.

Physical: When you have the feeling of being uncomfortable due to a physical pain, ask yourself what is the symptom – the first dart? Identify it. Give it time to be fully present and felt. See what thoughts start to surface beneath it. Try to identify the physical sensation for what it is and stop asking or predicting what it means or what it will become – second darts. Begin to separate the sensory experience from the rest. Can you simply begin to acknowledge that you are, in fact, uncomfortable but also fine?

Conclusion

As humans, our thought streams are continuous and often repetitive. The contents of our thoughts will dictate how we interact with our external as well as our internal environment. Our thoughts can make us prisoners or can be the keys that release us. Some aspects of pain may be out of our control; however, some are much more controllable than we may initially think. Shifting the perspective of ourselves first as clinicians and teachers will in turn help us to facilitate those working through the experience of pain.

The next two chapters will bring in the pain science side of our thoughts, beliefs and emotions and the direct way in which these impact the pain experience. As you read on, see if you can begin to relate the mindfulness practices of *and this too, real but not true* and *first and second darts* with ways to approach more medical or psychological concepts like catastrophization and fear avoidance. No need to fret: you don't have to have all this mastered yet – we will bring these mindfulness practices back again and again, because that is the practice.

References

1. Kabat-Zinn, J. Full Catastrophe Living. 2005, New York: Bantam Dell.

2. Rinpoche, T. Open Heart, Open Mind. 2012, New York: Harmony Books.

3. Bishop, S.R., M. Lau, S. Shapiro, et al. Mindfulness: A Proposed Operational Definition. Clinical Psychology, 2004. 11(3): 230–41.

4. Brach, T. True Refuge. 2016, New York: Bantam Books.

5. Kornfield, J. The Wise Heart. 2009, New York: Bantam Books.

6. Hanson, R. Buddha's Brain. 2009, Oakland, CA: New Harbinger Publications, Inc.

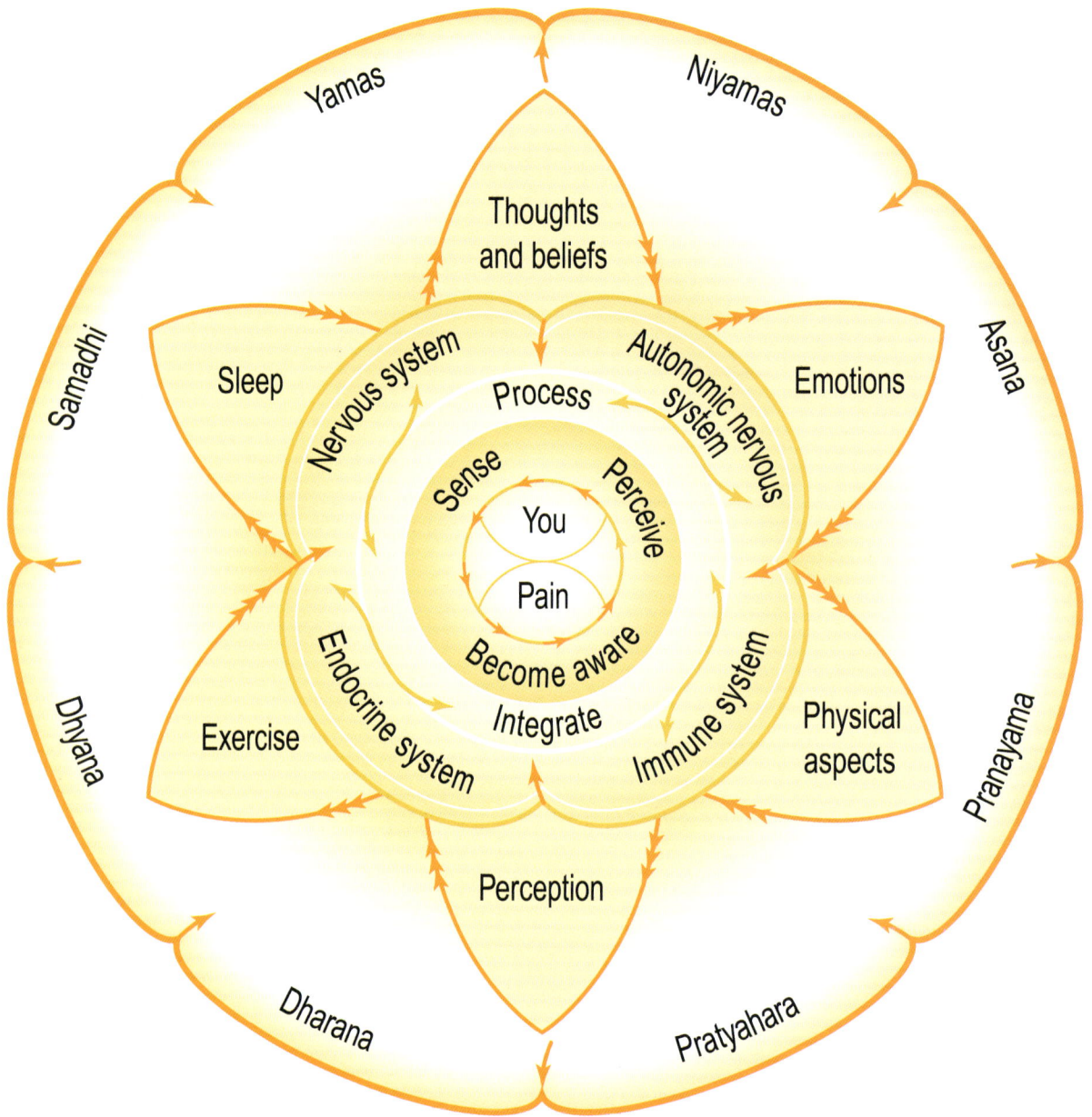

2

Case Study: Meeting Phillip

Phillip, an 18-year-old high-school senior and former baseball player (pitcher), attended for physiotherapy. As a 15-year-old he had been scouted for collegiate programs. Two years prior to meeting him, his life was changed by what seemed like a simple event on the playing field: he was hit on the back of the right hand with a moderately high-speed baseball.

When I met him two years on from the initial injury, his hand was intermittently swollen, at times very swollen, pale in color and cold to touch. The pain had spread up the arm into his shoulder and occasionally he reported a burning sensation around his face. His wrist was stiff and difficult to move, and he reported that it was increasingly difficult to move his elbow and shoulder. He described feeling as if his right arm wasn't actually part of him: "Kind of like it doesn't even belong to me anymore". The longer he was in pain, the more he felt like everything was beginning to hurt: "Like the right side of my trunk and the right side of my face even".

He had been seen by multiple sports medicine specialists and therapists. For the first year, most clinicians thought he was a dramatic teenager exaggerating his symptoms for attention, and some even accused him of drug-seeking. He was eventually diagnosed with complex regional pain syndrome (CRPS).

> CRPS is a complex and persistent pain condition, and some of the key features are pain, tissue color and temperature changes, disordered inflammation, heightened nervous system sensitization, and often changes in perception.

Phillip was previously under a great deal of stress. He was under pressure from his family to pursue a career in baseball and was struggling to fit in all the practice times required, as well as the study time to maintain the grades he wanted, as his dream was to be a surgeon. He was starting to live with a great deal of negative self-talk: he wasn't good enough, a disappointment to his friends and family. He had become withdrawn socially and his grades were declining. He was not sleeping well and was losing hope that his life would ever be 'normal' again.

We'll follow Phillip through the remaining chapters and explore how using science and yoga helped bridge the gap from pain back to a life that is fulfilling and hopeful for him.

Thoughts become things.

Bob Proctor

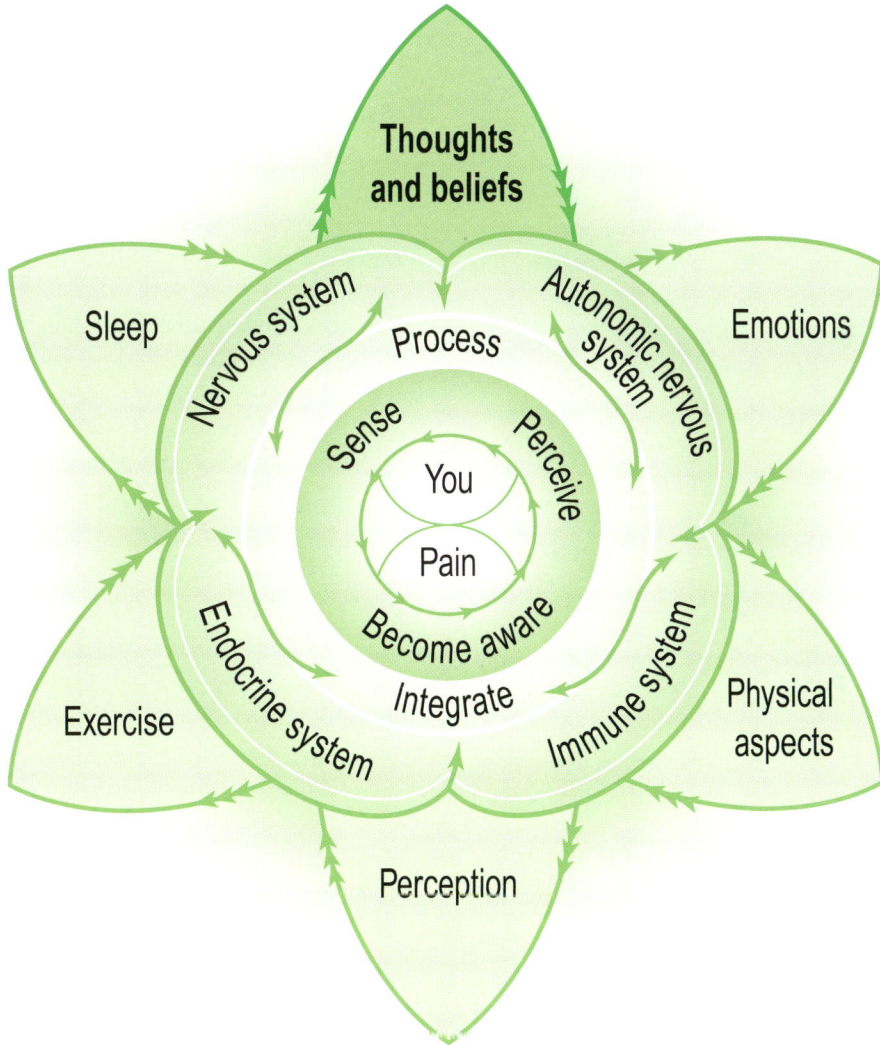

Figure 4.1

Pain Mandala – Thoughts and Beliefs. The way we think and the beliefs we hold will have an impact on the various systems of our body. These thoughts and beliefs can be integrated to improve the regulation of health and decrease pain experiences, or they can leave us in a negative feedback loop of suffering from poor health and pain.

Note: This mandala depicts aspects of the human experience of pain covered in Pain Science Yoga Life. *Other inputs, dimensions and body systems can contribute to pain than those noted here.*

Headspace
Painful Thoughts

Mike explains that his back pain is because of disc bulges and one day his back is going 'to go' and he will end up wheelchair-bound like his aunt. Claire twists her ankle and thinks she will never be able to dance again. Melissa's knee clicks and clunks, her scan shows arthritis and she believes that 'it is bone on bone in there.' Phillip (Case Study, p.51) believes he won't be able to play baseball or achieve his dream of becoming a surgeon. These are common thoughts expressed by the people we work with: thoughts and beliefs common in our society. "Marnie?", my friend Andrew inquires, "I've been on many mountain climbs and adventures with you, I've watched you twist your ankle, I've seen you graze the skin of your arms and legs, yet I rarely see you react in pain. Don't you feel pain?" "Of course I feel pain. I don't react because I believe I'm going to be OK. So, to be honest what I feel is discomfort of a skin scratch or an overstretched ankle and then my brain moves on." Both directions of these thoughts and beliefs will contribute to pain experiences.

Pain-related cognitions, how we think about pain, our understanding of what causes pain, and how pain affects our lives are 'inputs' that deeply impact the pain we experience. Claire and I both experience the *first dart* of an ankle twist; I recognize the physical sensation and am able to move on, while Claire jumps to a *second dart* of fear for the future. These second darts cause the next level of suffering we explored in Chapter 3 and are important players in pain neuroscience. Many of us will be familiar with the experience that people who are highly anxious or think the worst about their pain suffer more, and don't respond as well to the usual treatments. In contrast, we see people with considerable injuries being incredibly positive, seeming to have deep belief in their capacity to recover, going on to have positive health outcomes. Some of these traits and health factors such as

optimism and pessimism, stress and anxiety are well known, while others like pain catastrophizing, fear-avoidance and pain self-efficacy are less commonly recognized but very important, and have received a lot of focus in pain research. Let's look at what these latter constructs mean and how they become apparent.

Pain-Related Cognitions
Pain Beliefs

Pain beliefs are simply what we believe about pain, many of which are deeply ingrained and are generations old. They are also influenced by people we encounter including clinicians and teachers.[1,2] What we believe shapes how we behave; pain-related beliefs shape how we behave when we're in pain. For example, if I believe movement will be harmful, I will most likely be very protective of moving the painful area. This means that if the beliefs we have are helpful, we're more likely to behave in ways that support recovery. If the beliefs we hold are unhelpful, e.g. that we don't expect to recover, this can be detrimental.[3-5] Further, the strategies we might use to cope with pain are less likely to optimize recovery. One example is that if movement hurts, many conclude it must be harmful and should be avoided. While it is sensible to take things easier if you've had a recent injury, we know movement is good for reducing pain and promoting healing.[6,7] Avoiding movement totally is unhelpful. This is even more so for persistent pain, where pain equaling harm to tissues is much less likely and where avoiding movement can impede recovery.

Pain Catastrophizing

Pain catastrophizing can be thought of as thinking about the worst-case scenario about what pain means and feeling helpless about it. It is defined as "an exaggerated negative mental set brought to bear during actual or anticipated painful experience", and consists of three main elements: 1) rumination – "I can't stop thinking about how much it hurts"; 2) magnification – "I worry that something serious may happen"; and 3) helplessness –"There is nothing I can do to reduce the intensity of the pain."[8-10] We all think about consequences when we have pain, e.g. 'Will I be able to work/play football at the weekend?' Someone who catastrophizes quickly gets to 'I'll never be able to work again' or 'That's it for my sporting career.' We might all ask, 'What do I need to do about this problem?' These days we understand that a helpful response is to be proactive (e.g. actively take advice, do what you can to help yourself) whereas a catastrophizing response might be to feel very helpless and think 'I can't do anything because it hurts.'

> Take home message: What we believe shapes how we behave.

Pain-Related Fear

Pain-related fear is a close cousin of pain catastrophizing. We'll talk about fear and anxiety specifically in Chapter 5, but how we think about pain may drive fear and fear-related responses. One response is *fear-avoidance*. The fear-avoidance model describes how fear of pain, movement or re-injury can drive avoidance of activities resulting in higher levels of disability and pain.[11,12] Avoiding potentially painful activities is obviously sensible to some degree, particularly with recent injuries, but in persistent pain it's usually not helpful and becomes a barrier to returning to normal activities. It was originally considered that fear-avoidance was driven by pain catastrophizing, unhelpful health information and emotional distress;[11] however, more recent studies show that a linear process where thoughts lead to fear may not exist. Instead, fear-avoidance and negative cognitions (e.g. pain catastrophizing) co-exist and this cumulative load drives more disability and more pain.[13]

Another recent consideration of the fear-avoidance model is that protective behaviors are not so much about phobic reactions to movement, as once thought. Sam Bunzli and colleagues highlighted this when they investigated what explains fear-avoidance in people with persistent back pain and high fear-avoidance scores.[14] What they found was really interesting. Some reasons people gave for avoiding activities or fearing pain and further damage were things like: 1) their pain didn't make sense to them, and they were still seeking diagnostic certainty – looking for answers about the cause of pain; 2) they had poor control over pain and had experienced failed attempts at controlling pain; and 3) that pain was unpredictable.

Bunzli and team concluded that people were trying to 'make sense of pain,' and when pain didn't make sense, they feared it more and pain had greater impact. Therefore, as teachers and clinicians, if we can help individuals understand their pain, we may also help them escape this fear-avoidance cycle. This study uniquely highlights how human these responses are. Is it understandable to avoid something you might perceive as potentially harmful when you don't have a clear explanation for what is causing the pain, or why it behaves the way it does?

Pain Self-Efficacy

To move to more proactive constructs, pain self-efficacy has been well studied in persistent pain.[3] It relates to how well someone can continue normal activities despite being in pain, i.e. how well they cope with pain. Self-efficacy was historically defined as the confidence with which one can successfully execute a course of action to produce a desired outcome.[15] In the presence of pain, self-efficacy may be considered as the ability to engage in meaningful activities and activities that promote health and moving beyond pain. As such, it may affect the performance of actions necessary for pain care.[16] Lack of pain self-efficacy is the spiral of thoughts and beliefs such as 'I can't _____ because of my pain.'

Pain Acceptance

Really? Accept pain? It's counterintuitive, right? This idea might provoke resistance initially, but accepting pain may be more useful than it seems, as we'll see below. *Acceptance* forms part of a construct called *psychological flexibility*. General psychological flexibility is the ability to embrace unwanted experiences (pain, thoughts, memories, etc.) when they may be connected to our goals in life.[17] Acceptance of pain is a specific form of this general psychological flexibility.[18] It engenders willingness to engage in activity despite being in pain without always needing to control pain to be able to do so.[19] If we think back to Chapter 3 – *and this too* – these are the same concepts: being able to include, accept and hold space for different experiences, wanted or unwanted, without judgment or resistance. With pain acceptance and less resistance, people can engage in more of their meaningful, valued activities even in the presence of pain.[18,20,21]

> Take home message: Pain acceptance can mean greater engagement with meaningful, valued activities, even in the presence of pain.

Pain-Related Cognitions: Evidence from Clinical Populations

There are considerable amounts of data demonstrating that people with persistent pain frequently show high levels of pain catastrophizing and fear-avoidance, which correlate with greater pain and disability.[22,23] Pain-related fear also helps explain the relationship between pain and disability.[24,25] Both pain catastrophizing and fear-avoidance are predictors of poor prognosis in some pain conditions and adversely affect treatment response.[4, 26–35] They can even reduce the ability of people to maintain treatment gains following pain management programs.[36] Of course, these factors don't apply to everyone, but enough people are affected[37,38] that we should be asking people we work with: 'What does this mean for you?,' 'Does your pain make sense to you?,' 'What is your understanding of what's going on?' Only by starting this conversation will we begin to understand whether people are fearful and what beliefs they hold, and in turn, enable individuals to make sense of their pain. We'll see later how some of the ways we teach yoga can influence pain-related cognitions positively and negatively.

On the flip side, it may be worth considering more positive cognitive processes and appreciating their value. Higher levels of pain self-efficacy are associated with better functioning and less disability, less pain and lower depression rates in people with persistent pain, and are even more strongly associated with pain-related outcomes than factors like fear-avoidance.[3,32,39] Higher self-efficacy trumps high fear-avoidance, so to speak. Higher self-efficacy positively impacts prognosis, positively influences how much people with pain engage in physical activity and their work status,[32] and may affect how people respond to active treatments.[30] Further, if self-efficacy changes over the course of treatment, it influences changes in pain and disability as a result of that treatment.[40] Pain self-efficacy is modifiable, so when we use yoga in pain care, fostering an environment of 'I can, even with pain' and positive attitudes to recovery may benefit those with lower self-efficacy.

Remember pain acceptance: greater pain acceptance is associated with better health outcomes.[20] It is correlated with less pain interference (how pain interferes with life), greater quality of life, better physical function and less pain catastrophizing, frustration, depression, pain-related anxiety[41–43] and pain medication use.[44] A key intervention that promotes pain acceptance is Acceptance and Commitment Therapy, or ACT. Acceptance and engagement in values-based action both predict how well people with pain respond to ACT.[45] Further, pain-related acceptance partially explains changes in people's function following ACT.[46] These research findings ring true when we hear people's stories about their journey beyond pain. In the book *Pain Heroes*,[47] a number of people with long histories of debilitating pain tell their stories, and in almost every story a tipping point occurred when they accepted pain and re-engaged with much-loved activities anyway. When they understood their pain didn't mean more harm and were able to accept some physical sensations *(and this too),* they were able to move more and pain started to lose its hold on them. It seems ironic, but with greater acceptance of pain, and less resistance to pain, these pain heroes found their way back to meaningful living, and with that, pain lost its power and started to fade.

How Do Pain-Related Cognitions Affect Pain Processing?

In Chapter 1, we described how pain is the result of many inputs and processes. Inputs from bodily tissues can be relevant, but we saw how changing our perspective of pain from one where *'pain = tissue damage'* to *'pain = perceived need for protection'* shifts our attention towards looking at a person with pain from a broader perspective, conceptualized in the Pain Mandala (Figure 4.1).

Let's explore the idea that 'pain protects' in relation to thoughts and beliefs, and particularly the spiral of negative thoughts, by looking at a 'non-pain' example. Imagine that you have a fear of heights and while out hiking you come across a suspension bridge over a deep ravine. You panic, feel anxious (limbic system: emotional brain responses) and are hesitant about crossing; your sympathetic nervous system responds: your heart races, your breath quickens, you start to perspire. Scenario 1: you reassure yourself – you think logically: 'The bridge looks sturdy; it must be safe, otherwise it wouldn't be in a national park; lots of other people have crossed and they're safe.' This positive, reassuring self-talk (pre-frontal cortex: rational brain responses) calms your emotional brain and reduces your stress response enough to get you across

the bridge. Scenario 2: you panic, all you can think about is the bridge snapping and you falling into the ravine…it's like a rerun of an Indiana Jones movie. You can't think of anything else, that's it, you're done, you're not going any further. Panic wins today.

What does this have to do with pain? Take something we see almost daily in clinical practice and yoga: the avoidance of specific movements, postures or activities based on beliefs that 'it is bad for my condition.' Mike, whom we met at the start of the chapter, is a good example of this. He experiences low back pain on bending, and his MRI scan shows a couple of disc bulges – he's been told this is what's causing his pain. Now let's layer this up with some previous experiences and knowledge. When he used to go to the gym, he was told to keep his back straight when lifting weights to prevent damage to his discs. His work health and safety training emphasized how important it was not to slump when sitting or bend the spine when lifting to protect his spine. So now when he feels pain as he bends, isn't it reasonable for Mike to think that the pain is telling him to stop bending, avoid it, and that painful bending must mean he's harming 'vulnerable' discs? This is him 'making sense of his pain.' These thoughts provide a strong cue for the brain to protect. Isn't this like Scenario 2 at the bridge? That same panicked thinking that paralyzes us and stops us crossing the bridge can cause the brain to 'protect the spine' even more by producing more pain and more muscle activation, making movement stiffer and more guarded. It can also drive greater stress responses (more in Chapter 5). Can you see how these negative thought inputs produce other bodily responses (Figure 4.2), which in turn produce more 'inputs' into the system, as the Pain Mandala shows (see Figure 4.1)?

Now what if Mike is given really good evidence-based information about spines and pain (see Chapter 6): that findings on scans like disc bulges are common and don't always correlate with people's symptoms?[48,49] That

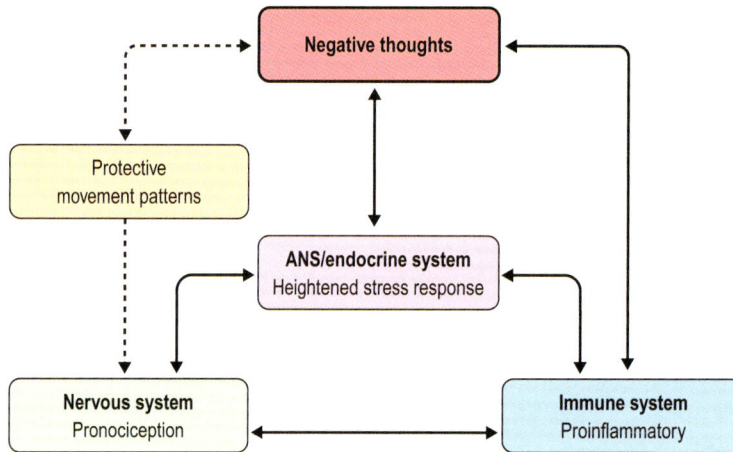

Figure 4.2

How thoughts and beliefs influence pain: possible mechanisms. Worrisome thoughts and beliefs can influence pain via effects on multiple systems. If you worry about arthritis in your knees developing, you may have increased pain and stiffness even without a change in the arthritis, due to the mechanisms depicted here. Thoughts can heighten stress responses (ANS and endocrine system) and facilitate a pro-nociceptive state (nervous system), both of which can impair immune system responses causing a pro-inflammatory state (immune system). The two-way arrows indicate two-way interactions between some of the elements included. *ANS,* autonomic nervous system.

spines, even with disc bulges, are well adapted to moving in all directions; that yes, in the early stages after a back injury it can be helpful to move gently and find ways to get pain relief, but as time moves on it's helpful to restore movement and find fluid ways of moving. What if Mike wasn't fearful that pain meant more damage to his discs, if he felt it was safe to move? This could look like Scenario 1 from the fear of heights example. Sure, the pain is still there, just like the anxiety is, but it's not so paralyzing. Importantly, these beliefs influence our pain experiences.

The Mechanisms

How do these thoughts and beliefs influence the mechanisms of pain? Take pain catastrophizing again, the cognitive interpretation that pain is very threatening. There is evidence to support two mechanisms by which pain catastrophizing affects pain processing. The first relates to descending

modulation of nociception. Remember that when cognitive centers of the brain appraise the situation as *threatening* they can signal to areas within the brain to *reduce* the release of neurotransmitters that calm nociception and therefore *more pain* may be experienced (Figure 4.3).[50–53] This is the pro-nociceptive state discussed in Chapter 1. Recent data show that rumination about pain (the repetitive focus on discomfort) also negatively affects this descending modulation.[54]

The second mechanism relates to nociceptive (warning signal) processing within the brain – activity in the 'pain neuromatrix' (Figure 4.4). Brain activity related to concentration, cognitions, emotions and memory is associated with pain perception and can enhance the pain experience.[51] For example, pain catastrophizing correlates with enhanced activity in brain areas associated with attention to pain, emotional responses to pain and anticipatory anxiety around pain – areas such as the anterior cingulate cortex (ACC) and dorsolateral pre-frontal cortex (PFC).[53,55] It even affects connectivity between sensory and emotional processing within the brain (somatosensory cortices (SI, SII) and insula).[55,56] For example, when healthy people were exposed to noxious stimuli, those with higher pain catastrophizing scores experienced more intense pain, which correlated with greater activity in the dorsal PFC.[57] Recent research also shows that the link between pain catastrophizing and pain hypersensitivity is partly driven by the way anticipating pain affects our brain. When people with fibromyalgia and high catastrophizing anticipated pain, activity in the lateral PFC was reduced – a part of the PFC important for anti-nociception or turning down warning signals.[58] Another way pain catastrophizing is linked with pain and pain hypersensitivity is through enhancing activity in the resting state of the brain,[53] called the 'default mode network.'[58] Just like your laptop on standby, the brain circuitry is primed and ready to go – it will be responsive to even small triggers. Finally, thoughts and beliefs influence emotional responses and hence the stress response, but we will discuss this in more detail in Chapter 5.

So, what does this mean for treating pain? Perhaps we can appreciate that if the cognitive centers of the brain appraise the situation as *less threatening*, they can signal to areas within the brain to release neurotransmitters that calm nociception, turning down warning signals, therefore producing *less pain*.[50, 51] By appraising the situation as not so threatening, there is less need for protection and therefore less need for pain. This is borne out in research showing that when people understand how pain works (pain neuroscience), they can achieve more pain relief.[59]

> Take home message: If you view a situation as less threatening, there will be less need to protect and thus the pain experience may be less.

Unfortunately, the understanding of pain for many people (including clinicians and teachers) is such that it is always interpreted as equating to tissue damage, injury or illness. This influences how we talk about pain and how we approach pain care. A major step in allowing the thinking brain to appraise the situation as non-threatening is to challenge the assumption that pain is always proportional to tissue damage. We need to reframe pain and consider all possible contributions to the pain experience. For many this will probably only be truly learned through *both* knowledge and experience. For Mike, as well as reconceptualizing pain and its meaning, he may need to *experience* bending more comfortably before he believes bending isn't harmful. Nonetheless, a key message here is that what we say and do as clinicians and teachers plays a role in influencing people's beliefs about pain. Our simplest interactions potentially influence thoughts and beliefs, enhancing proactive or protective behaviors, and thus enhancing or reducing people's pain experiences.

Hurt and Harm: The Link

Beliefs that pain is always caused by tissue damage and that identifying 'pathology' via medical imaging is key to getting the right health care are common.[60] This model of pain and damage has been around for centuries, so it's deeply ingrained. Advances in imaging techniques have brought enormous benefits. Scans (e.g. MRI, ultrasound, CT) are so sensitive that they pick up small abnormalities. This can be helpful but carries a downside. First, it drives many people, including clinicians, to focus on the findings of scans, ignoring the bigger picture. Second, many observations on imaging may be variations of normal and are common in healthy people.[48,49] For example, if you are over 40 you have a 50% chance of having a disc bulge on a spinal scan even if you don't have pain.[48] In people with back pain, knowing the results of scans leads to poorer outcomes than if they don't know the results.[61] Why? There are many reasons, such as imaging leading to unnecessary interventions, but

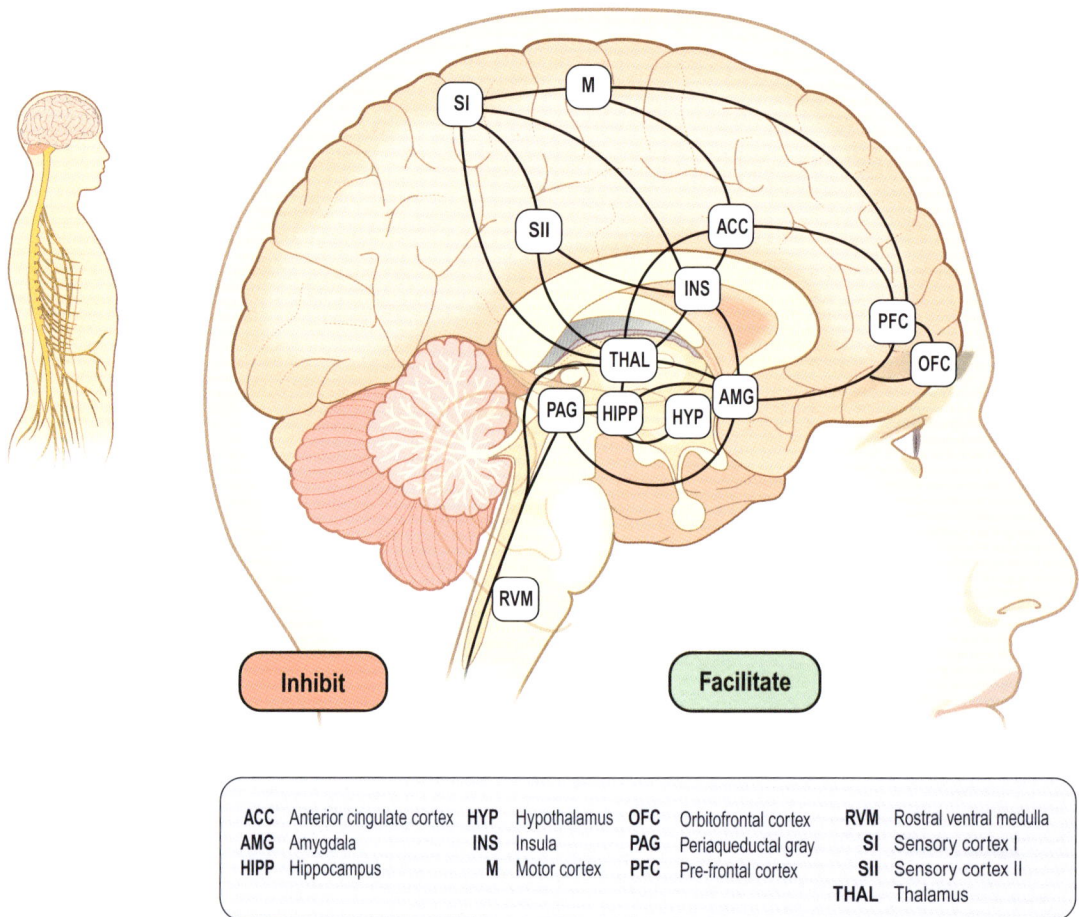

Figure 4.3

The nervous system: the 'brain's pharmacy' and descending modulation of nociception. The PAG/RVM can inhibit or facilitate nociception, turning the dial up or down on nociception. When neurotransmitters that inhibit nociception are released, nociceptive signals are turned down: result = less pain. When neurotransmitters that facilitate nociception are released, nociceptive signals are turned up: result = more pain.

relating to thought processes one might speculate that people will worry more about what has been found on the scans and treat their back in a way traditionally thought to protect it (e.g. don't bend, stop exercising) when these strategies might not be so helpful. Relying on tissue explanations for pain alone is limited, and ignoring the bigger picture is flawed. Because this hurt and harm link is often ingrained in our belief system,

it likely predates the onset of injury or pain without any real awareness. As clinicians or teachers, a challenging role in pain care is to begin to alter this belief.

Promoting Helpful Beliefs About Pain

What we as clinicians and teachers believe and say matters.[62] When people with persistent pain were asked what they thought about their pain and where

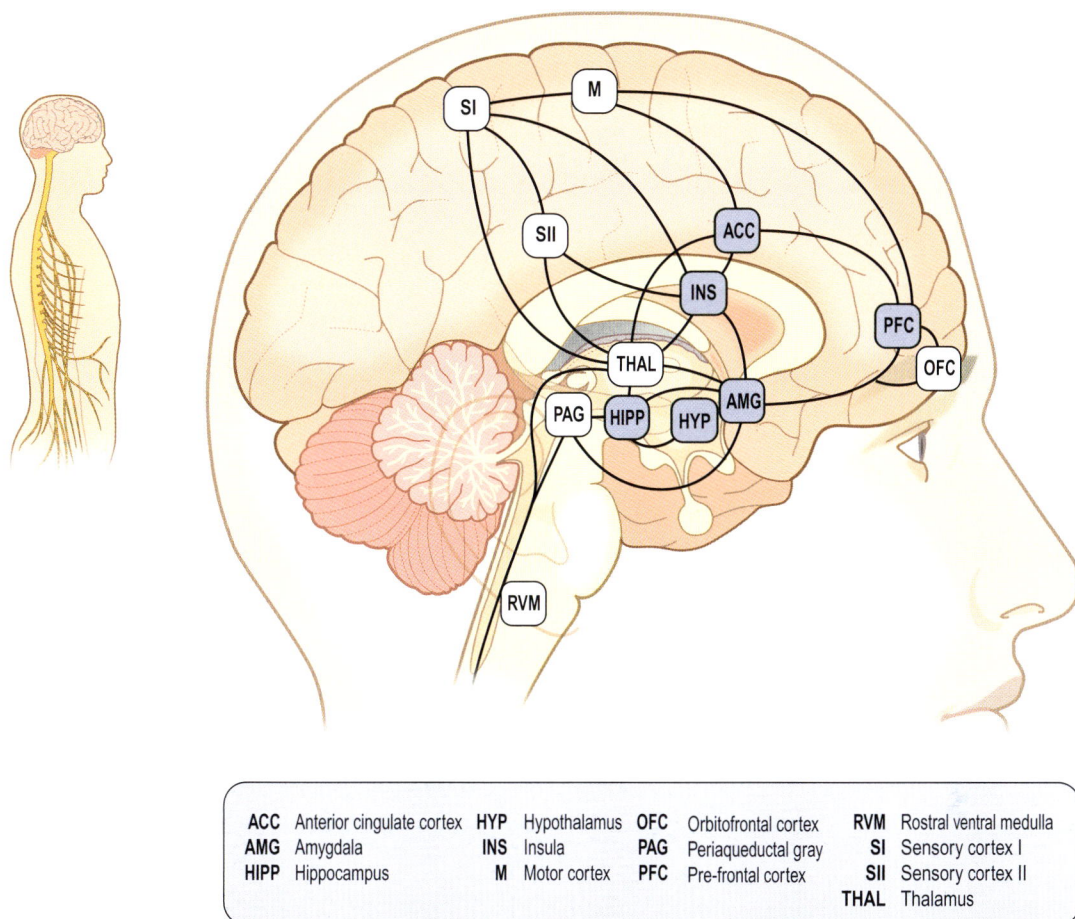

ACC	Anterior cingulate cortex	HYP	Hypothalamus	OFC	Orbitofrontal cortex	RVM	Rostral ventral medulla
AMG	Amygdala	INS	Insula	PAG	Periaqueductal gray	SI	Sensory cortex I
HIPP	Hippocampus	M	Motor cortex	PFC	Pre-frontal cortex	SII	Sensory cortex II
						THAL	Thalamus

Figure 4.4

The brain: a pain neuromatrix. Negative thoughts and beliefs can enhance activity in brain areas related to attention, emotional responses and anticipatory anxiety about pain.

those beliefs came from, the results were sobering.[1] Beliefs ranged from the rather common – 'I'm afraid to move in case I damage my back/pelvis' or 'My core is so weak' – to the extreme – 'I had an abortion because I didn't think I'd be able to carry the pregnancy.' Where did these beliefs come from? Health care providers mostly. No doubt, the clinician didn't say, 'You're so weak you won't be able to carry a baby,' but as clinicians and teachers, we need to be mindful

of what our words mean to different people. If someone is told repeatedly that their 'core is weak,' that can easily be interpreted as 'dangerously weak' and this thought can spiral. If someone is told, 'Look after your back, you've only got one,' that might be interpreted as 'Don't move, protect your spine and don't do anything painful,' when what may be meant is 'Do some exercise, find a healthy level of physical activity.' Other common phrases uttered by professionals are 'It's the

Chapter 4

worst I have ever seen' and 'At 45 you have the spine of a 70-year-old.' These expressions are unhelpful and may actually be harmful as they are likely to induce protective thoughts and anxiety leading to strong cues for protection – pain.

On a more positive note, many people with back pain hold positive attitudes about the health of their backs. Again, these thoughts and beliefs are often derived from clinicians promoting positive back pain beliefs and confidence around managing pain, reassuring people that this isn't the start of something awful, and encouraging people to keep moving and stay active.[1] We might reinforce how resilient the body is, or that the scan shows normal age-related changes, like gray hair and wrinkles – maybe not desirable but not something to worry about. We need to choose our words wisely and check in with how what we say is interpreted, knowing that our words can leave lasting impressions. With awareness and practice we can ensure these impressions are productive and positive.

Awareness of our word choices and the effects they can leave needs to be considered when teaching movements or asanas. Instructing in a rigid manner leading people to believe there is only one right way to move or position themselves may feed thoughts and beliefs around injury or risk of injury that could increase unnecessary protection. Again, these thoughts, beliefs and protective behaviors can influence present and future pain experiences.

Turning Knowledge Into Practice

As teachers and clinicians familiar with encouraging behavioral change, or even for those of us who have attempted to alter aspects of our own thoughts, emotions or behaviors, we know changing our perspective or thoughts and beliefs is no simple task. They can't be changed overnight or by following a recipe. The following are interventions that have addressed how we

think about pain or incorporated how we think about pain into a broader approach.

Pain Neuroscience Education

A cornerstone to making sense of one's pain comes from knowledge about modern pain neuroscience. This might be the first and most necessary step in creating change for many. Pain neuroscience education, i.e. learning about the biological processes that occur in the human body and brain to elicit the experience of pain, has seen growing attention thanks to key proponents like David Butler and Lorimer Moseley,[63] Adriaan Louw,[64] and others. While the effects of pain neuroscience education on pain itself may be limited, positive effects on pain catastrophizing and fear-avoidance are more substantial and relevant for people with persistent musculoskeletal pain.[65] In addition, pain education in combination with physiotherapy have been shown to have greater effects on measures of central sensitization and descending inhibition of nociception than physiotherapy alone.[66] Pain education on its own may not be the magic bullet that changes the experience of pain, but it can help change attitudes to pain, and where appropriate, help people reconceptualize pain and make sense of chronic pain.[65,67] Although we don't know this for sure yet, it's plausible that changing how we think about pain may allow us to be open to a broader approach to pain care rather than solely focusing on bodily structures, impairments and pathologies. Making sense of how pain works has become the cornerstone for many contemporary pain care approaches.

Modern pain science can be difficult to fully digest and often challenges what we think we have always known – long-held beliefs about body structures, for example. It takes time and effort for us and the people we work with to understand this. It may be helpful to create a slow transition toward change by first noticing your own beliefs. Consider how you talk to yourself about your own physical discomforts and injuries. Can you identify thoughts or beliefs of your own that may be less helpful? After turning this recognition inward, can you take note of how your students or patients talk? Is it possible to see opportunities in yourself and those you interact with to open a new place of understanding about pain and how we approach pain care?

Shifting our understanding of pain and reflecting on our thought processes is one thing but pain education on its own may not be sufficient to change thoughts and beliefs. It's likely to be more complex and involve experiential learning (experiencing change) before we understand pain and change how we think about it. For example, pain catastrophizing is modifiable but responds best to multimodal interventions like Cognitive Behavioral Therapy (CBT) and Acceptance and Commitment Therapy (ACT),[68] approaches that integrate cognitive, behavioral and emotional factors. Let's look at these a little more closely.

Cognitive Behavioral Therapy (CBT)

A part of psychology practice for over half a century, CBT is an active treatment that attempts to change unhelpful or distorted thoughts and by consequence, or in tandem, change behavior and feelings about the issue at hand. CBT has been extensively evaluated for persistent pain, and while the effects on pain intensity are small, the effects on disability, catastrophizing and mood are more impressive.[69] Recent iterations of CBT have changed the emphasis to shifting the *relationship* one has with unhelpful thoughts rather than changing the thoughts directly.[70,71] Rather than simply changing a negative thought into a positive one, this practice encourages a deeper inquiry with a goal of understanding what runs beneath the thought stream. The concept *real but not true* seems appropriate here. An instruction might be to name the emotion or belief that is driving the negative or unhelpful

thought pattern, and to let the emotion be felt without adding assumed meaning (or a *second dart*) to the experience. Rather than trying to force a change in thinking or feeling, it may be helpful to include thoughts, emotions and even pain sensations as they arise (*and this too*).

For Phillip (see p. 51), naming and including worked well for both his physical sensations and his catastrophic thoughts, as they often came and went together. When his hand symptoms increased, at times to the point where he felt like it was on fire, this would trigger his thoughts to spiral out of control into fears of loss of all of his goals in life and vice versa. He was encouraged to simply name the sensation, and make space for it while dampening the word choice: 'My hand feels hot, I have a sensation of burning.' He would take a few deep breaths and let this be there. If his thoughts started to spiral, he would label them, 'thinking', or label the emotion attached to them, 'fear.' He would return to his breath and use the mantra, '*and this too.*' Once he could pause and soften the intensity of thoughts and sensations, then he could often see that there was something else, like catastrophic thoughts or underlying beliefs, facilitating or intensifying these pain flares.

Acceptance and Commitment Therapy (ACT)

ACT, a form of CBT, is increasingly being used for persistent pain with considerable evidence of effectiveness. While the reduction in pain intensity tends to be small, greater change is demonstrated in pain interference, functionality, mood and distress, with ACT performing similarly or better than traditional CBT, and significantly better than more passive approaches.[72] Let's explore ACT to see how it sits with yoga for pain care.

ACT is an approach that fosters psychological flexibility and encourages mindful values-based action and living. While ACT for pain doesn't focus on reducing symptoms, often that is a reported outcome. There are six key features to ACT:[17,21]

1. Acceptance: being able to sit with pain and not allowing it to dominate your life – *and this too*.

2. Cognitive defusion: differentiating ourselves and our actual experiences from our thoughts. This is a matter of being able to step back from our thoughts and not cling to them so tightly – *real but not true*.

3. Flexible present-focused attention: tracking and being present in moment-to-moment experiences (the act of being mindful).

4. Self-as-context: being able to understand the 'observing self.' There are two different aspects to the mind: the thinking self and the observing self. Most people think of the mind as being the thinking self, the part that comes up with thoughts, beliefs, memories, and so on. Many people aren't aware of the observing self, the part of our mind able to step back and observe the thinking self and the rest of our being. This part of yourself is and always will be the same you (*the true self* or *the witness*), whereas our thinking self and physical self can change (Niyama – Svadhyaya).

5. Values: identifying our values, what's important for us and how we live our lives (Yama – Satya).

6. Committed action: taking values-congruent action, whereby we make behavior change based upon our values (Niyama – Tapas).

A key focus for ACT is the development of psychological flexibility.[17,21] When people experience pain they spend enormous effort (quite understandably) avoiding pain, seeking treatments to get rid of pain, checking their body for symptoms or thinking about pain. This focus often means they limit or stop living a meaningful life. They can become trapped in a cycle of 'I can't ____ because of my pain' or 'When my pain is gone, I'll do that.' Psychological flexibility fosters the opposite: a willingness to live life as fully as possible despite the unpleasantness. In other words, 'I will choose that I will, and can, even with pain in my life.'

From these core concepts we see how ACT and yoga resonate closely, and indeed how aspects of ACT are derived from mindfulness. Acceptance, cognitive defusion and self-as-context all relate to a mindful approach to living and are engendered in yoga: being content (santosha), staying present in the moment (truthfulness/saucha), not getting lost in distracted thoughts (pratyahara) or harmful thoughts (ahimsa), practicing mindfulness (dharna and dhyana). Committed action according to our values relates closely to tapas. Further, there are close links between the concept of psychological flexibility and the mindfulness approach of *and this too*. Ultimately, both foster acceptance of another dimension of life, whether it be pleasant or unpleasant, holding space for this dimension while pursuing a full and values-based life. Figure 4.5 outlines how these yoga practices potentially affect some of the mechanisms underlying pain.

Mindfulness and Meditation

Mindfulness, introduced in the simplest terms in Chapter 3, is moment-to-moment awareness.[73] We expanded this a little further with the idea of a directed focus on the present moment, while allowing and recognizing feelings, thoughts and sensations – 'What else is here?'[73–75] Mindfulness can be thought of as the ability to have control over your attention and reactions: "You can place your attention wherever you want and it stays there: when you want to shift it to something else, you can."[76] Mindfulness fosters acceptance of the moment as it arises, avoiding resistance to unwanted thoughts, feelings or sensations, allowing space for both wanted or unwanted experiences – *and this too*.

Within Buddhism, it is recognized that being mindful isn't enough: it isn't about walking around

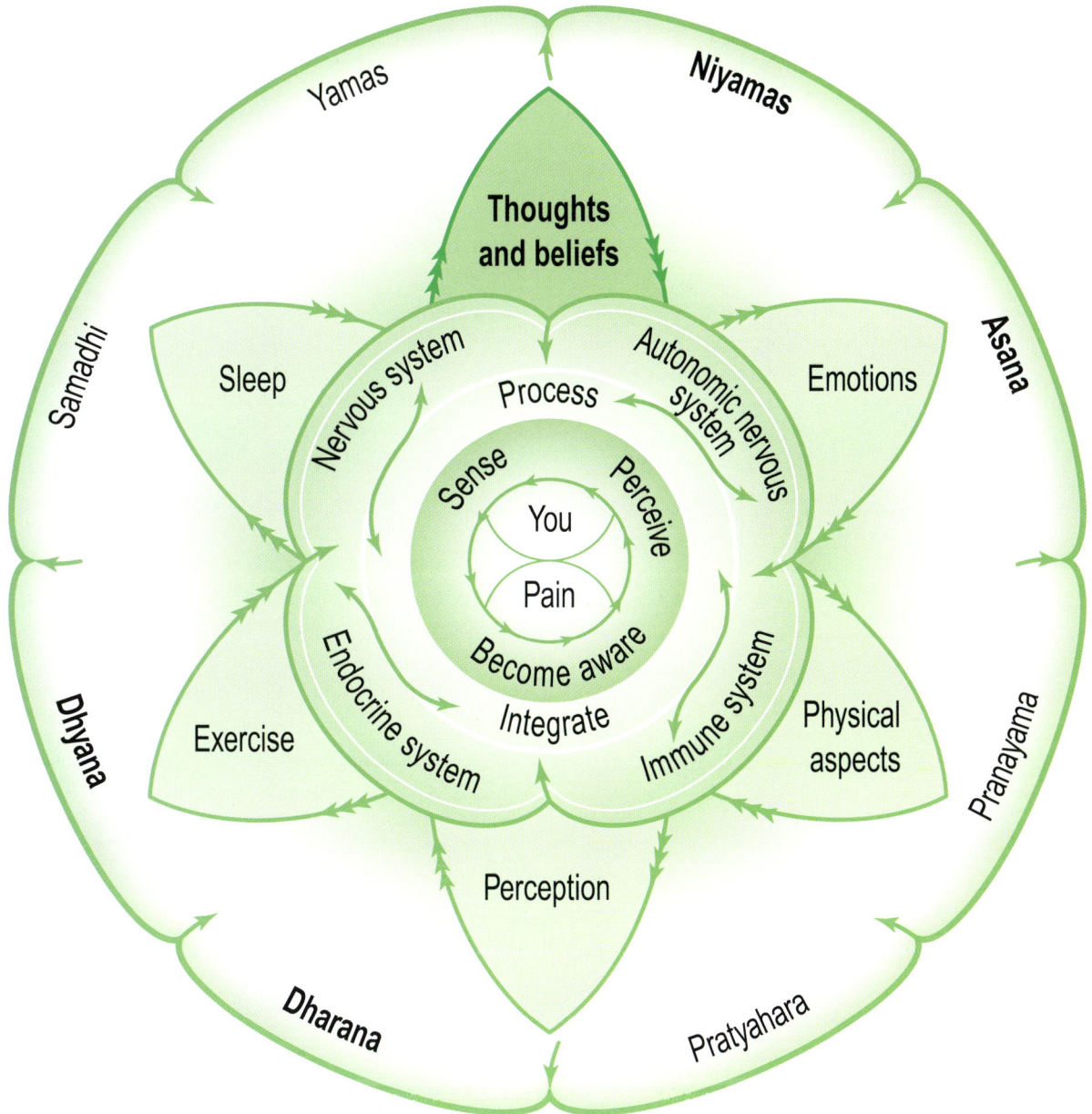

Figure 4.5
Pain and Yoga Mandala – Thoughts and Beliefs. These particular yoga practices – Dharana (focused attention), Dhyana (meditation), Niyama–Svadhyaya (self-study) and Asana (mindful movement) – allow us an opportunity for insight into our thoughts and beliefs about ourselves, our health and our painful experiences. When practiced along with pain science understanding, yoga may be useful in offering an alternate perspective, and with practice can reduce, or aid coping with, the experience of pain.

thinking, 'Focus on the present, be here now'; an actual focus is needed. Mantras like 'Here now' can be helpful to bring us back if our mind has wandered, but we need something to come back to. Thus, there are four foundations of mindfulness woven into Buddhist teachings, which can facilitate bringing us into the present: 1) mindfulness of body – noticing we have a body with all its abilities and difficulties; 2) mindfulness of feelings – identification of the emotions that are present; 3) mindfulness of thought – recognition of the conversation in our head, when the thinking brain has taken us away from the present moment; and 4) mindfulness of dharma, 'the way things are' – this is where we actually find the space of the here and now, where we look past the dualistic judgments of good and bad, right and wrong, and we rest in the space of what is.[75,77] Through awareness and practice is how we learn to prevent a downward spiral of *second dart* suffering.

In yoga, mindfulness relates mainly to dhyana. Dhyana is a key aspect of the quest of a yoga practitioner to find harmony within oneself and integrated connection to all living entities.[78] Awareness of the present moment allows for this, whether in daily life or through specific exercises. The Sixth Limb of yoga, dharana (holding attention), is also relevant as it calls us to bring focused attention to the present.

Mindful attention to any experience can be liberating. Mindfulness can bring perspective, balance and freedom from unhelpful thoughts and beliefs. If we can accept feelings that arise, we may investigate them without allowing these feelings to overwhelm us or drop us into automatic reactive responses.[77] This seems particularly applicable for pain. When we experience physical pain, how often do we get into an automatic negative thought spiral? 'I can't____because of my pain.' Mike thought that one day his back was going to give up and he would become wheelchair-bound. Phillip felt he was losing his dream of becoming a surgeon. These negative thought spirals can increase activity

in areas of our brain and worsen the pain experience. We are adding to our suffering with our *second darts*. In the practice section we will explore this with an exercise. What happens when we try to neutralize this second dart? Can we shift our experience? When working with pain this may be willingness to experience uncomfortable sensations without getting lost in a negative internal conversation about the sensations. It might also involve willingness to check in on reactive thoughts and emotions that arise as we experience pain, and willingness to adjust them.

Mindfulness-based interventions (MBIs) such as Mindfulness-Based Stress Reduction and Mindfulness-Based Cognitive Therapy are practices used in therapeutic settings, delivered as courses over 6–8 weeks. Over the last decade, research on MBIs has been on the rise. MBIs perform as well as traditional psychological therapies such as CBT and potentially offer more impact on outcomes like pain, pain interference, mood and disability compared with non-psychological multimodal treatment or simple relaxation interventions.[72] When people who had undertaken MBIs were interviewed about the effects of the intervention on their pain, they described several changes in their relationship with pain that researchers called "embodied awareness".[79] People re-appraised pain: no longer seeing pain as harmful or something they had to get rid of, but seeing pain and physical sensations more neutrally, as perceptions, that, like all perceptions and sensations, are ever-changing, and as such are less threatening. They also let go of the identity of pain, so that they no longer self-identified as their condition or as a sick person but rather as someone who happened to have a pain condition (*and this too*). Thus, they described being able to achieve wellness amidst their illness. They developed greater self-compassion and acceptance, allowing pain to have some space, not fighting it but learning to respond consciously rather than react automatically. They had greater connection with their body and started to become more aware of early warning signs like increased tension so found they could better manage pain.[79]

Cognitive Functional Therapy

A recent therapy that combines several different methods and is likely one of the most multidimensional approaches for managing musculoskeletal pain is Cognitive Functional Therapy. It is an adaptable, integrated behavioral approach, developed for persistent low back pain but potentially relevant for other conditions.[80] The intervention has four key components: 1) 'making sense of pain,' i.e. pain education in the context of the individual; 2) 'functional movement training,' addressing movement impairments and patterns, again specifically affecting the individual; 3) 'exposure with control,' facilitating improved confidence and control as an individual engages with movements and activities that provoke fear and/or pain; and 4) lifestyle change, integrating lifestyle factors important for facilitating greater recovery and preventing future recurrences (e.g. stress reduction, general physical activity, sleep retraining).

Important features of this approach are the seamlessness between the components delivered and the focus on empowering the individual. For example, the influence of thoughts and beliefs about pain is integrated with movement retraining and function. This approach is still under investigation but early research indicates its potential effectiveness in reducing pain and disability in people with persistent low back pain.[81] While this approach is best delivered on an individual basis with a suitably qualified musculoskeletal clinician, we can learn lessons from it for a broader yoga practice. We can reinforce a healthy, evidence-based understanding of pain and explore different themes in classes to help people explore multidimensional aspects of pain. We can explore movement and offer a forum for exposure to movement. Yoga can serve as a vehicle for lifestyle change in some people, offering a practice for physical activity, stress reduction and maybe even improved sleep.

Conclusion

Thoughts and beliefs have a powerful impact on pain and suffering. They affect our nociceptive processing and, importantly, shape how we behave when we're in pain. Research in the last two decades or more has incorporated addressing and shifting pain beliefs. This might be akin to reducing *second dart* suffering that becomes entwined with pain. While we don't have research evidence for all of this in yoga, potentially, if we teach mindfully, we can see the links between pain neuroscience and yoga practice, and nurture positive cognitions like self-efficacy, acceptance, cognitive defusion and self-compassion. We can reduce pain catastrophizing, fear and fear-avoidance. We can promote present moment awareness and help cultivate greater stress reduction and physical activity.

Since yoga encompasses a physical asana practice, people have exposure to experimenting with movement, an experience that can aid deeper learning. For Phillip, once he learned to pause to recognize and soften his fears and negative thought spirals, he was able to begin to move toward developing greater self-efficacy. He did this by first recognizing his achievement of being diligent in his efforts for sports and school; his successes had not come without hard work. He had to decide that he was going to apply this same discipline to his recovery. He began to accept that it was going to be a hard and potentially long term journey but he slowly gained confidence that he could have a purposeful life again.

Remember, as teachers and clinicians we might consider how *our* thoughts and beliefs about pain shape how we feel and behave in our interactions with individuals who suffer pain. We might reflect on how what we think influences what we say during a class or to an individual. Are we 'cueing for protection' and therefore increasing pain responses? If so, perhaps instead we could encourage people to explore variations of movement to find a way comfortable for them, and that by doing so they learn to trust their body and build self-efficacy with movement. We might also notice what feelings come up for us: are we fearful of causing a situation that might make someone's pain worse? Does this make us instruct in an overly protective way? Do we assume responsibility over an individual's response to a class or an exercise? We might notice the thoughts we hold about pain that are more difficult to shift, even with knowledge of pain science. The next step may be to ask, 'Why am I thinking this way?' Can you imagine how your behaviors or teaching style may change if you did not have certain thoughts or beliefs?

Out of the Head and Onto the Mat

> Transition to practice: These practice sections are not designed to be recipes for practices to give directly to a person participating in pain care. They are meant for you, the reader, to engage in experiential learning – to take the information from 'Headspace' onto your own mat and into life. As the subject, you can first explore the ideas presented, then consider how these might translate into practices for those with whom you work.

Below is an example of a practice that explores integration of thoughts, beliefs and behaviors on the mat. The goal is to experience and observe without seeking immediate answers or conclusions. For this practice, you might focus on asanas (physical postures or movements) that are uncomfortable for you, or if you don't have physical discomfort, maybe some that are mentally challenging.

- Choose an asana sequence (about five physical postures) either from Appendix 2: Asana, or one you are already familiar with. Go through the postures performing the following four rounds. During each round use the set of inquiries below to guide your focus. Let the observations build on

each other while allowing the focus to stay on the questions at hand.

- Start by sitting or lying in a comfortable position with eyes closed and the intention to turn your focus inward. Place one hand on your belly and one on your heart as a physical reflection of connection to your whole self. Take 5–10 slow, deep breaths.

- *Noticing:* When you feel a physical sensation, can you trace it from its perceived root (the tissue or physical place) back to the brain? Follow it into your own beliefs and the story the sensation holds for you, and then perhaps follow it to the emotions it evokes. Is it possible to make sense of the sensation? Can you look at these beliefs with your new understanding of pain science?

- *Setting an intention:* Establish an intention to shift relationships between thoughts and behaviors. Why do you think about your physical discomforts this way? Who would you be and what would you be able to do without these thoughts (not without the physical sensations but without the emotions and beliefs that run with the sensations)?

- *Being curious:* Focused curiosity and awareness of reactivity patterns. Notice any automatic responses. How do you react in thought, emotion, physical behavior (muscle tension, movement, breath)? Can you see the brief moment between the physical sensation and response? Can you choose to keep your awareness on the physical sensation and not drop into reactivity? Can you choose to respond from a place of calm, soothing, compassionate breath rather than bracing and splinting?

- *Choosing responses:* Putting it all together – choosing nurturing responses in the presence of discomfort. Try the practice one more time. Start with at least five breaths in a seated or lying position. Move softly and smoothly through each asana, maintaining a place of curiosity. If you observe spinning thoughts, emotions or reactive postures, try to nourish yourself with a relaxed breath.

- When you complete all four rounds, lie quietly in savasana.

- *Reflection:* Take time afterward to journal your discoveries. Gently remind yourself the primary purpose of pain is to offer protection and to call the body into action; however, protection and action are not always necessary, especially if pain has been present for longer periods of time. Our reactions may not be the best response to create an environment that allows us to return to optimal function.

- As you reflect try to lean deeper into your own experience. Where do your thoughts, fears and protective responses stem from? Close out the chatter from friends, neighbors, commercials and loved ones. Are the fears you feel yours or someone else's? Although presented with intent of helpfulness, often the beliefs of others can create another layer of misconception. Because others' pain will never be like yours, and your pain will never be like theirs, you need to lay out your own individualized path to becoming resilient. From these discoveries identify two reactions, psychological, emotional or physical behaviors, that you will take into the next practice section.

Off the Mat and Into Life

Can we now go one step further and put this into practice in daily life?

Hopefully, from the prior practice, you were able to identify at least two key thoughts, beliefs or behaviors associated with an uncomfortable sensation. Now begin to imagine one area of life that this physical discomfort (or mental challenge) gets in the way of. This can be as simple as walking down the stairs. Many people with persistent knee pain will alter the way they go down the stairs, turning sideways or holding

the handrail. Sometimes this is because it hurts, or because of fear it will hurt or do damage. It might take a day or two of mindful observation to notice these habits or reactions. Once you have an activity identified, try pausing for just a moment prior to performing the task and go through the rounds above: checking the root of the sensation and tracing it back to the brain, creating awareness around the reactive thought processes, emotional and physical/behavioral responses, then seeing the space between sensations and reactions and exploring whether you can choose a different response. Try not to force a physical change right away. Just observe what comes up and consider the ability to shift it. It is not uncommon for shifts to happen slowly and beneath our obvious awareness.

References

1. Darlow, B., S. Dean, M. Perry, et al. Easy to Harm, Hard to Heal: Patient Views About the Back. Spine, 2015. 40(11): 842–50.

2. Darlow, B., B.M. Fullen, S. Dean, et al. The Association Between Health Care Professional Attitudes and Beliefs and the Attitudes and Beliefs, Clinical Management, and Outcomes of Patients with Low Back Pain: A Systematic Review. European Journal of Pain, 2012. 16(1): 3–17.

3. Jackson, T., Y. Wang, Y. Wang, and H. Fan. Self-Efficacy and Chronic Pain Outcomes: A Meta-Analytic Review. Journal of Pain, 2014. 15(8): 800–14.

4. Wertli, M.M., E. Rasmussen-Barr, U. Held, et al. Fear-Avoidance Beliefs–A Moderator of Treatment Efficacy in Patients with Low Back Pain: A Systematic Review. Spine Journal, 2014. 14(11): 2658–78.

5. Hallegraeff, J.M., W.P. Krijnen, C.P. van der Schans, and M.H. de Greef. Expectations About Recovery from Acute Non-Specific Low Back Pain Predict Absence from Usual Work Due to

Chronic Low Back Pain: A Systematic Review. Journal of Physiotherapy, 2012. 58(3): 165–72.

6. Vuurberg, G., A. Hoorntje, L.M. Wink, et al. Diagnosis, Treatment and Prevention of Ankle Sprains: Update of an Evidence-Based Clinical Guideline. British Journal of Sports Medicine, 2018. 52(15): 956.

7. Dubois, B. and J.F. Esculier. Soft-Tissue Injuries Simply Need PEACE and LOVE. British Journal of Sports Medicine, 2020. 54: 72–3.

8. Osman, A., F.X. Barrios, B.A. Kopper, et al. Factor Structure, Reliability, and Validity of the Pain Catastrophizing Scale. Journal of Behavioural Medicine, 1997. 20(6): 589–605.

9. Sullivan, M., S. Bishop, and J. Pivik. The Pain Catastrophizing Scale: Development and Validation. Psychological Assessment, 1995. 7: 524–32.

10. Sullivan, M.J., B. Thorn, J.A. Haythornthwaite, et al. Theoretical Perspectives on the Relation between Catastrophizing and Pain. Clinical Journal of Pain, 2001. 17(1): 52–64.

11. Vlaeyan, J.W., A.M. Kole-Snijders, R.J. Boeren, and H. van Eek. Fear of Movement/(Re)Injury in Chronic Low Back Pain and Its Relation to Behavioral Performance. Pain, 1995. 62(3): 363–72.

12. Vlaeyen, J.W. and S.J. Linton. Fear-Avoidance Model of Chronic Musculoskeletal Pain: 12 Years On. Pain, 2012. 153(6): 1144–7.

13. Wideman, T.H., G.G. Asmundson, R.J. Smeets, et al. Rethinking the Fear Avoidance Model: Toward a Multidimensional Framework of Pain-Related Disability. Pain, 2013. 154(11): 2262–5.

14. Bunzli, S., A. Smith, R. Schutze, and P. O'Sullivan. Beliefs Underlying Pain-Related Fear and How They Evolve: A Qualitative Investigation in People with Chronic Back Pain and High Pain-Related Fear. BMJ Open, 2015. 5(10): e008847.

15. Bandura, A. Self-Efficacy: Toward a Unifying Theory of Behavioral Change. Psychological Review, 1977. 84(2): 191–215.

16. Lacker, J.M., A.M. Carosella, and M. Feuerstein. Pain Expectancies, Pain, and Functional Self-Efficacy Expectancies as Determinants of Disability in Patients with Chronic Low Back Disorders. Journal of Consulting and Clinical Psychology, 1996. 64(1): 212–20.

17. Feliu-Soler, A., F. Montesinos, O. Gutierrez-Martinez, et al. Current Status of Acceptance and Commitment Therapy for Chronic Pain: A Narrative Review. Journal of Pain Research, 2018. 11: 2145–59.

18. de Boer, M.J., H.E. Steinhagen, G.J. Versteegen, et al. Mindfulness, Acceptance and Catastrophizing in Chronic Pain. PLoS One, 2014. 9(1): e87445.

19. Vowles, K.E., L.M. McCracken, C. McLeod, and C. Eccleston. The Chronic Pain Acceptance Questionnaire: Confirmatory Factor Analysis and Identification of Patient Subgroups. Pain, 2008. 140(2): 284–91.

20. McCracken, L.M. and J. Zhao-O'Brien. General Psychological Acceptance and Chronic Pain: There Is More to Accept Than the Pain Itself. European Journal of Pain, 2010. 14(2): 170–5.

21. McCracken, L.M. and K.E. Vowles. Acceptance and Commitment Therapy and Mindfulness for Chronic Pain: Model, Process, and Progress. American Psychologist Journal, 2014. 69(2): 178–87.

22. Zale, E.L., K.L. Lange, S.A. Fields, and J.W. Ditre. The Relation Between Pain-Related Fear and Disability: A Meta-Analysis. Journal of Pain, 2013. 14(10): 1019–30.

23. Alamam, D., N. Moloney, A. Leaver, et al. Pain Intensity and Fear Avoidance Explain Disability Related to Chronic Low Back Pain in a Saudi Arabian Population. Spine, 2019. 44(15): E889-E898.

24. Lee, H., M. Hubscher, G.L. Moseley, et al. How Does Pain Lead to Disability? A Systematic Review and Meta-Analysis of Mediation Studies in People with Back and Neck Pain. Pain, 2015. 156(6): 988–97.

25. Odole, A., E. Ekediegwu, E.N.D. Ekechukwu, and C. Uchenwoke. Correlates and Predictors of Pain Intensity and Physical Function Among Individuals with Chronic Knee Osteoarthritis in Nigeria. Musculoskeletal Science and Practice, 2019. 39: 150–6.

26. Wertli, M.M., E. Rasmussen-Barr, S. Weiser, et al. The Role of Fear Avoidance Beliefs as a Prognostic Factor for Outcome in Patients with Nonspecific Low Back Pain: A Systematic Review. Spine Journal, 2014. 14(5): 816–36.e4.

27. Robinson, J.P., B.R. Theodore, E.J. Dansie, et al. The Role of Fear of Movement in Subacute Whiplash-Associated Disorders Grades I and Ii. Pain, 2013. 154(3): 393–401.

28. Alhowimel, A., M. AlOtaibi, K. Radford, and N. Coulson. Psychosocial Factors Associated with Change in Pain and Disability Outcomes in Chronic Low Back Pain Patients Treated by Physiotherapist: A Systematic Review. SAGE Open Medicine, 2018. 6: 2050312118757387.

29. Burns, L.C., S.E. Ritvo, M.K. Ferguson, et al. Pain Catastrophizing as a Risk Factor for Chronic Pain after Total Knee Arthroplasty: A Systematic Review. Journal of Pain Research, 2015. 8: 21–32.

30. De Baets, L., T. Matheve, M. Meeus, et al. The Influence of Cognitions, Emotions and Behavioral Factors on Treatment Outcomes in Musculoskeletal Shoulder Pain: A Systematic Review. Clinical Rehabilitation, 2019: 269215519831056.

31. Martinez-Calderon, J., M.P. Jensen, J.M. Morales-Asencio, and A. Luque-Suarez. Pain Catastrophizing and Function in Individuals with Chronic Musculoskeletal Pain: A Systematic Review and Meta-Analysis. Clinical Journal of Pain, 2019. 35(3): 279–93.

32. Martinez-Calderon, J., F. Struyf, M. Meeus, and A. Luque-Suarez. The Association Between Pain Beliefs and Pain Intensity and/or Disability in People with Shoulder Pain: A Systematic Review. Musculoskeletal Science and Practice, 2018. 37: 29–57.

33. Sorel, J.C., E.S. Veltman, A. Honig, and R.W. Poolman. The Influence of Preoperative Psychological Distress on Pain and Function After Total Knee Arthroplasty: A Systematic Review and Meta-Analysis. Bone and Joint Journal, 2019. 101-b(1): 7–14.

34. Urquhart, D.M., P.P. Phyomaung, J. Dubowitz, et al. Are Cognitive and Behavioural Factors Associated with Knee Pain? A Systematic Review. Seminars in Arthritis and Rheumatism, 2015. 44(4): 445–55.

35. Smith, A.D., G.A. Jull, G.M. Schneider, et al. Low Pain Catastrophization and Disability Predict Successful Outcome to Radiofrequency Neurotomy in Individuals with Chronic Whiplash. Pain Practice, 2016. 16(3): 311–19.

36. Moore, E., P. Thibault, H. Adams, and M.J.L. Sullivan. Catastrophizing and Pain-Related Fear Predict Failure to Maintain Treatment Gains Following Participation in a Pain Rehabilitation Program. Pain Reports, 2016. 1(2): e567.

37. Ostelo, R.W., I.J. Swinkels-Meewisse, D.L. Knol, et al. Assessing Pain and Pain-Related Fear in Acute Low Back Pain: What Is the Smallest

Detectable Change? International Journal of Behavioural Medicine, 2007. 14(4): 242–8.

38. Sieben, J.M., J.W. Vlaeyen, S. Tuerlinckx, and P.J. Portegijs. Pain-Related Fear in Acute Low Back Pain: The First Two Weeks of a New Episode. European Journal of Pain, 2002. 6(3): 229–37.

39. Thompson, D.P., D. Antcliff, and S.R. Woby. Cognitive Factors Are Associated with Disability and Pain, but Not Fatigue Among Physiotherapy Attendees with Persistent Pain and Fatigue. Physiotherapy, 2019. EPub Ahead of Print.

40. Karasawa, Y., K. Yamada, M. Iseki, et al. Association between Change in Self-Efficacy and Reduction in Disability among Patients with Chronic Pain. PLoS One, 2019. 14(4): e0215404.

41. Semeru, G.M. and M.S. Halim. Acceptance Versus Catastrophizing in Predicting Quality of Life in Patients with Chronic Low Back Pain. Korean J Pain, 2019. 32(1): 22–9.

42. McCracken, L.M. and K.E. Vowles. A Prospective Analysis of Acceptance of Pain and Values-Based Action in Patients with Chronic Pain. Health Psychology, 2008. 27(2): 215–20.

43. Vowles, K.E., L.M. McCracken, and C. Eccleston. Patient Functioning and Catastrophizing in Chronic Pain: The Mediating Effects of Acceptance. Health Psychology, 2008. 27(2s): S136–43.

44. Kratz, A.L., F. Murphy Jr. 3rd, C.Z. Kalpakjian, and P. Chen. Medicate or Meditate? Greater Pain Acceptance Is Related to Lower Pain Medication Use in Persons with Chronic Pain and Spinal Cord Injury. Clinical Journal of Pain, 2018. 34(4): 357–65.

45. Vowles, K.E. and L.M. McCracken. Acceptance and Values-Based Action in Chronic Pain: A Study of Treatment Effectiveness and Process. Journal of Consulting and Clinical Psychology, 2008. 76(3): 397–407.

46. Akerblom, S., S. Perrin, M. Rivano Fischer, and L.M. McCracken. The Mediating Role of Acceptance in Multidisciplinary Cognitive-Behavioral Therapy for Chronic Pain. Journal of Pain, 2015. 16(7): 606–15.

47. Sim, A. Pain Heroes: Stories of Hope and Recovery. 2018, Australia.

48. Brinjikji, W., P.H. Luetmer, B. Comstock, et al. Systematic Literature Review of Imaging Features of Spinal Degeneration in Asymptomatic Populations. American Journal of Neuroradiology, 2015. 36(4): 811–16.

49. Englund, M., A. Guermazi, D. Gale, et al. Incidental Meniscal Findings on Knee MRI in Middle-Aged and Elderly Persons. New England Journal of Medicine, 2008. 359(11): 1108–15.

50. Lumley, M.A., J.L. Cohen, G.S. Borszcz, et al. Pain and Emotion: A Biopsychosocial Review of Recent Research. Journal of Clinical Psychology, 2011. 67(9): 942–68.

51. De Felice, M. and M.H. Ossipov. Cortical and Subcortical Modulation of Pain. Pain Management, 2016. 6(2): 111–20.

52. Weissman-Fogel, I., E. Sprecher, and D. Pud. Effects of Catastrophizing on Pain Perception and Pain Modulation. Experimental Brain Research, 2008. 186(1): 180–90.

53. Malfliet, A., I. Coppieters, P. Van Wilgen, et al. Brain Changes Associated with Cognitive and Emotional Factors in Chronic Pain: A Systematic Review. European Journal of Pain, 2017. 21(5): 769–86.

54. Kucyi, A., M. Moayedi, I. Weissman-Fogel, et al. Enhanced Medial Prefrontal Default Mode Network Functional Connectivity in Chronic Pain and Its Association with Pain Rumination. Journal of Neuroscience, 2014. 34(11): 3969–75.

55. Galambos, A., E. Szabo, Z. Nagy, et al. A Systematic Review of Structural and Functional MRI Studies on Pain Catastrophizing. Journal of Pain Research, 2019. 12: 1155–78.

56. Lazaridou, A., J. Kim, C.M. Cahalan, et al. Effects of Cognitive-Behavioral Therapy (CBT) on Brain Connectivity Supporting Catastrophizing in Fibromyalgia. Clinical Journal of Pain, 2017. 33(3): 215–21.

57. Seminowicz, D.A. and K.D. Davis. Cortical Responses to Pain in Healthy Individuals Depends on Pain Catastrophizing. Pain, 2006. 120(3): 297–306.

58. Loggia, M.L., C. Berna, J. Kim, et al. The Lateral Prefrontal Cortex Mediates the Hyperalgesic Effects of Negative Cognitions in Chronic Pain Patients. Journal of Pain, 2015. 16(8): 692–9.

59. Lee, H., J.H. McAuley, M. Hubscher, et al. Does Changing Pain-Related Knowledge Reduce Pain and Improve Function through Changes in Catastrophizing? Pain, 2016. 157(4): 922–30.

60. Jenkins, H.J., M.J. Hancock, C.G. Maher, et al. Understanding Patient Beliefs Regarding the Use of Imaging in the Management of Low Back Pain. European Journal of Pain, 2016. 20(4): 573–80.

61. Webster, B.S., A.Z. Bauer, Y. Choi, et al. Iatrogenic Consequences of Early Magnetic Resonance Imaging in Acute, Work-Related, Disabling Low Back Pain. Spine (Phila Pa 1976), 2013. 38(22): 1939–46.

62. Bigos, S.J., J. Holland, C. Holland, et al. High-Quality Controlled Trials on Preventing Episodes of Back Problems: Systematic Literature Review in Working-Age Adults. Spine Journal, 2009. 9(2): 147–68.

63. Butler, D. and L.G. Moseley. Explain Pain. 2003, Adelaide: Noigroup Publications.

64. Louw, A. and E.J. Puentedura. Therapeutic Neuroscience Education: Teaching Patients About Pain - A Guide for Clinicians. 2013, Minneapolis: International Spine and Pain Institute.

65. Watson, J.A., C.G. Ryan, L. Cooper, et al. Pain Neuroscience Education for Adults with Chronic Musculoskeletal Pain: A Mixed-Methods Systematic Review and Meta-Analysis. Journal of Pain, 2019. 20(10): 1140.e1–1140.e22.

66. Malfliet, A., J. Kregel, I. Coppieters, et al. Effect of Pain Neuroscience Education Combined with Cognition-Targeted Motor Control Training on Chronic Spinal Pain: A Randomized Clinical Trial. JAMA Neurology, 2018. 75(7): 808–17.

67. Traeger, A.C., H. Lee, M. Hubscher, et al. Effect of Intensive Patient Education Vs Placebo Patient Education on Outcomes in Patients with Acute Low Back Pain: A Randomized Clinical Trial. JAMA Neurology, 2018. 76(2): 161–9.

68. Schutze, R., C. Rees, A. Smith, et al. How Can We Best Reduce Pain Catastrophizing in Adults with Chronic Noncancer Pain? A Systematic Review and Meta-Analysis. Journal of Pain, 2018. 19(3): 233–56.

69. Pike, A., L. Hearn, and A.C. Williams. Effectiveness of Psychological Interventions for Chronic Pain on Health Care Use and Work Absence: Systematic Review and Meta-Analysis. Pain, 2016. 157(4): 777–85.

70. Hassett, A.L. and R.N. Gevirtz. Nonpharmacologic Treatment for Fibromyalgia: Patient Education, Cognitive-Behavioral Therapy, Relaxation Techniques, and Complementary and Alternative Medicine. Rheumatic Disease Clinics of North America, 2009. 35(2): 393–407.

71. Hayes, S.C., M. Villatte, M. Levin, and M. Hildebrandt. Open, Aware, and Active: Contextual Approaches as an Emerging Trend in the Behavioral and Cognitive Therapies. Annual Review of Clinical Psychology, 2011. 7: 141–68.

72. Veehof, M.M., H.R. Trompetter, E.T. Bohlmeijer, and K.M. Schreurs. Acceptance- and Mindfulness-Based Interventions for the Treatment of Chronic Pain: A Meta-Analytic Review. Cognitive Behavioural Therapy, 2016. 45(1): 5–31.

73. Kabat-Zinn, J. Full Catastrophe Living. 2005, New York: Bantam Dell.

74. Bishop, S.R., M. Lau, S. Shapiro, et al. Mindfulness: A Proposed Operational Definition. Clinical Psychology, 2004. 11(3): 230–41.

75. Rinpoche, T. Open Heart, Open Mind. 2012, New York: Harmony Books.

76. Hanson, R. and R. Medius. Buddha's Brain. 2009, Oakland, CA: New Harbinger Publications, Inc.

77. Kornfield, J. The Wise Heart. 2009, New York: Bantam Books.

78. Iyengar, B.K.S. Light on Yoga. 2015, London: Harper Thorsons.

79. Doran, N.J. Experiencing Wellness within Illness: Exploring a Mindfulness-Based Approach to Chronic Back Pain. Qualitative Health Research, 2014. 24(6): 749–60.

80. O'Sullivan, P.B., J.P. Caneiro, M. O'Keeffe, et al. Cognitive Functional Therapy: An Integrated Behavioral Approach for the Targeted Management of Disabling Low Back Pain. Physical Therapy, 2018. 98(5): 408–23.

81. Vibe Fersum, K., P. O'Sullivan, J.S. Skouen, et al. Efficacy of Classification-Based Cognitive Functional Therapy in Patients with Non-Specific Chronic Low Back Pain: A Randomized Controlled Trial. European Journal of Pain, 2013. 17(6): 916–28.

We must care for our suffering the way we would care for our own baby.

Thich Nhat Hanh

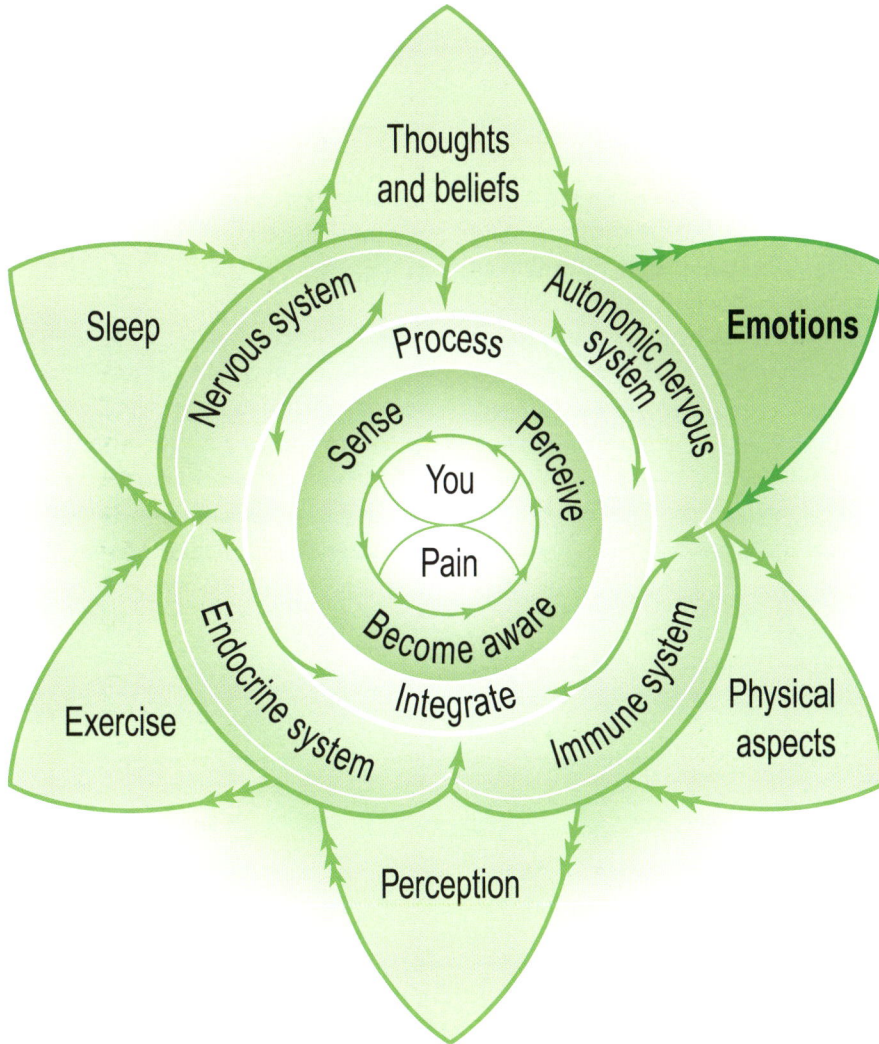

Figure 5.1

Pain Mandala – Emotions. How we feel emotionally will directly impact how we feel physically. Our mood, fear, anxiety and stress all drive our need for protection, and in turn elicit responses from our immune, endocrine and nervous systems, potentially elevating our pain experiences. However, the alternate is also true – when we learn how to regulate our emotional reactions, we can also regulate these systems' responses and begin to modulate the output of pain.

Note: This mandala depicts aspects of the human experience of pain covered in Pain Science Yoga Life. *Other inputs, dimensions and body systems can contribute to pain than those noted here.*

Headspace

Pain and Mood: A Synergistic Relationship

It's common for people with persistent pain to experience considerable emotional distress. When people tell their stories of painful struggles, their language is often loaded with emotion, distress and hopelessness, the anguish evident in their body and postures. Persistent pain is itself a form of chronic stress, emotionally, physically and physiologically. In a vicious circle, pain and distress feed one another, each increasing the risk of the other.[1–3] It's staggering to think that up to 60% of people with persistent pain report depressive symptoms.[4–6] More shockingly, up to 46% report suicidal ideation.[7] And people with clinical depression frequently report significant pain.[8,9] Stress and anxiety are also linked with pain, although interestingly, they are less consistently linked with pain than depression.[10,11] Unfortunately, the fact that psychological factors and pain go hand in hand is often misinterpreted as 'pain is all in one's head'. However, as the Pain Mandala indicates (Figure 5.1), important interactions between our emotions, physiology and behavioral responses strongly influence our pain experiences.

> Scope of practice consideration: If a mood disorder is present, a referral to an appropriately qualified health care provider is warranted.

Refresher: Interactions Between Pain Processing, Thoughts and Mood

In Chapter 1 we described descending modulation of nociception (warning signals): how brain activity influences how much the brain's pharmacy releases natural painkillers like endorphins, serotonin and GABA, turning the dial on pain up or down. We then explored how thoughts and beliefs influence descending modulation. Thinking the worst about pain, not understanding it, becoming hypervigilant and focusing high levels of attention on bodily sensations, can impair our ability to turn down the dial on pain by preventing the release of natural painkillers. Further, negative thoughts can cause the release of sensitizing neurotransmitters, turning up the dial on pain. As we consider mood and pain, bear in mind that our thoughts and beliefs interact with our emotions. Negative thoughts lower our mood and cause anxiety and stress, and vice versa. In this chapter we'll explore the effects of stress, anxiety and depression on pain, look at mechanisms that explain some of these effects, and see how yoga can help this aspect of pain care. Let's start with our body under stress.

Our Body Under Stress

Fear, anxiety and stress are designed to protect us from harm and ensure survival[12] by actioning a 'stress response'. This 'stress response' – our 'fight, flight or freeze' response – involves defensive behaviors and physiological changes driven by our hormonal and autonomic systems. Stress responses to acute short-lived threatening events are helpful. However, if stress responses become excessive or prolonged, significant health issues, including persistent pain, can arise.[13]

While fear, anxiety and stress all produce a 'stress response' and are related, noting the subtle differences may aid understanding when we explore helpful and unhelpful responses. Both fear and anxiety activate 'fear circuitry' in the brain, and both can produce stress responses. Fear is our response when we perceive we are *immediately* in danger, while anxiety relates more to *anticipated* threats.[14] For example, while on holiday recently, my partner and I went for a cycle through some orange groves. Our leisurely meander came to an abrupt end when a pack of dogs appeared and started snarling at us. I froze until my partner, in his flight, yelled at me to get out of there, at which point I kicked into action and speedily pedaled away. We both had a strong stress response – our fight, flight, freeze response appropriate at that moment. The next day we contemplated going for a walk but I was hesitant because of our dog encounter, anticipating danger and feeling somewhat anxious.

This was probably healthy – adaptive. However, if I developed high anxiety every time I anticipated going for a walk or every time I came across a dog, this vigilance and apprehension, states of high alert, could cause repeated or persistent 'stress responses'.[15]

Stress is a broader concept originally defined as a non-specific response to potentially harmful stimuli.[16] Stressors might be physical, e.g. from manual work, exposure to infection or noise; or psychological, e.g. the result of an unhappy relationship, financial worries or high work demands. Importantly, whether stress is considered positive, facilitating learning and growth (eustress), or negative (distress) is thought to reflect an interaction between the stress we're exposed to and our perceived ability to cope with that stress.[17] Importantly, chronic distress can lead to higher levels of anxiety.[18] The purpose of highlighting this is that acute fear and acute stress responses can be very helpful. But when we experience high or repeated anxiety, or sustained, chronic stress, our normally helpful 'stress responses' can become unhelpful and contribute to pain.

The Stress Response

Tom, a single father, is facing a deadline at work, forcing long, tedious workdays. His teenage son is struggling in school and acting out, while his mum has recently been diagnosed with dementia and may need increasing care. Years of stress-induced headaches have returned with a vengeance, making concentrating difficult and feeling patient with his family nearly impossible. So, what's happening in Tom's body?

When our brain interprets that we are under stress, or facing threat, it activates two systems: the sympathetic nervous system (or sympatho-adrenal medullary (SAM) axis) (Figure 5.2A) and the hypothalamic–pituitary–adrenal (HPA) axis (Figure 5.2B).[19,20] These axes govern the body's subsequent stress responses, which incorporate nervous, immune and endocrine system activity.

The SAM and HPA systems have overlapping but slightly different downstream effects on the body.[21,22] The SAM system belongs to the autonomic nervous system, which has two parts: the sympathetic (SAM) and parasympathetic nervous systems. Classic responses of the SAM are the flight, fight or freeze responses listed in Table 5.1. The parasympathetic nervous system governs our relaxation response (rest and digest). It's associated with recovery, balancing the effects of sympathetic nervous system activity (see Table 5.1).[20] Note that both influence the immune system and inflammatory responses (more about this in a moment).

Our instantaneous response to *acute* stress is sympathetic nervous system activity under the control of the hypothalamus and brain stem (as well as other brain areas like the amygdala), causing the release of neurotransmitters (chemical messengers) that drive the stress response.[20] These neurotransmitters work in two main ways. First, they activate neurons that communicate directly with target tissues, e.g. the heart and lungs. Second, sympathetic neurons signal to the adrenal gland (sitting on top of our kidneys) to release neurotransmitters into the bloodstream. These then circulate, leading to widespread effects.[20] The neurotransmitters employed by the autonomic nervous system (both sympathetic and parasympathetic) include adrenaline and noradrenaline (epinephrine and norepinephrine) and acetylcholine. These chemicals produce the physical effects of the stress response. But, as we'll see, they also influence nociception.

Once the stressor has been removed, the hypothalamus and brain stem signal the sympathetic nervous system to reduce its activity and call the parasympathetic nervous system to action.[20] As such, the sympathetic and parasympathetic nervous systems need to balance to promote appropriate stress and recovery responses, appropriately turning on and turning off responses in each system.[23]

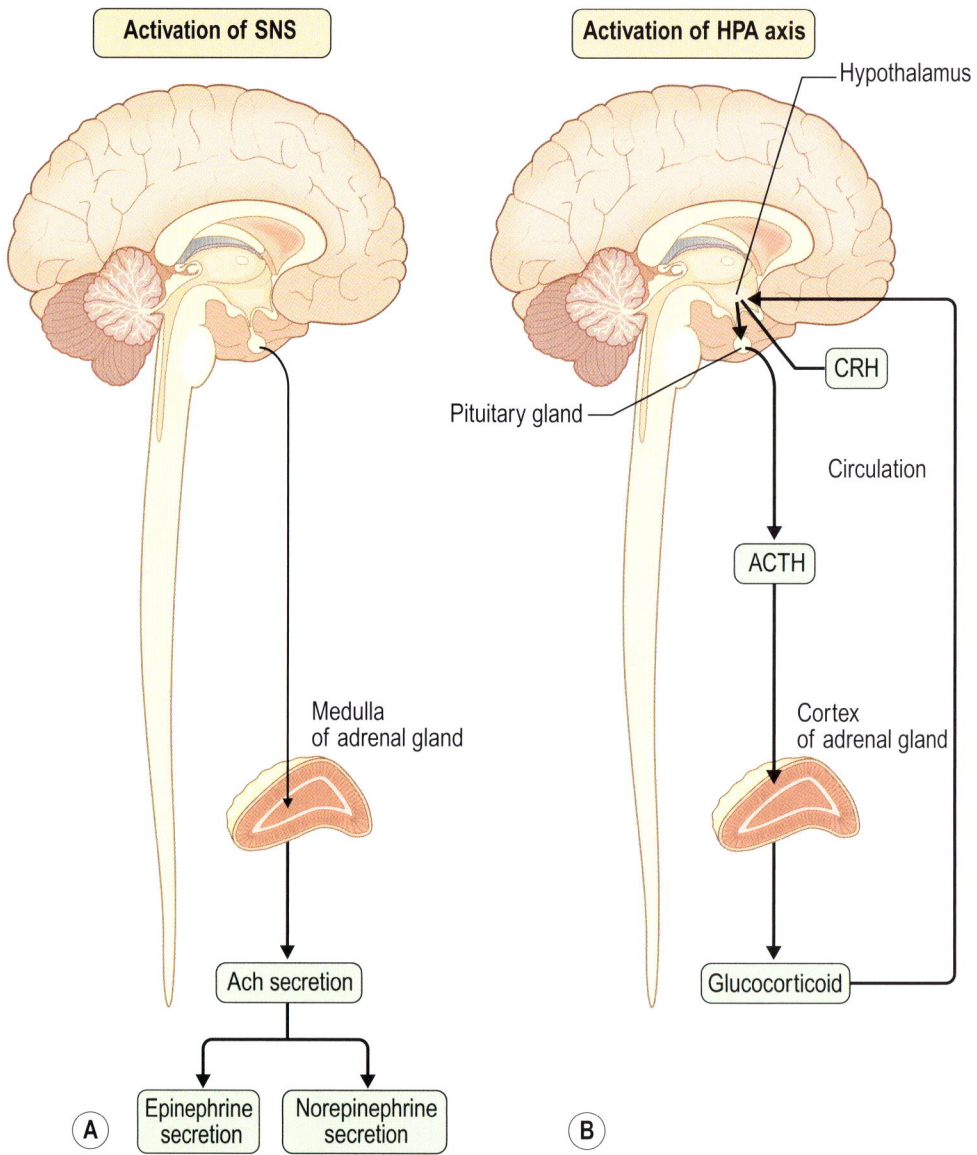

Figure 5.2
Stress systems. **(A)** Sympathetic nervous system (or sympatho-adrenal medullary axis); part of the autonomic nervous system. **(B)** Hypothalamus–pituitary–adrenal (HPA) axis; part of the endocrine system. Once the brain determines a situation of stress, or threat is present, it activates these two systems to control the body's subsequent stress responses. These responses incorporate nervous, immune and endocrine system activity through hormone release. Although often helpful, these responses can become altered in pain states and contribute to the persistence of pain. *Ach*, acetylcholine; *ACTH*, adrenocorticotropic hormone; *CRH*, corticotropin-releasing hormone; *SNS*, sympathetic nervous system.

Table 5.1 Effects of the autonomic nervous system

Sympathetic nervous system responses	Parasympathetic nervous system responses
Increased blood flow to our muscles and away from our internal organs, preparing muscles for action but reducing internal functions like digestion	Reduced blood flow to muscles and increased blood flow to internal organs
	Improved gastric and intestinal motility and secretion to improve absorption of nutrients
	Contraction of the urinary bladder which results in urination
Increased muscle tension	Reduced muscle tension
Increased heart rate and blood pressure	Reduced heart rate and blood pressure
Increased respiratory rate	Reduced respiratory rate
Increased perspiration to help thermoregulation associated with physical activity	Reduced perspiration
Increased alertness and reduced sleepiness	Reduced alertness and increased restfulness and sleepiness
Increased release of stress hormones and chemical messengers such as adrenaline, noradrenaline and cortisol	Reduced release of stress hormones and chemical messengers such as adrenaline, noradrenaline and cortisol
Immune system responses	Immune system responses

The HPA axis response is similar but tends to be slower to respond than the sympathetic nervous system and thus is linked with prolonged stress.[22] It works like this: first, the hypothalamus releases corticotropin-releasing hormone (CRH) to initiate a stress response within the brain. It stimulates release of adrenocorticotropic hormone (ACTH) from the pituitary gland (within the brain). From there, signals sent to the adrenal glands cause the release of glucocorticoids into the bloodstream.[22,24] Glucocorticoids are corticosteroids (anti-inflammatories) and steroid hormones. Cortisol is one you may have heard of and is commonly measured as a marker of stress. Chemicals like cortisol contribute to many bodily functions: one of the most important for our discussion is that cortisol helps terminate inflammation as it is a powerful anti-inflammatory.[25]

These stress systems have inbuilt feedback loops to prevent over-shooting of stress responses.[24] For example, when cortisol is released into the bloodstream, a signal is relayed to the hypothalamus to stop it releasing more CRH (see Figure 5.2B). Critically, this depends on removal of the stressor, e.g. when Tom meets his deadline. But there is scope for the stress response to become dysfunctional if the stressor is sustained, e.g. if Tom becomes the caregiver for his mum and struggles to cope.

Interestingly, the other way this system can get out of kilter is if the response by the body isn't strong enough, e.g. if insufficient cortisol is released.[26] Insufficient release has been demonstrated in some health conditions, including persistent pain. One theory is that with sustained stress, cortisol levels become depleted, while another is that the problem is with the receptors for cortisol rather than the amount of cortisol per se.[26,27] Either way, the trigger to stop the 'stress response' never gets relayed back to the brain. This can result in prolonged 'stress responses' as well as dysregulated inflammatory responses.[28,29]

So, the SAM and HPA systems regulate stress and relaxation responses. How do these interact with our pain experience?

Stress and Immune System Interactions

The first way stress and pain are linked is by immune system activation, via effects on inflammation.[24] The initial, acute stress response causes a pro-inflammatory response.[30-32] This is a defensive action to prevent infection or stimulate healing of an injury and is a normal, healthy and beneficial response. Adrenaline and noradrenaline, the SAM chemical messengers, regulate immune responses influencing the onset, maintenance and termination of inflammation.[24,31-33] Under normal circumstances, the release of cortisol, that powerful anti-inflammatory, will signal a termination of inflammation.[25] However, cortisol levels can become dysregulated with persistent stress and persistent pain.[25,26] It is beyond the scope of this chapter to explain these in detail but, simply, if the stress response is prolonged, too severe or not sufficient in the first place, cortisol levels can become dysregulated.[25,26] The result can be a pro-inflammatory state,[34] which can drive more nociception. It can also mean poorer tissue healing, again important for pain.[25]

Stress and Neural System Interactions

Both the HPA and SAM axes interact with the nervous system, particularly affecting descending modulation of nociception. As well as communicating within the HPA and SAM axes and communicating with the immune system, adrenaline and noradrenaline are chemical messengers within the nervous system.[24,35] Different versions of adrenaline and noradrenaline exist and, depending on their expression, can actually have pro- or anti-nociceptive effects – they can turn up or turn down the dial on pain.[36] Our clever nervous system adjusts, but it can be a little Jekyll and Hyde in behavior. With sustained stress, these chemicals can become pro-nociceptive, turning up nociception and increasing the potential for more pain.[35-37]

Stress: An Integrated System

Here is the clever part: in mounting responses to protect us, there is a three-way conversation between hormonal, immune and nervous systems. In a detailed review, Chapman and colleagues[24] describe interactions between these systems, each system communicating with and regulating the other (Figure 5.3). While there are feedback systems *within* each system telling it to switch on and off, feedback loops also exist *between* systems, with information from one system telling other systems when to switch on and off. Dysfunction of any one system can lead to inappropriate responses in all systems. Dysfunction could arise with: 1) sustained stress; 2) a very strong initial stress response; or 3) a stress response that was inadequate in the first place.

Remember, the stressors initiating or maintaining the stress response can be physical or emotional. Dysfunction could also arise with sustained illness. As shown by the Pain Mandala (see Figure 5.1), appreciating interactions between stress, immune and nervous systems helps us to understand how pain has many inputs – including emotions, thoughts or physical stressors that potentially produce stress responses. For Tom, we can see how his current combination of stressors means he has many inputs potentially influencing his pain.

> Take home message: Stressors initiating or maintaining a stress response can be physical or emotional.

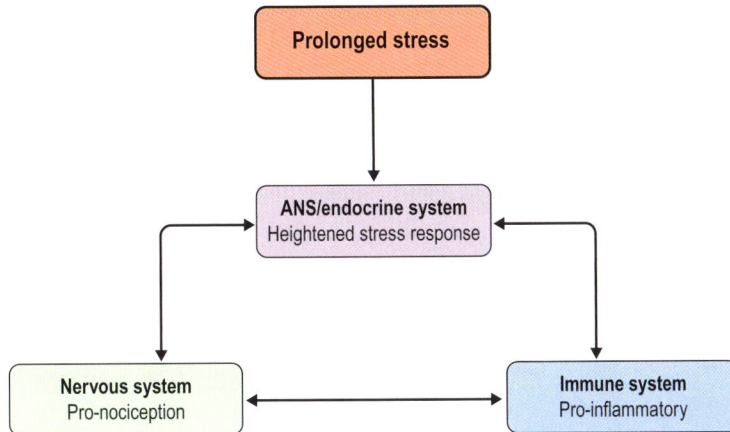

Figure 5.3

Stress response and integration with other systems: integration between stress, immune and nervous systems. You've been under pressure at work or home for months. You've had three colds in a row and now your back hurts: what's happening in your body? Prolonged stress heightens physiological stress responses activated by the autonomic nervous system and endocrine system. The resultant chemical shifts can create a pro-inflammatory state and a pro-nociceptive state, meaning your immune system struggles to fight off any more bugs and you're more susceptible to experiencing pain. The two-way arrows indicate that each system can influence the other, e.g. prolonged inflammation can also influence heightened stress responses and a pro-nociceptive state.

Stress and Pain: Clinical Evidence

What is the evidence for these 'inputs' in the people we see in pain? Most studies that investigate stress responses in people with persistent pain demonstrate some degree of altered stress response with increased sympathetic nervous system activity and reduced parasympathetic nervous system activity, both associated with altered neural and immune responses.[38] The interactions between stress responses and neural and immune responses may be important in pain, as demonstrated by markers of deficient parasympathetic nervous system activity after physical stress (e.g. reduced heart rate recovery) being associated with findings of increased pro-inflammatory markers.[39] Lower parasympathetic nervous system function is associated with higher pain sensitivity and poorer modulation of nociception in people with widespread pain,[40–43] while altered cortisol levels (too much or too little) are associated with persistent pain.[26,38,44,45] The interactions between stress responses, inflammation and pain may explain why some painful autoimmune conditions are linked with stress, e.g. multiple sclerosis and rheumatoid arthritis.[34]

> Take home message: With stronger stress responses, prolonged stress and poorer recovery, the dial gets turned up on warning signals, and the brain's pharmacy becomes less effective.

So, stress responses are important in pain, but remember, how closely pain and stress are related isn't clear-cut. There are studies that link stress responses closely to pain and pain persistence,[46,47] and others showing it's not so relevant.[48] Maybe this is where we acknowledge that each individual's pain picture is different, and when stress is present, it has the *potential* to influence pain but may not always do so. This perhaps asks us, and the people we work with, to just become curious about its impact – observe without judgment first.

And from there, start to make some gentle shifts when appropriate.

Our Brain Under Stress

Let's transition back into the brain and how the brain joins the body during stress to influence pain experiences and modulation of nociception.[14,18,49] Let's look at fear, anxiety and stress together before exploring depression.

Fear, Anxiety and Stress Drive Increased Brain Activity

When the brain perceives threat, it calls on the 'fear circuitry' to coordinate activity in brain areas (Figure 5.4A), which ultimately drives our stress responses. Like the pain neuromatrix, the 'fear circuitry' includes multiple brain areas: the amygdala, hippocampus, pre-frontal cortex (PFC), anterior cingulate cortex (ACC), thalamus, periaqueductal gray (PAG) and rostral ventromedial medulla (RVM):[14] in short, areas of emotional and cognitive regulation, decision-making, sensation and descending modulation of nociception. Can you see the overlap with the pain neuromatrix (Figure 5.4B)? Activity in these areas is also controlled by inhibitory circuits, to calm down activity within the fear circuit.[50]

Let's discuss one area, the amygdala, in more detail. The amygdala is key for emotional processing, particularly fear-based responses. By communicating with the hypothalamus and areas of the brain stem, it is pivotal in driving stress responses.[51,52] Importantly for pain processing, the amygdala integrates sensory, emotional and cognitive aspects of pain.[50,53,54] The amygdala receives inputs from many brain areas and the spinal cord,[54] including nociceptive inputs (warning signals). In fact, the amygdala has nuclei that respond preferentially to nociception from the tissues.[55] The amygdala's job is to attach emotional context to this sensory information. During experiments, people with pain demonstrate greater amygdala activity than healthy controls,[56,57] and this has been linked to greater emotional responses to pain as well as pain unpleasantness and pain catastrophizing.[18]

The amygdala also has an important role in communicating with other parts of the brain. Connections with brain areas such as the ACC, insula and PFC are important for integrating emotions and cognitions.[54] The amygdala's connections with other brain areas such as the insula, hypothalamus and the PAG[50] are also recognized as influencing pain and related behaviours.[50,53,54] In Phillip's case (Case Study, p. 51), this may be reflected in how his sense of loss or grief about his future career as a surgeon interacts with negative, worrisome thoughts and influences his behaviors, causing him to 'put his life on hold'. He also became aware of a physical sense of almost constant armoring; he noted increased muscle tension generally, and increased heart and breath rate, as well as a change in his desire for food – all symptoms of a stress response.

Like all of our nervous system, amygdala neurons are plastic and can become sensitized in response to exposure – firing more easily and for longer. When we experience fear, this sensitization is fundamental to learning, enhancing future protection and survival; but it can also be unhelpful, contributing to persistent pain.[50] If the fearful stimulus is unexpected – like when I was confronted by the pack of dogs – greater sensitization is more likely than if the stimulus is expected.[14,58,59] That helps me to learn quickly that I should be careful while out in those orange groves.

Studies show that anxiety can feed this sensitization too. Remember Mike from Chapter 4 who had back pain and was anxious about bending? Say he has a back spasm. His amygdala will receive inputs about his body's tissues and must process this information, adding emotional context to it. Because he is anxious about becoming wheelchair-bound, it's likely his amygdala is more active and becomes more sensitized or responsive. As for many people, his spasms seem unpredictable and difficult to control.[60] This unpredictability (unexpected stimuli) compounds sensitization of amygdala neurons, in turn producing greater fear responses and ultimately increasing the potential for more pain.

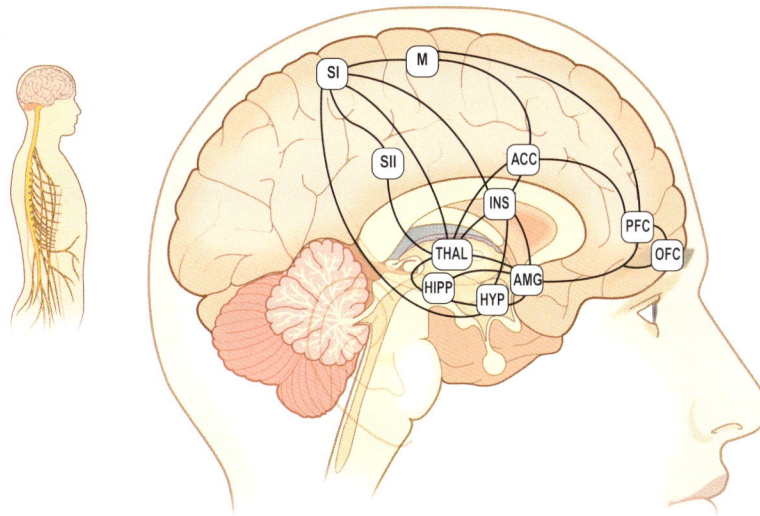

ACC	Anterior cingulate cortex	HYP	Hypothalamus	OFC	Orbitofrontal cortex	SII	Sensory cortex II
AMG	Amygdala	INS	Insula	PFC	Pre-frontal cortex	THAL	Thalamus
HIPP	Hippocampus	M	Motor cortex	SI	Sensory cortex I		

(A)

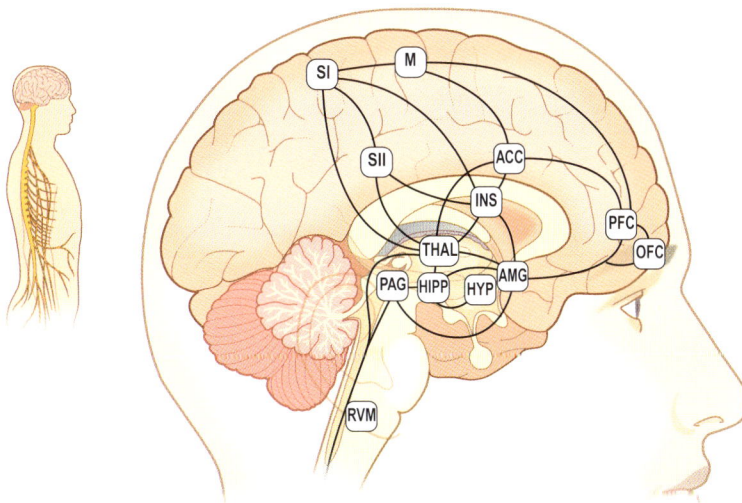

ACC	Anterior cingulate cortex	HYP	Hypothalamus	OFC	Orbitofrontal cortex	RVM	Rostral ventral medulla
AMG	Amygdala	INS	Insula	PAG	Periaqueductal gray	SI	Sensory cortex I
HIPP	Hippocampus	M	Motor cortex	PFC	Pre-frontal cortex	SII	Sensory cortex II
						THAL	Thalamus

(B)

Figure 5.4

Brain circuitry in **(A)** fear and **(B)** pain. Can you see the commonality between these neuromatrices utilized to process perceptions of threat in order to determine the most appropriate response, be it physical pain or emotional states – fear, anxiety or stress?

Chapter 5

The Brain's Control System

The brain has a control system to help balance this type of activity and subsequent responses: the inhibitory systems mentioned earlier, involving chemical messengers like GABA. The amygdala is under this control as well. For example, under normal circumstances the medial PFC (which regulates thoughts and meaning) inhibits amygdala activity.[50,61] Firing of the medial PFC can cause amygdala cells to signal safety and reduce anxiety.[61] However, hyperactivity in the amygdala, e.g. when its neurons are sensitized, has a feed-forward effect on the medial PFC, stifling its inhibitory effect. In a classic vicious circle this loss of inhibition on the amygdala in turn facilitates greater amygdala activity. Importantly, this sensitization and loss of inhibition can enhance future fear and anxiety responses.[50,53]

Let's consider Mike again: because Mike is anxious and thinking the worst about his pain (becoming wheelchair-bound) there is likely to be less inhibition from the medial PFC, thus enhancing the amygdala's fear-based responses. As well as contributing to the overall pain experience, this activity in the amygdala can both reduce Mike's natural pain relief and increase his stress responses.[62] Conversely, if Mike understood that the spasm didn't mean more damage (the pain and stiffness were just related to muscle over-activation), the pain experience would likely play out differently. There would still be nociception from his muscles, which would trigger activity in the amygdala, but now his medial PFC has a better chance of calming his amygdala's response, moderating both stress and pain responses. We can see how different factors are feeding into Mike's Pain Mandala, and how addressing some of these factors, such as his thoughts and emotions, could potentially influence his movement and other aspects of his overall pain experience.

We've discussed the amygdala, but other brain areas are important too. Anxiety, including pain-related

anxiety, increases ACC activity, which is associated with increased pain and pain sensitivity.[49,63] Some studies also highlight the importance of the hippocampus in anxiety. The hippocampus is important for memory,[64] so perhaps ties in with anxiety being about *anticipating* threats, or related to memories of previous negative experiences. For pain, aspects of the initial onset may drive activity in the hippocampus and contribute to what may appear as unpredictable triggers of pain, such as driving or hearing the sounds of a car after a severe whiplash injury.

> Take home message: Memories and emotional connections are important inputs that can elicit a pain response.

Stress and Anxiety Impact the Brain's Pharmacy

How we feel emotionally affects our brain's pharmacy. The limbic system (emotional brain) communicates with the PAG and RVM, brain areas responsible for modulating nociception, turning up or turning down warning signals (Figure 5.5). Interestingly, fear and stress can both increase and decrease pain sensitivity.

Acute stress can have pain-relieving effects: stress-induced *hypo*algesia.[65-67] This involves the opioid system (releases endorphins) and non-opioid systems (release chemicals like GABA, endocannabinoids, serotonin, dopamine and noradrenaline).[12,65-68] Remember when I was confronted by a dog pack while on holiday? At the time, I was pregnant and had some pelvic girdle pain. But in that moment, as I speedily cycled away, I can safely say there was no pain! The sudden fight, flight, freeze response caused stress-induced **hypoalgesia**. But emotional distress can also promote pain, increasing pain sensitivity: stress-induced **hyperalgesia**. We know different types of noradrenaline and its receptors exist, some of which turn up nociception.[37,69] Serotonin demonstrates

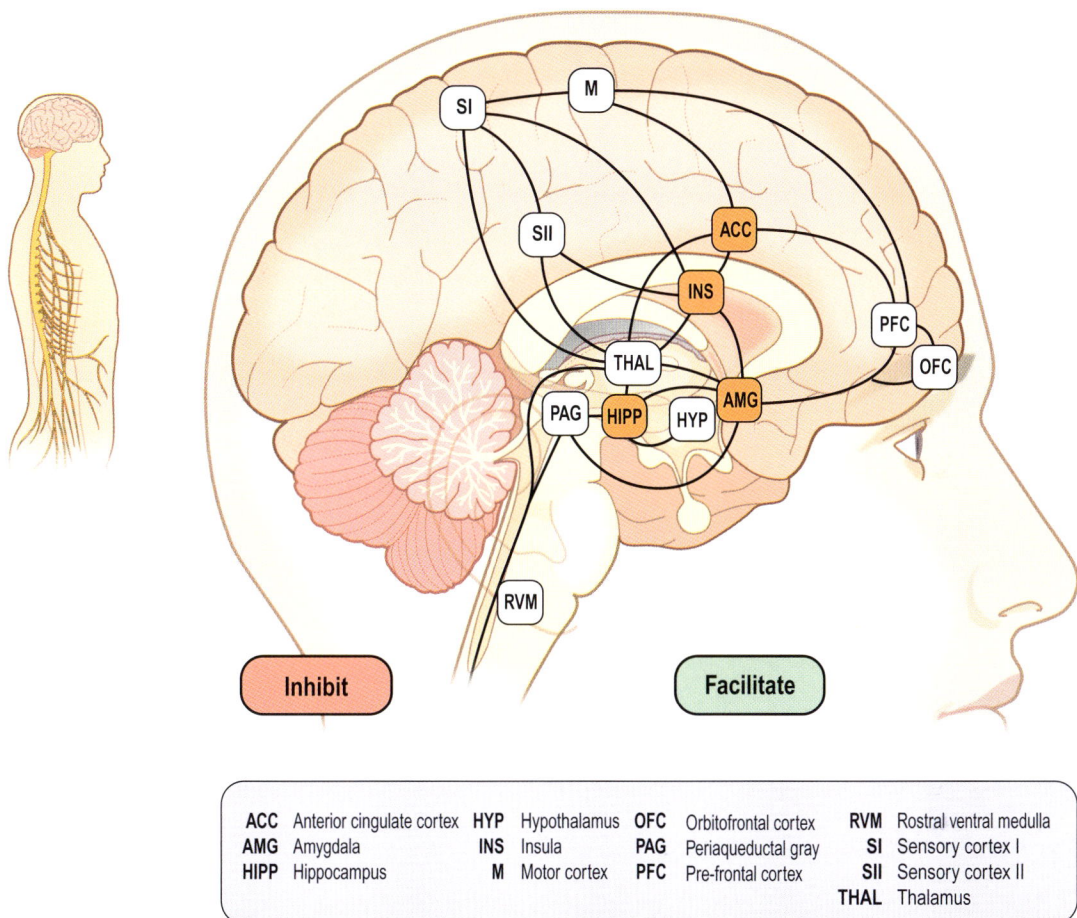

Figure 5.5

The nervous system: the 'brain's pharmacy' and descending modulation of nociception. The PAG/RVM can inhibit or facilitate nociception, turning the dial up or down on nociception. When neurotransmitters that inhibit nociception are released, nociceptive signals are turned down: result = less pain. When neurotransmitters that facilitate nociception are released, nociceptive signals are turned up: result = more pain.

ACC	Anterior cingulate cortex	**HYP**	Hypothalamus	**OFC**	Orbitofrontal cortex
AMG	Amygdala	**INS**	Insula	**PAG**	Periaqueductal gray
HIPP	Hippocampus	**M**	Motor cortex	**PFC**	Pre-frontal cortex

RVM	Rostral ventral medulla
SI	Sensory cortex I
SII	Sensory cortex II
THAL	Thalamus

similar properties.[60,70] Instead of calming nociception, stress can cause normally pain-relieving chemicals to switch and turn up the dial on pain.

For Phillip, until his injury, exceling in baseball and pursuing medicine were his 'life's missions'. He felt called to both of these internally and through pressures from his family and surrounding culture.

His injury placed two valued areas of his life under threat. Potentially, fearing the assumed loss of these ventures promoted stress responses that turned up his sensitivity to warning signals.

> Stress-induced hypoalgesia: reduced pain from a stimulus that normally provokes pain following exposure to stress.

Stress-induced hyperalgesia: increased pain from a stimulus that normally provokes pain following exposure to stress.

It seems that, normally, our body strives to maintain a delicate balance of nociception modulation in response to distress, but sometimes the balance shifts towards poorer pain relief.[71] Why this happens is unclear, but may relate to higher brain activity as previously discussed.[72] Animal studies tell us that chronic mild stress, repeated stress, social defeat and early life or maternal stress may predispose to stress sensitivity and heightened stress-induced hyperalgesia, and therefore may be important inputs to pain in humans.[71] And while preliminary, some recent human studies support this, showing that with those with higher stress sensitivity reporting higher pain levels during experimental pain tests.[63,73,74] While further research is needed before we have a full understanding of how stress-induced hyperalgesia works in humans, it's worth reflecting on how stress is contributing to pain in those we work with. How does their pain behave when they're under stress? How does their body respond (e.g. more muscle tension)? This might also include reflection on previous life events and acknowledging that these might have laid a foundation for stress sensitivity, potentially contributing to pain.

Pain and Depression

We all know what it's like to feel low, to lack interest and motivation, or to gain less pleasure from things we normally find enjoyable. Often these are passing episodes but when these feelings become pervasive, persist and affect our quality of life, it is called depression.[75] Like fear, anxiety and stress, relationships between depression and pain exist, associated with shared neural circuitry and neurotransmitters within the nervous system. Highlighting interactions

between different inputs, this relationship is also influenced by how we cope, whether we catastrophize,[76-78] or whether we tend toward positive outlooks.[79-81] It's also influenced by how well we sleep, as we explore in Chapter 9.

Shared Brain Neural Circuitry and Shared Neurotransmitters

The story here is similar to that previously discussed for fear, anxiety and stress (Figure 5.6). Depression is associated with dysregulation of areas important for emotional and cognitive processing, including emotional memory (e.g. PFC, ACC, nucleus accumbens, hippocampus and amygdala).[72,82-86] These findings correlate with greater anticipation of pain and greater perceived helplessness in people with depression and pain. This possibly relates to greater monitoring of negative information like uncomfortable sensations and feeling helpless about them.[87] Increased activity in these brain areas has been identified in response to painful stimuli in those with clinical depression,[87] while overlap between neural networks in emotional distress and physical pain has also been identified.[88]

Depressed mood also impairs modulation of nociception.[18] Pain and depression share similarities in the dysregulation of neurotransmitters involved in regulating nociception, and cognitive and emotional processing (e.g. glutamate, noradrenaline, dopamine, serotonin and endocannabinoids).[85,89] One line of thinking is that reduced 'central inhibition' is a common mechanism underpinning both pain and depression.[90] With less inhibition or calming of neuronal activity, the nervous system is more sensitized and reactive. The result: greater emotional reactivity, sensitization of nociceptive pathways, and poorer modulation of nociception.[18,90] Medications are often used to address these chemical imbalances,[91-95] but non-pharmacological

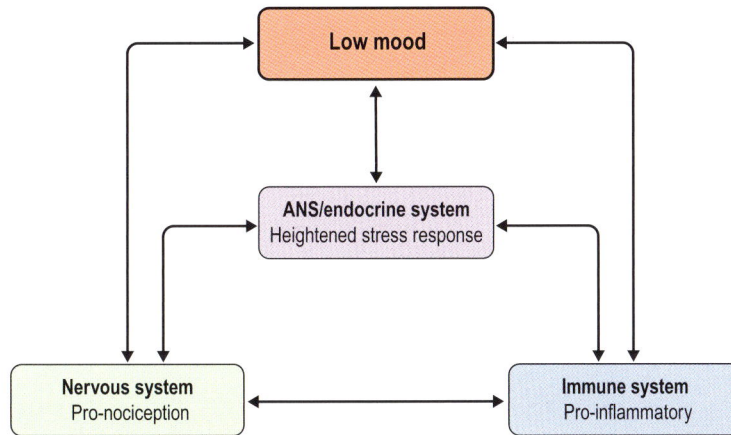

Figure 5.6
Effects of low mood on pain mechanisms. You've been going through a bad patch, feeling really low. Your body aches all over, you feel really reactive and can't sleep. What's happening in your body? Low mood can influence pain by effects on multiple systems. Low mood can heighten stress responses (ANS and endocrine system), can influence a pro-nociceptive state (nervous system) and impair immune system responses, causing a pro-inflammatory state (immune system). This can lead to more pain and can also lead to more emotional reactivity and poorer sleep. The two-way arrows indicate that all systems can influence one another. *ANS*, autonomic nervous system.

approaches (e.g. meditation, exercise) influence these neurotransmitters too.[96,97]

Hopefully the science of emotions is becoming clearer: when we're in any kind of distress, there is integration between our nervous, immune and endocrine systems that influence our mood and thus pain. As Phillip's pain sensitivity increased, he became more withdrawn and depressed. This led to less tolerance, physically and emotionally, of even simple activities. The cycle of increased pain and helplessness feeding depression, and thus depression feeding pain, was not hard to see with his case. With this understanding, the question arises whether it is possible for us to consciously influence these systems. Can we use yoga to shift our responses, potentially gaining an element of control over our emotions and pain?

Adjusting Emotional Responses

Several approaches exist in psychology, yoga and mindfulness to support moderating emotional responses to adversity such as persistent pain, stress, anxiety and depression, shifting cognitive–emotional evaluation and judgments as well as reactive thoughts, emotions and behaviors. If Mike was able to see his worry of becoming wheelchair-bound as that – a worrisome thought, but just a thought nonetheless – he might shift his response to his spasm away from a fear-based reaction. Like the practice in Chapter 4, he might be able to hold space for the discomfort and recognize his worries about becoming wheelchair-bound, but see the space where he can choose different responses: perhaps with reassuring thoughts that he will be OK, that 'this is just a spasm', and by softening his breath and relaxing his body. Encompassing the principle of *and this too* he might

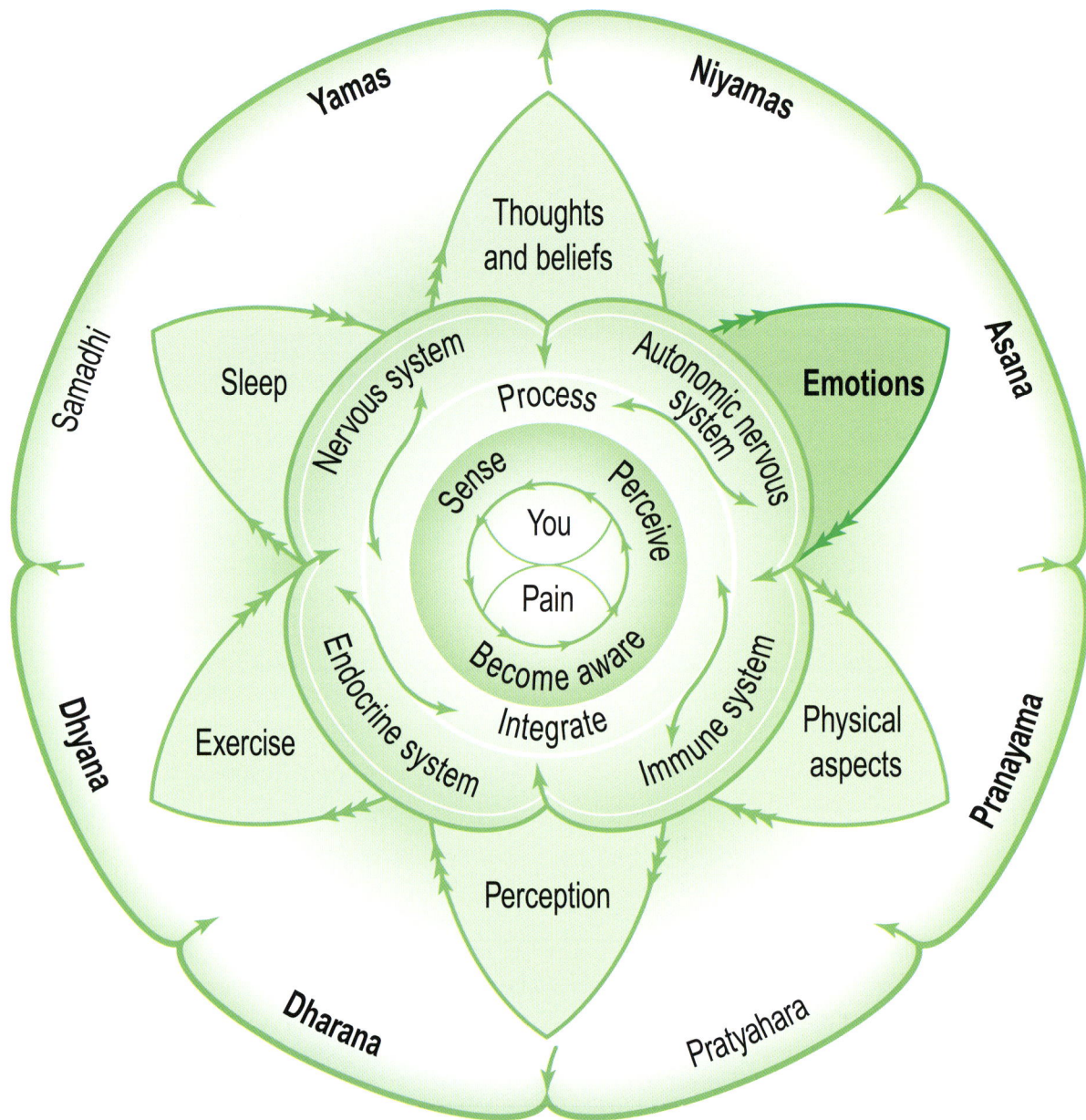

Figure 5.7

Pain and Yoga Mandala – Emotions. Gaining awareness of emotional reactivity, developing skills to bring a deeper sense of calm and improving self-compassion, may have great value in shifting our body's system responses and pain experiences. The yoga practices of Dhyana (meditation), Dharana (focused attention), Pranayama (breath practice), Asana (mindful movement), Yama–Aparigraha (non-grasping) and Niyama–Santosha (contentment) all support the ability to cultivate this awareness and the skills needed for greater calm and self-compassion.

allow himself to experience the discomfort without adding *second dart* suffering by becoming anxious.

When we hold space for life's experiences – pain, comfort, stress, joy, happiness, sadness, etc. – and attempt to experience each with equanimity, we live more mindfully and arguably with greater contentment and less distress. Our ability to find comfort may stop depending on the absence of pain. We may find contentment more easily, and with it, less suffering. In yoga philosophy, santosha (contentment) and aparigraha (non-grasping or non-attachment) engender this. Indeed, these aspects of yoga are quite connected in that when we lack contentment, as when in pain, we often also grasp at a different situation, e.g. avoiding or getting rid of pain. Adopting the principles of santosha and aparigraha does not mean we cannot be ambitious for our health and journey beyond pain. It just means we accept pain's ups and downs and choose to learn from them, rather than spiraling into more suffering. Remember Kyle, the Australian rules football player (Chapter 3)? By deciding to include his pain rather than trying to just be rid of it, he was able to learn to use his body more effectively. Moreover, he was able to use the compassion and patience he began to practice with his own physical limitations to improve his personal relationships.

Using Yoga and Mindfulness to Adjust Emotional Responses

In Chapters 3 and 4 we explored how mindfulness can reduce suffering by fostering perspective and present-moment awareness, prevent *second-dart* suffering by arresting negative thoughts, and encourage pain acceptance and psychological flexibility: in other words, adjusting cognitive factors that influence pain. So, what about exploring and adjusting emotional responses? Yoga and mindfulness may have value here for pain care, and are thought to work by reducing emotional reactivity, improving self-compassion and awareness of our own thoughts and emotions.[98]

Specifically, for pain, research supports the following: 1) emotional regulation including reappraisal of pain sensations and experiences; 2) improved body awareness; and 3) reduced stress responses. As well as improving pain, extensive research shows Mindfulness-Based Interventions (MBIs) improve mood in people with depression and pain and are as effective as other evidence-based interventions.[99–101] Meditative movement practices like yoga have small but significant effects on pain,[102] but potentially greater effects on depression and anxiety.[103,104] As described in Chapter 4, mindfulness practices positively influence pain experiences[105] and stimulate our natural pain-relieving system.[96] Let's delve further into these effects on pain.

Emotional and Cognitive Regulation

It's common for people with persistent pain to feel a loss of control and confidence over their body and their emotions or a loss of connection between body and mind, so gaining control over emotional responses holds potential benefits. This is key in mindfulness, where monitoring and reducing reactive thoughts, emotions and behaviors, and approaching experiences in a non-judgmental way are fundamental practices. In people undertaking MBIs for pain, some evidence supports these changes. When interviewed, participants reported reduced emotional reactivity and greater pain acceptance.[106] Similarly, in a pilot study of comprehensive yoga for people with fibromyalgia, people in the yoga group improved their pain acceptance and experienced improved mood compared to controls.[107]

The topic of trauma is vast and outside the scope of this book. However, it is certainly relevant for many with persistent pain and some approaches used for trauma care may hold value in pain care. While using yoga as part of trauma care has produced mixed results so far,[108,109] those studies that show promise involved trauma-sensitive yoga delivered by professionals qualified in trauma care as an adjunct to treatment, where people were encouraged to explore their internal experience of the physical practice.[110] Approaches that might be helpful to extend into pain care include exploring movement sensitively, tuning into emotions that arise through the practice, and fostering a greater sense of connection between mind and body as well as fostering a sense of agency over the body that might have been lost or compromised. All of these aspects might be considered part of self or emotional regulation.

Brain imaging potentially supports assertions that mindfulness and yoga can affect cognitive and emotional regulation. They show consistent trends in structural and functional (activity) changes in brain areas in response to mindfulness practices – areas associated with emotional responses and cognitive regulation (e.g. ACC, medial PFC, amygdala, orbitofrontal cortex).[111,112] Better integration between brain areas has also been shown in response to mindfulness practice, which is thought to explain improved connections between emotions, body awareness, attention and higher-order thinking.[111,112] We don't know for sure how brain imaging findings relate to improving pain, but it's possible findings are consistent with changing how we think about pain, greater pain acceptance and reduced emotional reactivity. While the responses to meditative movement practices like yoga are less well known, preliminary data show meditative movement can also have positive effects on brain areas associated with awareness and emotional regulation.[113]

Improved Body Awareness

Mindfulness practices can include specific exercises to enhance body awareness: for example, breath awareness, focused attention on the body, and open monitoring of physical sensations. Meditative movements like asana practice can also promote body awareness. For pain, this might involve allowing sensations and emotions to be experienced non-judgmentally, and observing the changing nature of sensations and emotions. Again, qualitative research suggests this is possible, with participants of an MBI reported as being able to experience pain and physical discomfort while

controlling emotional responses.[106] Brain imaging supports this, showing alterations in the insula and sensory cortex in response to mindfulness practices, areas associated with our body perception.[111,112] This may be relevant for pain care where changing how we sense our body may be related to better pain-related outcomes (explored further in Chapter 7).

Improved Stress Responses

Research tells us yoga and mindfulness practices change our stress responses. Results from 42 studies of healthy people and clinical populations on the effects of yoga and/or MBIs compared with controls demonstrate significant improvements on HPA axis and autonomic nervous system function.[114] Some of these findings correlate with reductions in reported stress.[103] Whether or not these changes correlate with changes in pain remains to be seen, with early studies indicating mixed results.[115,116]

Does the Type of Meditation Matter?

As we explore this topic, it may be worthwhile considering different types of meditation, as one large review found that they have different effects.[111] For example, *focused attention* and *open monitoring* styles of meditation were associated with greater activity in brain areas involved in thought regulation. Interoceptive sensory regulation was increased in *focused attention,* but decreased in *open monitoring. Mantra meditation* was associated with activity in areas involved in practiced motor behaviors, but a reduction of activity in the insula – associated with sensory and emotional processing. *Loving-kindness meditation* was associated with greater activity in the ACC, somatosensory cortex II and the insula.

How can we use this information? Angela was a lady who came to see me for persistent widespread pain. She also had high anxiety. During an open monitoring body scan (described later), she noticed a lot of physical sensations (*first dart*) and became very anxious, thinking about her 'damaged body' (*second dart*). Although this exercise provided useful insight, due to the potential to increase her anxiety I decided to leave it for later. I leaned on the evidence mentioned above and trialed a non-body-related activity of focused attention meditation (also described later) to encourage greater control of this emotional response. This allowed Angela to develop skills in breath and attentional control, before controlling emotional responses to general thoughts arising during meditation practice. With these skills in place she was able to return later to a body scan and work on reducing her automatic anxious response to bodily sensations, preventing *second-dart* suffering.

Using the Breath to Adjust Emotional Responses

As we have been discussing, our emotions directly and indirectly affect pain and physiological processes, and vice versa – inputs and outputs. Breathing follows this same trend, a fascinating spiral back and forth. Persistent pain can leave a person feeling out of control physically and emotionally. Breath-focused practices, such as pranayama, may provide a great tool for adjusting emotional responses and potentially pain. Let's peer into the science of breath in relation to pain as well as emotional responses and how pranayama might facilitate regaining a little control.

Pain and Breath Responses

Pain has a measurable effect on our breathing. You know that gasp of breath when you cut your finger on a knife, and how you gasp even when you think you have cut yourself and then realize that the knife is too dull to break the skin. Acute pain of this nature elicits a reflexive response of increased inspiratory flow, increasing the rate and volume of the inhalation.[117] Pain, or, indeed, anticipation of pain, leads to an automatic change of breath. When pain is more persistent, we tend towards hyperventilation, or too much airflow.[118] Hyperventilation occurs with anticipation of pain even without a physical stimulus. These observations are consistent with suggestions that hyperventilation is

the respiratory system's stress response during times of fear, pain and emotional distress (see Jafari et al.[118] for review). It is suggested that these respiratory responses don't only depend on stimulation of nociceptors; instead, they may reflect the influence of emotional states and the sense of uncontrollability in response to potential threats, such as pain.[118] If this is true, offering the ability to 'control' the breath may be beneficial, emotionally and physically. For Phillip, using focused breathing and other pranayama practices helped soothe him during times of increased stress which also stimulated pain, such as exams. This gave him a greater sense of control over his responses and these situations.

How Does Breath Control Influence Pain?

Breathing happens regardless of our awareness and yet with breath awareness we can consciously change it. How does this breath control influence pain? Potentially, breath control acts to enhance the voluntary regulation of parasympathetic activity and brain activity, and reduce emotional distress.[119] We can use the breath to adjust stress responses and associated cardiovascular effects like heart rate and blood pressure. And by doing so we may influence brain areas involved in emotions and pain.

When we breathe there is an oscillation in heart rate (heart rate variability) along with breathing cycle (the combination of heart rate variability with breathing is called respiratory sinus arrhythmia). The magnitude of heart rate variability and respiratory sinus arrhythmia is dependent on the breathing pattern: stronger fluctuations in heart rate are seen with slower, deeper breathing.[118,119] As we saw earlier in the chapter, heart rate variability is a measure of parasympathetic nervous system activity: greater heart rate variability is associated with greater parasympathetic nervous system activity. Slow deep breathing (SDB) has been used as a specific breath practice for pain,[118,119] a strategy with the potential to change the stress response and increase parasympathetic nervous system activity, which, as we've seen, can influence pain.

A mechanism responsible for the variability of heart rate and blood pressure is known as the *baroreflex*. The baroreflex is a homeostatic feedback loop adjusting heart rate and blood pressure.[120] The baroreflex is dependent on baroreceptors, pressure sensors in blood vessel walls that detect heart rate and blood pressure.[121] As discussed earlier, the brain can drive heart rate and blood pressure as part of the stress or relaxation responses.[120,122,123] The baroreflex also has a direct branch to the brain, communicating information regarding heart rate and blood pressure to brain areas involved in emotional regulation and pain perception (e.g. insula, hippocampus, amygdala, ACC and thalamus).[119,120] Thus, through this reflex and its link to autonomic areas in the brain, breathing and the resulting cardiovascular responses may influence nociception and emotional regulation as well as pain.[120] So how do we consciously influence a reflex? As noted above, a practice known as SDB is being studied as one potential tool.

Evidence of Slow Deep Breathing

The most common rate investigated for SDB in moderating stress responses is using approximately six breaths per minute, with some evidence that strategies like nostril breathing increases effects.[119] However, inconsistencies across studies make it difficult to make strong claims that SBD in isolation can effectively reduce physical or emotional distress.[119] Perhaps its potential benefit lies in combination with emotional and cognitive practices such as mindfulness/meditation,[124] CBT or a holistic yoga practice.

For pain, SDB has shown that a reduction in pain and measures of pain sensitivity such as the nociceptive reflex is possible,[118] but investigations remain limited and vary in the actual breath practice studied, thus leaving findings inconsistent. There may also be benefit to combining SDB with cues for relaxation to reduce pain.[125] Again, a rate of about six breaths per minute,[118] and in one study, specific practice techniques involving breath retention, seem to have positive effects on pain.[126]

Conclusion

Emotional distress and its responses are intimately connected to pain. This happens through neural circuitry in the brain, influences on descending modulation of nociception, and the way stress responses interact with our immune and nervous systems. As illustrated by the Pain Mandala (see Figure 5.1), appreciating these interactions urges us to consider strategies that incorporate adjusting emotional responses to move beyond pain. And the evidence suggests we may be able to influence these using elements of yoga. Phillip continued much of his practice discussed in Chapter 4 to address his mood as well. When he found himself feeling irritated and hopeless, he would pause, name the emotion and often move toward gratitude to help promote a greater sense of wellbeing. When his anxiety and pain symptoms escalated, he would begin to notice his stress response and use breath awareness and mindfulness to help soften the response. Mindfulness became possible for him because he had adopted a regular meditation practice. This controlled practice afforded him the skills needed to be present during stressful times with his pain, fears and anxieties.

Let's put all of this into practice.

Out of the Head and Onto the Mat

Transition to practice: These practice sections are not designed to be recipes for practices to give directly to a person participating in pain care. They are meant for you, the reader, to engage in experiential learning – to take the information from 'Headspace' onto your own mat and into life. As the subject, you can first explore the ideas presented, then consider how these might translate into practices for those with whom you work.

Scope of practice consideration: Because meditation practices ask the practitioner to 'go within', they can sometimes bring suppressed memories and emotions to the surface. This commonly occurs in cases of unresolved trauma where dissociation was used as a coping mechanism but resulted in a fragmented traumatic memory network. Unexpectedly accessing this network during meditation may be distressing and may require the assistance of a psychologist or multidisciplinary team.

We have outlined five meditations below: the first two are pranayama (breath practice), the others guided meditations. Simple pranayama practices can be a nice way to help settle into other meditations. If you or someone you are working with struggles to find stillness, or is reactionary with laughter, fidgeting or even talking, using the breath can be a great way to change the pattern, even if it needs to happen mid-session. Pranayama can also be a good bridge to come out of meditation. Using either a stimulating practice like kapalbjhati (breath of fire) or a soothing balanced practice like alternate nostril breathing can be helpful depending on what you want your tone to be as you exit the meditation session. In Appendix 1: Meditation and Pranayama, we offer full instructions and other traditional pranayama practices.

Pranayama

Find a comfortable position to sit, lie or stand. Assume a posture that is relaxed yet alert.

Simple Breath Awareness

- Bring your attention to your breath. Without trying to change anything about your breath, just notice it. Focus on the tip of your nose, sensing the air as it enters your nose, fills up your lungs and then leaves your body.

- Alternatively, bring your attention to your abdomen, rising as you breathe in and falling as you breathe out.

- Spend a few moments observing your breath, keeping your attention on your point of focus. If thoughts come, as they always do, just acknowledge each one and bring your attention back to your breath.

- Now spend a few moments allowing your breath to slow down and become a little deeper or fuller. The goal is to maintain a rate and depth that is soft and intentional but not effortful.

Squaring the Breath

- Start this practice with a few rounds of breath awareness as described above; if able, try to keep the breath flowing through the nostrils.

- When you feel ready, start to stretch the breath out a little further, feeling the inhalation first in the belly, then in the ribs, then into the chest. Pause for a moment with the breath held in, then as you exhale do so gradually; note the breath first leave the chest, then the ribs and finally the depths of the belly.

- Pause again at the bottom of the exhalation before inhaling again. Take care not to strain through any of this. If the pauses with the breath held in or out are met with resistance initially, it is fine to leave the pauses out until you are more comfortable with the breath practice.

- Once you have settled, start a simple breath count to establish the square. It looks like this:

   o Inhale: belly, ribs, chest, counting 1-2-3-4

   o Pause: hold the breath in, counting 1-2-3-4

   o Exhale: chest, ribs, belly, counting 1-2-3-4

   o Pause: hold the breath out, counting 1-2-3-4*

- You can repeat this for as long as you feel comfortable. If you lose your place or become distracted, simply come back to the inhalation and start the

---

* The four-count practice should keep you around the six breaths per minute protocol used in some of the studies discussed above.

count again. You may find you need to start this process over a number of times before you sink into a sustainable rhythm.

- If you like, you can play with slowly increasing these counts to 6, 8 or longer. If the count simply feels too long or too slow, just start where you feel comfortable –maybe a count of 2 is better for you; you can always progress from there when you are ready.

Meditation Practice

Begin each meditation from a comfortable posture and commitment to be present with the practice. Again, a little breath awareness is a great way to set the scene.

Focused Attention Meditation (or One-Pointed Concentration)

- Light a candle and place it in front of you (in yoga, candle meditation is called *trataka*).

- Sit or stand in front of the candle. Close your eyes or drop your gaze and bring your awareness to your breath.

- When you are ready, bring your gaze to the candle flame. Allow your eyes to softly focus on the flame, absorbing the quality of the light and following it as it dances. Use the flame to absorb your attention, allowing its image and movement to imprint on your mind. Notice when your attention drifts away and without judgment bring your attention back to the flame.

- After a few minutes, close your eyes and hold the impression of the candle flame in your mind's eye, the quality of the light, its movement as it dances. Notice when your attention drifts away and again bring it back to the image of the candle flame.

- After a few minutes let go of the image. When you're ready to end, bring your attention to your breath for a few moments, then into the room you are in, finally opening your eyes.

Open Monitoring Meditation – Modified for Emotions and Stress Responses

Note: *This practice of open monitoring can also be incorporated into an asana practice. The prompts to include all sensations, thoughts and emotions are the same: allowing the presence of all sensations without judgment or reaction – 'and this too', approaching the asana practice with curiosity.*

- Find a comfortable place and position.

- Close your eyes or drop your gaze and bring your attention to your breath as described above. Spend a few minutes on breath awareness.

- Now allow yourself to come to a state of awareness and openness, letting all that is present be included. Allow the mind to be calm and relaxed, not focused on anything in particular. Become present and open to take note without analysis or judgment.

- When thoughts arise, notice them but simply let them pass through your mind. If you do find yourself following those thoughts, acknowledge them, maybe name them, e.g. 'thinking', 'planning', and come back to your breath or other focal point for a moment before allowing your mind to open to full awareness once again.

- When emotions arise, again notice, acknowledge and choose to include them without further analysis. If you find yourself tracking or engaging in an emotion, recognize it, and maybe name it. You can name it simply 'feeling' or you can name what it is you are feeling – 'sad', 'anxious', 'uncertain'. You may notice the emotion being present in an area of the body; again, simply include it. Come back to a focal point (e.g. breath) and then open to all again.

- If you notice physical sensations, acknowledge them as well and stay open with your focus. If you hone in on the physical sensation, recognize that you are doing so, and name what you are feeling – itch, ache, burning.

- Continue to do these again and again as you need, recognize, name and include, and then come back to the open focus.

- Allow the mind to be present and all-inclusive. Reassure yourself it's OK to think this, it's OK to feel this.

- Continue this practice for several minutes. When you're ready to end, bring your attention back to your breath for a few moments, then back into the room you are in, before opening your eyes.

Loving-Kindness Meditation – Modified for Pain

- Find a comfortable position.

- Close your eyes or drop your gaze and bring your attention to your breath. Spend a few minutes on breath awareness.

- Allow your attention to come into your body, particularly any area of discomfort or pain. Notice what you feel, how that part of your body feels: try to name the feeling or sensation without placing a meaning on it – 'I feel sore,' 'I feel tender.' How does this physical sensation make you feel? Again, name the emotion that is present: fear, sadness, uncertainty. If you wander down the path of catastrophic thoughts, acknowledge them as such and shift them back to naming the sensation and the emotion without allowing the rest to become attached or part of a story.

- When you are ready, allow these phrases to come to mind:

    May I be filled with loving kindness
    May I be free from suffering
    May I be well in body and mind
    May I be at ease and happy

- Take your time, and allow each phrase to settle, listening to any thoughts, feelings and bodily sen-

sations as you do. There is no need to judge what arises; simply acknowledge it and allow it to be. It is not unusual to have self-doubt or lack of faith in these phrases when you first begin them. That is OK. This too can be included and recognized, and then return to the practice of reciting the phrases to yourself.

- Play with this meditation for pain or emotions specifically by extending it directly to any particular area of struggle. For example:

    May I fill my – knee, back, anxious mind, tender heart – with loving kindness
    May my – knee, back, mind, heart – be free of suffering
    May my – knee, back, mind, heart – be well
    May I be at ease with my – knee, back, mind, heart – and be happy

- To close this practice, bring your attention back to your breath for a few moments and then drop your attention into your body, once more noticing the area of your body that troubles you. Finish with a few deep breaths. Bring your attention back to the room you are in and finish your practice.

Off the Mat and Into Life

With the common focus on physical stressors for pain, many of us are unaware that our emotional states are contributing, so paying attention to this and the broader Pain Mandala can provide deeper insights into possible triggers.

Mindfulness fosters a move from a 'doing' (planning, analyzing, critiquing, problem solving) to a 'being' state of mind. Several characteristics differentiate the two modes (see Williams and Penman[127] for more information):

- Automatic pilot versus conscious choice.

- Analyzing versus sensing.

- Striving versus accepting.

- Seeing thoughts as solid and real versus treating them as transient events.

- Avoiding versus approaching.

- Mental time travel versus remaining in the present moment.

- Depleting versus nourishing activities.

Here are three focuses designed to explore your 'doing' versus 'being' modes in relation to pain. From this you might choose to focus on some elements to incorporate more mindfulness in your daily life.

Twenty-Four-Hour Observation

Over a day observe your physical discomfort or your mood. You might want to perform this on different days, changing the focus from your body to your mood. In italics at the end of each of the following sections are guides towards choosing a different response.

- *Automatic pilot versus conscious choice.* When you experience physical or emotional discomfort:

  o Do you have a tendency towards certain thoughts or automatic emotional reactions?

  o Do you expect to feel your pain at certain times or in relation to certain activities?

  o Have your responses become automatic?

  o *If so, can you shift them towards more conscious responses or move away from 'expecting' pain?*

- *Seeing thoughts as solid and real versus treating them as transient events: 'real but not true'.* When you experience physical or emotional discomfort:

  o What thoughts do you have about your discomfort? Do you treat these as fixed and factual?

  o *If so, can you hold space for thoughts to be 'real but not true'?*

  o *And can you hold space for changing perspective about how you see or interpret your pain or discomfort?*

- *Avoiding versus approaching: 'and this too'.* When you experience physical or emotional discomfort:

  o Do you avoid further physical or emotional discomfort?

  o Is this making you avoid valued activities?

  o *If so, can you engage in valued activities whilst also being in pain or discomfort? Can you allow yourself to experience discomfort, reassuring yourself that it's OK to experience pain and discomfort, even if it is unpleasant?*

References

1. Parreira, P., C.G. Maher, D. Steffens, et al. Risk Factors for Low Back Pain and Sciatica: An Umbrella Review. Spine Journal, 2018. 18(9): 1715–21.

2. Pinheiro, M.B., M.L. Ferreira, K. Refshauge, et al. Symptoms of Depression and Risk of New Episodes of Low Back Pain: A Systematic Review and Meta-Analysis. Arthritis Care and Research (Hoboken), 2015. 67(11): 1591–603.

3. Hilderink, P.H., H. Burger, D.J. Deeg, et al. The Temporal Relation between Pain and Depression: Results from the Longitudinal Aging Study Amsterdam. Psychosomatic Medicine, 2012. 74(9): 945–51.

4. Rayner, L., M. Hotopf, H. Petkova, et al. Depression in Patients with Chronic Pain Attending a Specialised Pain Treatment Centre: Prevalence and Impact on Health Care Costs. Pain, 2016. 157(7): 1472–9.

5. De La Torre Canales, G., M.B. Camara-Souza, V.R.M. Munoz Lora, et al. Prevalence of Psychosocial Impairment in Temporomandibular

Disorder Patients: A Systematic Review. Journal of Oral Rehabilitation, 2018. 45(11): 881–9.

6. Bair, M.J., R.L. Robinson, W. Katon, and K. Kroenke. Depression and Pain Comorbidity: A Literature Review. Archives of Internal Medicine, 2003. 163(20): 2433–45.

7. McCracken, L.M., S. Patel, and W. Scott. The Role of Psychological Flexibility in Relation to Suicidal Thinking in Chronic Pain. European Journal of Pain, 2018. 22(10): 1774–81.

8. Aguera-Ortiz, L., I. Failde, J.A. Mico, et al. Pain as a Symptom of Depression: Prevalence and Clinical Correlates in Patients Attending Psychiatric Clinics. Journal of Affective Disorders, 2011. 130(1–2): 106–12.

9. Lee, P., M. Zhang, J.P. Hong, et al. Frequency of Painful Physical Symptoms with Major Depressive Disorder in Asia: Relationship with Disease Severity and Quality of Life. Journal of Clinical Psychiatry, 2009. 70(1): 83–91.

10. Bair, M.J., E.L. Poleshuck, J. Wu, et al. Anxiety but Not Social Stressors Predict 12-Month Depression and Pain Severity. Clinical Journal of Pain, 2013. 29(2): 95–101.

11. Poleshuck, E.L., M.J. Bair, K. Kroenke, et al. Psychosocial Stress and Anxiety in Musculoskeletal Pain Patients with and without Depression. General Hospital Psychiatry, 2009. 31(2): 116–22.

12. Finn, D.P. Endocannabinoid-Mediated Modulation of Stress Responses: Physiological and Pathophysiological Significance. Immunobiology, 2010. 215(8): 629–46.

13. Asmundson, G.J. and J. Katz. Understanding the Co-Occurrence of Anxiety Disorders and Chronic Pain: State-of-the-Art. Depression and Anxiety, 2009. 26(10): 888–901.

14. Tovote, P., J.P. Fadok, and A. Luthi. Neuronal Circuits for Fear and Anxiety. Nature Reviews Neuroscience, 2015. 16(6): 317–31.

15. Kornfield, J. The Wise Heart. 2009, New York: Bantam Books.

16. Selye, H. What Is Stress? Metabolism, 1956. 5(5): 525–30.

17. Rudland, J.R., C. Golding, and T.J. Wilkinson. The Stress Paradox: How Stress Can Be Good for Learning. Medical Education, 2020. 54(1): 40–5.

18. Knudsen, L., G.L. Petersen, K.N. Norskov, et al. Review of Neuroimaging Studies Related to Pain Modulation. Scandinavian Journal of Pain, 2018. 2(3): 108–20.

19. Micale, V. and F. Drago. Endocannabinoid System, Stress and HPA Axis. European Journal of Pharmacology, 2018. 834: 230–9.

20. McCorry, L.K. Physiology of the Autonomic Nervous System. American Journal of Pharmaceutical Education, 2007. 71(4): 78.

21. Padgett, D.A. and R. Glaser. How Stress Influences the Immune Response. Trends in Immunology, 2003. 24(8): 444–8.

22. Tsigos, C. and G.P. Chrousos. Hypothalamic-Pituitary-Adrenal Axis, Neuroendocrine Factors and Stress. Journal of Psychosomatic Research, 2002. 53(4): 865–71.

23. McEwen, B.S. Protective and Damaging Effects of Stress Mediators. New England Journal of Medicine, 1998. 338(3): 171–9.

24. Chapman, C.R., R.P. Tuckett, and C.W. Song. Pain and Stress in a Systems Perspective: Reciprocal Neural, Endocrine, and Immune Interactions. Journal of Pain, 2008. 9(2): 122–45.

25. Hannibal, K.E. and M.D. Bishop. Chronic Stress, Cortisol Dysfunction, and Pain: A

Psychoneuroendocrine Rationale for Stress Management in Pain Rehabilitation. Physical Therapy, 2014. 94(12): 1816–25.

26. Tak, L.M., A.J. Cleare, J. Ormel, et al. Meta-Analysis and Meta-Regression of Hypothalamic-Pituitary-Adrenal Axis Activity in Functional Somatic Disorders. Biological Psychology, 2011. 87(2): 183–94.

27. Woda, A., P. Picard, and F. Dutheil. Dysfunctional Stress Responses in Chronic Pain. Psychoneuroendocrinology, 2016. 71: 127–35.

28. Bote, M.E., J.J. Garcia, M.D. Hinchado, and E. Ortega. Inflammatory/Stress Feedback Dysregulation in Women with Fibromyalgia. Neuroimmunomodulation, 2012. 19(6): 343–51.

29. Geiss, A., N. Rohleder, and F. Anton. Evidence for an Association between an Enhanced Reactivity of Interleukin-6 Levels and Reduced Glucocorticoid Sensitivity in Patients with Fibromyalgia. Psychoneuroendocrinology, 2012. 37(5): 671–84.

30. Nance, D.M. and V.M. Sanders. Autonomic Innervation and Regulation of the Immune System (1987–2007). Brain Behavior and Immunity, 2007. 21(6): 736–45.

31. Pongratz, G. and R.H. Straub. The Sympathetic Nervous Response in Inflammation. Arthritis Research and Therapy, 2014. 16(6): 504.

32. Scheiermann, C., Y. Kunisaki, D. Lucas, et al. Adrenergic Nerves Govern Circadian Leukocyte Recruitment to Tissues. Immunity, 2012. 37(2): 290–301.

33. Powell, N.D., E.K. Sloan, M.T. Bailey, et al. Social Stress Up-Regulates Inflammatory Gene Expression in the Leukocyte Transcriptome Via Beta-Adrenergic Induction of Myelopoiesis.

Proceedings of the National Academy of Sciences USA, 2013. 110(41): 16574–9.

34. Straub, R.H., J.W. Bijlsma, A. Masi, and M. Cutolo. Role of Neuroendocrine and Neuroimmune Mechanisms in Chronic Inflammatory Rheumatic Diseases – the 10-Year Update. Seminars in Arthritis and Rheumatism, 2013. 43(3): 392–404.

35. Dawson, L.F., J.K. Phillips, P.M. Finch, et al. Expression of Alpha1-Adrenoceptors on Peripheral Nociceptive Neurons. Neuroscience, 2011. 175: 300–14.

36. De Felice, M. and M.H. Ossipov. Cortical and Subcortical Modulation of Pain. Pain Management, 2016. 6(2): 111–20.

37. Lockwood, S.M., K. Bannister, and A.H. Dickenson. An Investigation into the Noradrenergic and Serotonergic Contributions of Diffuse Noxious Inhibitory Controls in a Monoiodoacetate Model of Osteoarthritis. Journal of Neurophysiology, 2019. 121(1): 96–104.

38. Maletic, V. and C.L. Raison. Neurobiology of Depression, Fibromyalgia and Neuropathic Pain. Frontiers in Bioscience (Landmark Ed), 2009. 14: 5291–338.

39. Ackland, G.L., G. Minto, M. Clark, et al. Autonomic Regulation of Systemic Inflammation in Humans: A Multi-Center, Blinded Observational Cohort Study. Brain Behavior and Immunity, 2018. 67: 47–53.

40. Nahman-Averbuch, H., E. Sprecher, G. Jacob, and D. Yarnitsky. The Relationships between Parasympathetic Function and Pain Perception: The Role of Anxiety. Pain Practice, 2016. 16(8): 1064–72.

41. Nahman-Averbuch, H., Y. Granovsky, E. Sprecher, et al. Associations between Autonomic

Dysfunction and Pain in Chemotherapy-Induced Polyneuropathy. European Journal of Pain, 2014. 18(1): 47–55.

42. Reyes del Paso, G.A., S. Garrido, A. Pulgar, and S. Duschek. Autonomic Cardiovascular Control and Responses to Experimental Pain Stimulation in Fibromyalgia Syndrome. Journal of Psychosomatic Research, 2011. 70(2): 125–34.

43. Barakat, A., N. Vogelzangs, C.M. Licht, et al. Dysregulation of the Autonomic Nervous System and Its Association with the Presence and Intensity of Chronic Widespread Pain. Arthritis Care and Research (Hoboken), 2012. 64(8): 1209–16.

44. Generaal, E., N. Vogelzangs, G.J. Macfarlane, et al. Reduced Hypothalamic-Pituitary-Adrenal Axis Activity in Chronic Multi-Site Musculoskeletal Pain: Partly Masked by Depressive and Anxiety Disorders. BMC Musculoskeletal Disorders, 2014. 15: 227.

45. McBeth, J., Y.H. Chiu, A.J. Silman, et al. Hypothalamic-Pituitary-Adrenal Stress Axis Function and the Relationship with Chronic Widespread Pain and Its Antecedents. Arthritis Research and Therapy, 2005. 7(5): R992-R1000.

46. McBeth, J., A.J. Silman, A. Gupta, et al. Moderation of Psychosocial Risk Factors through Dysfunction of the Hypothalamic-Pituitary-Adrenal Stress Axis in the Onset of Chronic Widespread Musculoskeletal Pain: Findings of a Population-Based Prospective Cohort Study. Arthritis and Rheumatism, 2007. 56(1): 360–71.

47. Nees, F., M. Loffler, K. Usai, and H. Flor. Hypothalamic-Pituitary-Adrenal Axis Feedback Sensitivity in Different States of Back Pain. Psychoneuroendocrinology, 2018. 101: 60–6.

48. Generaal, E., N. Vogelzangs, G.J. Macfarlane, et al. Biological Stress Systems, Adverse Life Events, and the Improvement of Chronic Multisite Musculoskeletal Pain across a 6-Year Follow-Up. Journal of Pain, 2017. 18(2): 155–65.

49. Lumley, M.A., J.L. Cohen, G.S. Borszcz, et al. Pain and Emotion: A Biopsychosocial Review of Recent Research. Journal of Clinical Psychology, 2011. 67(9): 942–68.

50. Thompson, J.M. and V. Neugebauer. Amygdala Plasticity and Pain. Pain Research and Management, 2017. 2017: 8296501.

51. Dampney, R.A. Central Mechanisms Regulating Coordinated Cardiovascular and Respiratory Function During Stress and Arousal. American Journal of Physiology–Regulatory, Integrative and Comparative Physiology, 2015. 309(5): R429–43.

52. Herman, J.P., J.M. McKlveen, S. Ghosal, et al. Regulation of the Hypothalamic-Pituitary-Adrenocortical Stress Response. Comprehensive Physiology, 2016. 6(2): 603–21.

53. Neugebauer, V. Amygdala Pain Mechanisms. Handbook of Experimental Pharmacology, 2015. 227: 261–84.

54. Thompson, J.M. and V. Neugebauer. Cortico-Limbic Pain Mechanisms. Neuroscience Letters, 2019. 702: 15–23.

55. Bourbia, N. and A. Pertovaara. Involvement of the Periaqueductal Gray in the Descending Antinociceptive Effect Induced by the Central Nucleus of Amygdala. Physiological Research, 2018. 67(4): 647–55.

56. Simons, L.E., I. Elman, and D. Borsook. Psychological Processing in Chronic Pain: A Neural Systems Approach. Neuroscience and Biobehavioral Reviews, 2014. 39: 61–78.

57. Simons, L.E., E.A. Moulton, C. Linnman, et al. The Human Amygdala and Pain: Evidence from

Neuroimaging. Human Brain Mapping, 2014. 35(2): 527–38.

58. Belova, M.A., J.J. Paton, S.E. Morrison, and C.D. Salzman. Expectation Modulates Neural Responses to Pleasant and Aversive Stimuli in Primate Amygdala. Neuron, 2007. 55(6): 970–84.

59. Johansen, J.P., J.W. Tarpley, J.E. LeDoux, and H.T. Blair. Neural Substrates for Expectation-Modulated Fear Learning in the Amygdala and Periaqueductal Gray. Nature Neuroscience, 2010. 13(8): 979–86.

60. Bunzli, S., A. Smith, R. Schutze, and P. O'Sullivan. Beliefs Underlying Pain-Related Fear and How They Evolve: A Qualitative Investigation in People with Chronic Back Pain and High Pain-Related Fear. BMJ Open, 2015. 5(10): e008847.

61. Likhtik, E., J.M. Stujenske, M.A. Topiwala, et al. Prefrontal Entrainment of Amygdala Activity Signals Safety in Learned Fear and Innate Anxiety. Nature Neuroscience, 2014. 17(1): 106–13.

62. Rhudy, J.L., J.L. DelVentura, E.L. Terry, et al. Emotional Modulation of Pain and Spinal Nociception in Fibromyalgia. Pain, 2013. 154(7): 1045–56.

63. Ochsner, K.N., D.H. Ludlow, K. Knierim, et al. Neural Correlates of Individual Differences in Pain-Related Fear and Anxiety. Pain, 2006. 120(1–2): 69–77.

64. Strange, B.A., M.P. Witter, E.S. Lein, and E.I. Moser. Functional Organization of the Hippocampal Longitudinal Axis. Nature Reviews Neuroscience, 2014. 15(10): 655–69.

65. Butler, R.K. and D.P. Finn. Stress-Induced Analgesia. Progress in Neurobiology, 2009. 88(3): 184–202.

66. Ford, G.K. and D.P. Finn. Clinical Correlates of Stress-Induced Analgesia: Evidence from Pharmacological Studies. Pain, 2008. 140(1): 3–7.

67. Yilmaz, P., M. Diers, S. Diener, et al. Brain Correlates of Stress-Induced Analgesia. Pain, 2010. 151(2): 522–9.

68. Nakamura, T., M. Tomida, T. Yamamoto, et al. The Endogenous Opioids Related with Antinociceptive Effects Induced by Electrical Stimulation into the Amygdala. The Open Dentistry Journal, 2013. 7: 27–35.

69. Pertovaara, A. Noradrenergic Pain Modulation. Progress in Neurobiology, 2006. 80(2): 53–83.

70. Zhuo, M. Descending Facilitation. Molecular Pain, 2017. 13: 1744806917699212.

71. Jennings, E.M., B.N. Okine, M. Roche, and D.P. Finn. Stress-Induced Hyperalgesia. Progress in Neurobiology, 2014. 121: 1–18.

72. Baliki, M.N., P.Y. Geha, H.L. Fields, and A.V. Apkarian. Predicting Value of Pain and Analgesia: Nucleus Accumbens Response to Noxious Stimuli Changes in the Presence of Chronic Pain. Neuron, 2010. 66(1): 149–60.

73. Dodo, N. and R. Hashimoto. The Effect of Anxiety Sensitivity on Psychological and Biological Variables During the Cold Pressor Test. Autonomic Neuroscience, 2017. 205: 72–6.

74. Vaegter, H.B., T.E. Andersen, M. Harvold, et al. Increased Pain Sensitivity in Accident-Related Chronic Pain Patients with Comorbid Post-traumatic Stress. Clinical Journal of Pain, 2018. 34(4): 313–21.

75. World Health Organisation, International Classification of Diseases. 2018; Available from: https://icd.who.int/en.

76. Morasco, B.J., T.I. Lovejoy, M. Lu, et al. The Relationship between PTSD and Chronic

Pain: Mediating Role of Coping Strategies and Depression. Pain, 2013. 154(4): 609–16.

77. Penacoba Puente, C., L. Velasco Furlong, C. Ecija Gallardo, et al. Self-Efficacy and Affect as Mediators between Pain Dimensions and Emotional Symptoms and Functional Limitation in Women with Fibromyalgia. Pain Management Nursing, 2015. 16(1): 60–8.

78. Wood, B.M., M.K. Nicholas, F. Blyth, et al. Catastrophizing Mediates the Relationship between Pain Intensity and Depressed Mood in Older Adults with Persistent Pain. Journal of Pain, 2013. 14(2): 149–57.

79. Finan, P.H., A.J. Zautra, and M.C. Davis. Daily Affect Relations in Fibromyalgia Patients Reveal Positive Affective Disturbance. Psychosomatic Medicine, 2009. 71(4): 474–82.

80. Zautra, A.J., L.M. Johnson, and M.C. Davis. Positive Affect as a Source of Resilience for Women in Chronic Pain. Journal of Consulting and Clinical Psychology, 2005. 73(2): 212–20.

81. Hassett, A.L., L.E. Simonelli, D.C. Radvanski, et al. The Relationship between Affect Balance Style and Clinical Outcomes in Fibromyalgia. Arthritis and Rheumatology, 2008. 59(6): 833–40.

82. Russo, S.J. and E.J. Nestler. The Brain Reward Circuitry in Mood Disorders. Nature Reviews Neuroscience, 2013. 14(9): 609–25.

83. Nestler, E.J. Role of the Brain's Reward Circuitry in Depression: Transcriptional Mechanisms. Int Rev Neurobiol, 2015. 124: 151–70.

84. Zhu, X., L. Helpman, S. Papini, et al. Altered Resting State Functional Connectivity of Fear and Reward Circuitry in Comorbid PTSD and Major Depression. Depression and Anxiety, 2017. 34(7): 641–50.

85. Doan, L., T. Manders, and J. Wang. Neuroplasticity Underlying the Comorbidity of Pain and Depression. Neural Plasticity, 2015. 2015: 504691.

86. Hashmi, J.A., M.N. Baliki, L. Huang, et al. Shape Shifting Pain: Chronification of Back Pain Shifts Brain Representation from Nociceptive to Emotional Circuits. Brain, 2013. 136(Pt 9): 2751–68.

87. Strigo, I.A., A.N. Simmons, S.C. Matthews, et al. Association of Major Depressive Disorder with Altered Functional Brain Response During Anticipation and Processing of Heat Pain. Archives of General Psychiatry, 2008. 65(11): 1275–84.

88. Meerwijk, E.L., J.M. Ford, and S.J. Weiss. Brain Regions Associated with Psychological Pain: Implications for a Neural Network and Its Relationship to Physical Pain. Brain Imaging and Behavior, 2013. 7(1): 1–14.

89. Huang, W.J., W.W. Chen, and X. Zhang. Endocannabinoid System: Role in Depression, Reward and Pain Control (Review). Molecular Medicine Reports, 2016. 14(4): 2899–903.

90. Klauenberg, S., C. Maier, H.J. Assion, et al. Depression and Changed Pain Perception: Hints for a Central Disinhibition Mechanism. Pain, 2008. 140(2): 332–43.

91. Cipriani, A., T. La Ferla, T.A. Furukawa, et al. Sertraline Versus Other Antidepressive Agents for Depression. Cochrane Database Systematic Reviews, 2010. 4: CD006117.

92. von Wolff, A., L.P. Holzel, A. Westphal, et al. Selective Serotonin Reuptake Inhibitors and Tricyclic Antidepressants in the Acute Treatment of Chronic Depression and Dysthymia: A Systematic Review and Meta-Analysis. Journal of Affective Disorders, 2013. 144(1–2): 7–15.

93. Yohn, C.N., M.M. Gergues, and B.A. Samuels. The Role of 5-HT Receptors in Depression. Molecular Brain, 2017. 10(1): 28.

94. Chopra, K. and V. Arora. An Intricate Relationship between Pain and Depression: Clinical Correlates, Coactivation Factors and Therapeutic Targets. Expert Opinion on Therapeutic Targets, 2014. 18(2): 159–76.

95. Khouzam, H.R. Psychopharmacology of Chronic Pain: A Focus on Antidepressants and Atypical Antipsychotics. Postgraduate Medicine, 2016. 128(3): 323–30.

96. Sharon, H., A. Maron-Katz, E. Ben Simon, et al. Mindfulness Meditation Modulates Pain through Endogenous Opioids. Am J Med, 2016. 129(7): 755–8.

97. Sluka, K.A., L. Frey-Law, and M. Hoeger Bement. Exercise-Induced Pain and Analgesia? Underlying Mechanisms and Clinical Translation. Pain, 2018. 159 Suppl 1: S91-S97.

98. Guendelman, S., S. Medeiros, and H. Rampes. Mindfulness and Emotion Regulation: Insights from Neurobiological, Psychological, and Clinical Studies. Frontiers in Psychology, 2017. 8: 220.

99. Goldberg, S.B., R.P. Tucker, P.A. Greene, et al. Mindfulness-Based Interventions for Psychiatric Disorders: A Systematic Review and Meta-Analysis. Clinical Psychology Review, 2018. 59: 52–60.

100. Goyal, M., S. Singh, E.M. Sibinga, et al. Meditation Programs for Psychological Stress and Well-Being: A Systematic Review and Meta-Analysis. JAMA Internal Medicine, 2014. 174(3): 357–68.

101. Veehof, M.M., H.R. Trompetter, E.T. Bohlmeijer, and K.M. Schreurs. Acceptance- and Mindfulness-Based Interventions for the Treatment of Chronic Pain: A Meta-Analytic Review. Cognitive Behavior Therapy, 2016. 45(1): 5–31.

102. Langhorst, J., P. Klose, G.J. Dobos, et al. Efficacy and Safety of Meditative Movement Therapies in Fibromyalgia Syndrome: A Systematic Review and Meta-Analysis of Randomized Controlled Trials. Rheumatology International, 2013. 33(1): 193–207.

103. Zou, L., A. Yeung, C. Li, et al. Effects of Meditative Movements on Major Depressive Disorder: A Systematic Review and Meta-Analysis of Randomized Controlled Trials. Journal of Clinical Medicine, 2018. 7(8).

104. Cramer, H., R. Lauche, J. Langhorst, and G. Dobos. Yoga for Depression: A Systematic Review and Meta-Analysis. Depression and Anxiety, 2013. 30(11): 1068–83.

105. Bilevicius, E., T.A. Kolesar, and J. Kornelsen. Altered Neural Activity Associated with Mindfulness During Nociception: A Systematic Review of Functional MRI. Brain Science, 2016. 6(2).

106. Doran, N.J. Experiencing Wellness within Illness: Exploring a Mindfulness-Based Approach to Chronic Back Pain. Qualitative Health Research, 2014. 24(6): 749–60.

107. Brown, C.A. and A.K. Jones. Meditation Experience Predicts Less Negative Appraisal of Pain: Electrophysiological Evidence for the Involvement of Anticipatory Neural Responses. Pain, 2010. 150(3): 428–38.

108. Gallegos, A.M., H.F. Crean, W.R. Pigeon, and K.L. Heffner. Meditation and Yoga for Posttraumatic Stress Disorder: A Meta-Analytic Review of Randomized Controlled Trials. Clinical Psychology Reviews, 2017. 58: 115–24.

109. Nguyen-Feng, V.N., C.J. Clark, and M.E. Butler. Yoga as an Intervention for Psychological Symptoms Following Trauma: A Systematic Review

and Quantitative Synthesis. Psychological Services, 2019. 16(3): 513–23.

110. van der Kolk, B.A., L. Stone, J. West, et al. Yoga as an Adjunctive Treatment for Posttraumatic Stress Disorder: A Randomized Controlled Trial. Journal of Clinical Psychiatry, 2014. 75(6): e559–65.

111. Fox, K.C., M.L. Dixon, S. Nijeboer, et al. Functional Neuroanatomy of Meditation: A Review and Meta-Analysis of 78 Functional Neuroimaging Investigations. Neuroscience Biobehavioral Reviews, 2016. 65: 208–28.

112. Fox, K.C., S. Nijeboer, M.L. Dixon, et al. Is Meditation Associated with Altered Brain Structure? A Systematic Review and Meta-Analysis of Morphometric Neuroimaging in Meditation Practitioners. Neuroscience and Biobehavioural Reviews, 2014. 43: 48–73.

113. Wadden, K.P., N.J. Snow, P. Sande, et al. Yoga Practitioners Uniquely Activate the Superior Parietal Lobule and Supramarginal Gyrus During Emotion Regulation. Frontiers in Integrative Neuroscience, 2018. 12: 60.

114. Pascoe, M.C., D.R. Thompson, Z.M. Jenkins, and C.F. Ski. Mindfulness Mediates the Physiological Markers of Stress: Systematic Review and Meta-Analysis. Journal of Psychiatry Research, 2017. 95: 156–78.

115. Ebnezar, J., R. Nagarathna, B. Yogitha, and H.R. Nagendra. Effect of Integrated Yoga Therapy on Pain, Morning Stiffness and Anxiety in Osteo arthritis of the Knee Joint: A Randomized Control Study. International Journal of Yoga, 2012. 5(1): 28–36.

116. Grossman, P., G. Deuring, H. Walach, et al. Mindfulness-Based Intervention Does Not Influence Cardiac Autonomic Control or the Pattern of Physical Activity in Fibromyalgia

During Daily Life: An Ambulatory, Multimeasure Randomized Controlled Trial. Clinical Journal of Pain, 2017. 33(5): 385–94.

117. Green, D.A., J. Bowtell, and D.L. Turner. Electrical Percutaneous Tibial Stimulation Modulates Within-a-Breath Respiratory Drive in Man. Respiratory Physiology and Neurobiology, 2008. 161(2): 214–17.

118. Jafari, H., I. Courtois, O. Van den Bergh, et al. Pain and Respiration: A Systematic Review. Pain, 2017. 158(6): 995–1006.

119. Zaccaro, A., A. Piarulli, M. Laurino, et al. How Breath-Control Can Change Your Life: A Systematic Review on Psycho-Physiological Correlates of Slow Breathing. Frontiers in Human Neuroscience, 2018. 12: 353.

120. Duschek, S., N.S. Werner, and G.A. Reyes Del Paso. The Behavioral Impact of Baroreflex Function: A Review. Psychophysiology, 2013. 50(12): 1183–93.

121. Wehrwein, E.A. and M.J. Joyner. Regulation of Blood Pressure by the Arterial Baroreflex and Autonomic Nervous System. Handbook of Clinical Neurology, 2013. 117: 89–102.

122. Gianaros, P.J., I.C. Onyewuenyi, L.K. Sheu, et al. Brain Systems for Baroreflex Suppression During Stress in Humans. Human Brain Mapping, 2012. 33(7): 1700–16.

123. Reyes del Paso, G.A., C. Montoro, C. Munoz Ladron de Guevara, et al. The Effect of Baroreceptor Stimulation on Pain Perception Depends on the Elicitation of the Reflex Cardiovascular Response: Evidence of the Interplay between the Two Branches of the Baroreceptor System. Biological Psychology, 2014. 101: 82–90.

124. Vollestad, J., M.B. Nielsen, and G.H. Nielsen. Mindfulness- and Acceptance-Based Interventions

for Anxiety Disorders: A Systematic Review and Meta-Analysis. British Journal of Clinical Psychology, 2012. 51(3): 239–60.

125. Busch, V., W. Magerl, U. Kern, et al. The Effect of Deep and Slow Breathing on Pain Perception, Autonomic Activity, and Mood Processing – An Experimental Study. Pain Medicine, 2012. 13(2): 215–28.

126. Reyes del Paso, G.A., C. Munoz Ladron de Guevara, and C.I. Montoro. Breath-Holding During Exhalation as a Simple Manipulation to Reduce Pain Perception. Pain Medicine, 2015. 16(9): 1835–41.

127. Williams, M. and D. Penman. Mindfulness: A Practical Guide to Finding Peace in a Frantic World. 2011, London: Piatkus.

The body is like a living book, it should be read every day.

Traditional Ayurvedic medicine principle

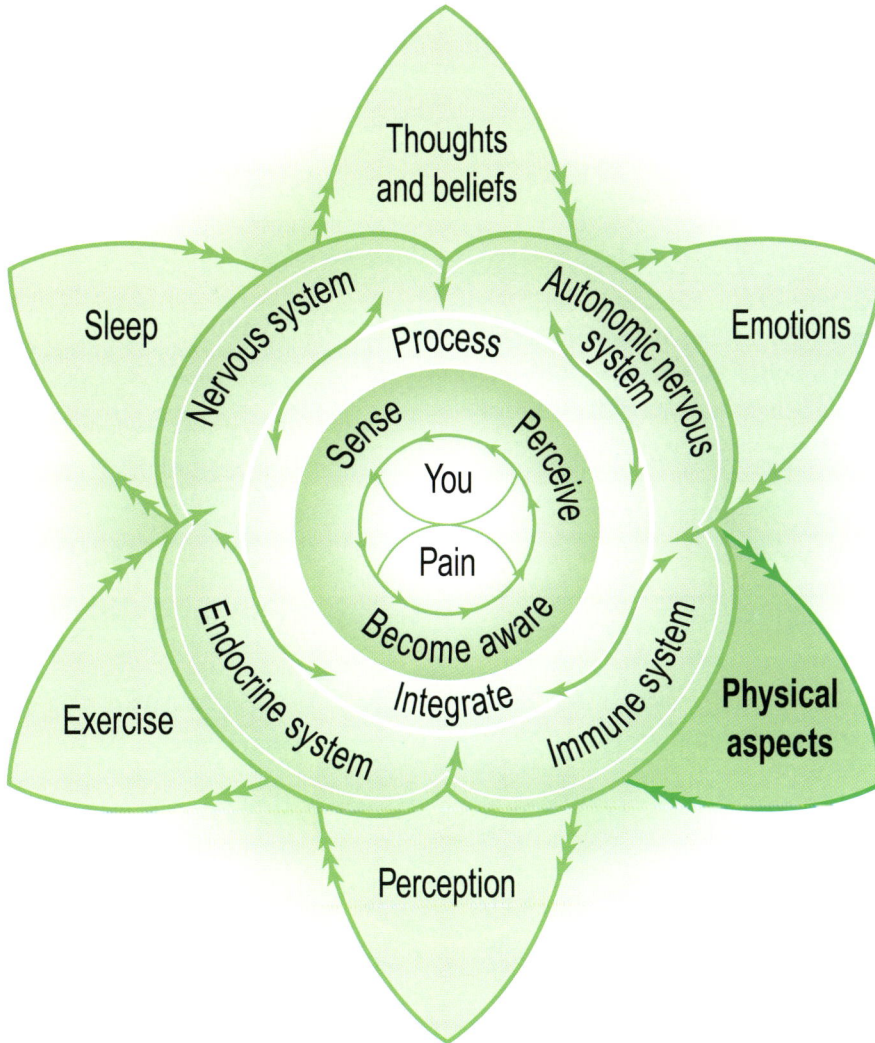

Figure 6.1

Pain Mandala – Physical Aspects. The physical aspects of pain include inputs from injured or sensitive tissues, as well as inputs from how we move. These inputs and potentially protective movements have the ability to influence our body systems, our processing and our awareness, particularly if the way we move in pain has become an unhelpful or avoidance response. The role of pathology and alignment may be less important in many cases of pain, particularly persistent pain. Understanding tissue sensitivity and helpful versus unhelpful movement adaptations may allow the person in pain to develop a more accurate way to consider the role of tissue inputs in their whole pain experience.

Note: This mandala depicts aspects of the human experience of pain covered in Pain Science Yoga Life. *Other inputs, dimensions and body systems can contribute to pain than those noted here.*

Headspace
Our Bodies in Pain

When we experience pain, it is easy to notice the physical manifestation. We perceive pain in our body, such as stomachache, headache and backache. For centuries, our go-to explanation for pain has been to identify the source of pain in our tissues (muscles, tendons, ligaments, joints, viscera). Vast resources and time are invested in examining tissues and performing diagnostic imaging (MRI, ultrasound, X-ray). When seeking professional help, people want to know what is causing the pain and what can be done to fix it. They are usually focused on a physical, tissue source. Our tissues can contribute to pain and we will cover some of these important inputs, but our understanding about how much tissue pathology contributes to pain has shifted. As outlined in Chapter 1, tissue inputs don't reflect the full picture of the multidimensionality of pain. The first part of this chapter explores tissue inputs and how shifts in thinking about pathology may influence pain care.

Yoga asana practice asks us to consider *how* we move. This is the focus for the second part of this chapter. How we move matters, both when we are in pain and when we are recovering from pain, but movement approaches that rigidly adhere to principles of 'ideal' alignment are being challenged by research over the last decade. We'll discuss teaching and assessing movement in a way that accommodates the individual, and which considers whether their movement strategies are helpful or unhelpful.

> Scope of practice consideration: Tissue injuries can span a broad range of severity, from minor strains and sprains to significant injuries or conditions. While yoga may support injury management, evaluation by an appropriately qualified health care provider may be necessary.

Part 1: Inputs from the Tissues

In Chapter 1 we introduced the concept of nociception or danger detection. Nerves from our tissues send signals to the spinal cord and brain. These signals inform the brain about changes in tissue chemistry, pressure, position and temperature. While some peripheral nerve fibers relay 'noxious' information (e.g. too much pressure, very high temperatures),[1] we don't have pain receptors, nor do the nerves from our tissues send pain signals per se. But they can send warning signals: this is nociception. In understanding pain, it's important to recognize that *one input* contributing to pain is nociception or warning signals from the body's tissues.

Can you think of a time you had a painful injury, tweaked a joint or strained a muscle? How did our brain know something might be wrong and what was happening in the tissues? Let's begin to explore what actually happened to the tissues when the baseball impacted Phillip's hand (Case Study, p. 51).

Acute Pain Conditions and Injuries

Acute (meaning recent-onset) injuries or pain can occur when tissues are overloaded from a sudden movement, load or impact that is outside something they are accustomed to. For example, Phillip's hand was struck suddenly by a baseball. Injuries can also occur gradually, with prolonged loads eventually exceeding the tissue's tolerance, e.g. such as for waiting staff, stressing the wrist carrying heavy trays every night, or long-distance runners straining calf muscles due to increased miles. Recent muscle strains, joint/ligament sprains, or disc and cartilage injuries can all generate inflammation, changing tissue chemistry, potentially sensitizing free nerve endings and receptors, and initiating nociception. Let's explore these responses to physical stress on tissues more specifically.

Inflammation

Inflammation is a natural response to tissue stress and is crucial for tissue healing and recovery. It is broken

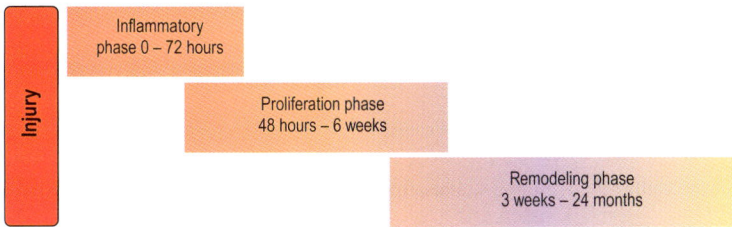

Figure 6.2

Stages of inflammation. There are three primary stages of inflammation: (1) inflammatory response, (2) proliferation stage and (3) remodeling phase. All of these phases overlap. While we consider most healing to have occurred within 3 months of injury, note how remodeling can continue up to 24 months post injury.

down into stages which have considerable overlap, rather than distinctive start and end points (Figure 6.2)[2]:

- Stage 1: Bleeding (0–6 hours). Small capillaries in the tissues tear and leak fluid. This stimulates the immune system to initiate inflammation.[2]

- Stage 2: Inflammatory response (0–72 hours). Inflammation causes the release of inflammatory cells required for healing, including macrophages which clean up the mess, absorbing damaged tissue. Cells, such as fibroblasts, myoblasts and tenoblasts, move into the area in preparation for tissue healing. Certain inflammatory chemicals, like bradykinin, sensitize nerve endings, making it easier to generate warning signals (nociception). This 'cue for protection' increases the likelihood of pain as a response from the brain and nervous system, to help protect the area from excessive stress while early healing occurs.[2]

- Stage 3: Proliferation (48 hours–6 weeks). Fibroblasts, myoblasts and tenoblasts start the process of scar formation and regeneration. Different types of collagen are formed by each cell type: e.g. fibroblasts produce connective tissue, chondrocytes produce cartilage and tenocytes produce tendon. For bone healing, osteoblasts and osteoclasts produce new bone cells.[2]

- Stage 4: Remodeling (weeks–months). Newly formed tissues undergo changes so that healed tissues can adapt to the loads that will be placed

upon them. This mainly occurs in the first three months post injury; however, tissue remodeling can continue for many months.[2]

So, for Phillip, when his hand was struck by the baseball, it is likely that he had swelling and bruising as a result of the bleeding from the contused tissue. It is also expected that he would have sensitivity and stiffness from this chemical response as a means to protect him and allow the tissues time to heal. At this stage inflammation and pain are a very good thing! They are necessary for him to heal.

General care for acute soft tissue injuries (sprains and strains) has changed a little in recent years. Table 6.1 demonstrates the current soft tissue injury guide of PEACE and LOVE, which builds on the previous PRICE (protect, rest, ice compress and elevation) model by advising that anti-inflammatory modalities are used with caution, and advocating progressive loading.[3]

Table 6.1 Acute soft tissue management with PEACE and LOVE

Protect	Load
Elevate	Optimism
Avoid (inappropriate*) anti-inflammatory modalities	Vascularization: Through mobilization and aerobic activity
Compress	Exercise
Educate	

*Careful consideration is advocated with using anti-inflammatory modalities. PEACE is advocated for immediate management of a recent soft tissue injury, while LOVE is needed for rehabilitation once the first few days have passed.[1]

Movement in Early Tissue Healing

Tissues need LOVE: load (i.e. physical stress), optimism, vascularization (through mobilization and aerobic exercise) and exercise specific to the tissues.[3] Appropriate, gradual increases in tissue load stimulate collagen to remodel optimally, preparing repaired tissue to withstand future demands.[2] 'Appropriate' is a key word to focus on here. While relative rest is required immediately after injury, prolonged rest impairs recovery and contributes to secondary effects such as stiffness, weakness and reduced function.[2] Too much load too early in recovery can also delay healing.[2] Therefore, adjusting load for the degree of injury and stage of healing is important across rehabilitation.

Common Misunderstandings About Tissue Healing: Real But Not True

- *Real:* You need to rest. *Not true*: You need to rest *completely.*
  Most acute injuries from ankle sprains[4] to back pain[5] don't recover optimally with complete rest. Gently moving within pain tolerance, then gradually progressing activity, is needed. Complete rest with the expectation of returning to activities at pre-injury level is unrealistic and risks re-injury.[6]

- *Real:* You should modify activity when injured. *Not true:* You need to be pain-free before you return to usual activities.
  While pain is a reasonable guide in acute injuries, performing exercises and movement within pain tolerance limits is appropriate. It obviously makes sense to increase activities gradually.

Expectations About Tissue Healing

Consider your injury again. How long did it take to heal? Were you surprised by how long it took to recover? Many people want or expect an instant recovery, so to ease their anxiety or encourage more patience and optimize the healing process, I often explain that rather than a straight line of improvement, the road to recovery is more like a winding road, which can sometimes get a bit bumpy.

In my 20s I experienced significant back pain and sciatica. I was surprised by the expectations of healing expressed by my friends and family. For example, when I met my running coach to let him know I'd be out for a while, he expected me back in a couple of weeks. When I replied that it would be probably more like a couple of months (2–3 months is normal recovery time for back pain with sciatica), he was shocked and uttered "Wow, must be really bad." This was echoed by many I encountered who were not medically trained. It left me with a deep impression that generally people might not appreciate typical recovery times. These interactions didn't cause me much angst but I understand how they might for someone without a full understanding of normal recovery times, not to mention the part played by thoughts, beliefs and emotional inputs (see Chapters 4 and 5). Since back pain and disc injuries are quite common, let's take a side step and look at these for a moment.

Discs Are Tissues Too

Discs are worth a special mention as they are blamed for a lot of back pain, and cause considerable fear and uncertainty about management. Here are some notes to consider.

- For about 90% of back pain, a specific structure is hard to identify as the cause of pain.[7] Intervertebral discs, trunk muscles, spinal joints and ligaments are all structures with a nerve supply capable of generating nociception when injured or inflamed. Discs are probably blamed for a lot more than they're responsible for.

- Discs never slip. The disc is strongly adhered to the bone around it and is surrounded by a vast array of ligaments and spinal muscles. Discs do bulge and protrude, and sometimes when they do, they can stimulate inflammation, which can irritate nearby nerves. Occasionally, when disc protrusions are large, nearby spinal nerves can become compressed.

- Disc bulges and degeneration are common even if you don't have pain[8] – a part of ageing that isn't necessarily associated with pain and doesn't always predict future pain.[9] Think of this like skin: it gets wrinkly as it gets older but for most of us it still works, offering protection for what lies beneath.

- Discs heal: inflammation settles and protrusions reduce or disappear for most people who have disc protrusions associated with their pain.[10,11]

- Discs don't need to be protected any more than other tissues in the body: gradually increasing movement and load is important for healing. During rehabilitation, restoring normal function is important. We will discuss helpful and unhelpful movement strategies later, but it's worth noting that advising someone to move in a guarded way to 'protect their back' over the longer term is not evidence-based advice and may prove to be harmful rather than helpful.[12]

If we again consider Phillip, he expected to recover within a relatively short time, certainly within a few months. However, that was not the case; he then became increasingly sensitive and life became more and more challenging for him. Let's look at why might that be from a tissue perspective.

Chronic Conditions

Conditions that last beyond the expected healing time, usually more than three months, are often referred to as persistent or chronic. All pain experiences are multifactorial but this is particularly the case for chronic conditions: tissue inputs are just one part to consider. We'll explore how some tissue changes can contribute to persistent nociception next.

Some conditions can drive sustained or repeated nociception. Classic examples include osteoarthritis[13] and rheumatoid arthritis,[14] whereby joint changes are associated with recurrent or persistent inflammation. In turn, this can cause repeated nociception and perpetuate a vicious cycle – inputs becoming outputs. Recurrent or persistent inflammation (input) can negatively impact joint structure and nearby soft tissues (ligaments/muscles), causing more pathology and inflammation (output) and therefore increasing the potential for a protective pain response (output).[14] Recurrent or persistent inflammation can sensitize the nervous system, thus becoming more deeply entrenched as inflammation and sensitization persist.[15] This may make reversing pain more difficult for some.

Persistent nociception may also arise from compromised soft tissues, e.g. in persistent tendon pain. Common tendinopathies such as tennis elbow, patellar and Achilles tendinopathies can become persistent, making management challenging. While not completely understood, repeated tendon overload and changes within tendon make-up and function (histology and physiology) may be ongoing sources of nociception.[16,17]

Persistent nociception may arise from more idiopathic (meaning specific pathology is hard to identify) conditions like non-specific neck or back pain, repetitive strain and overuse disorders. While defining a specific source of nociception is difficult, possible inputs may arise from joints, nerves and soft tissues in the area. This may result from sustained low-level repetitive load or high physical loads, which may cause a low-grade inflammatory process.[18-21]

It is also worth noting that tissue inputs might also arise from low-grade inflammation that is more systemic. There is growing awareness that systemic low-grade inflammation is an important contributor to pain and can result from poor diet,[22] obesity, low physical activity,[22] poor sleep[23,24] or psychological factors.[25,26] The Pain Mandala (see Figure 6.1) highlights some of these interactions; the links between stress responses and immune system responses such as inflammation have already been discussed. We'll also delve into these a little more in Chapter 9.

For Phillip, his poor recovery and transition into persistent pain may partly be explained by disordered inflammation that became a source of persistent/recurrent nociception. Some of these changes can be driven by or interact with broader factors like autonomic nervous system and peripheral/central nervous system sensitization. These were in turn likely heightened by thoughts, beliefs, fears and stress (which can promote ongoing inflammation). His Pain Mandala is growing in its layers and connections.

Nociception and Nerves

Nerve pain warrants a special mention because it is often difficult to manage and carries a higher risk of becoming persistent.

- Pain can spread, and often when pain spreads people talk about it being related to a trapped or pinched nerve; however, that is only the case some of the time. Joints, discs, cartilage and muscle all have referral zones and can cause a spread of pain, particularly with peripheral and central sensitization.

- Nerve (neuropathic) pain refers to a "lesion or disease of the somatosensory nervous system".[27] Nerve pain is often accompanied by burning sensations, pins and needles, and numbness. However, the diagnosis is not made on symptoms alone and a full examination of the nervous system is required to identify true nerve pathology and pain.[27]

- Injured (compressed) or irritated nerves can be potent sources of nociception and can trigger excessive inflammation[28] and nervous system sensitization.[15,29]

- Treatment can range from simple strategies like wearing splints and rest, to surgery and comprehensive programs including neuropathic pain medication,[30] physical therapies,[31,32] and psychological and self-management strategies.[33]

- Nerve pain has a tendency to be irritable, and so early management by a suitably qualified health care provider is necessary.

- Yoga asanas may be helpful once the individual has a good understanding of management of their condition. It's important that mobilization and stretching are done very gradually, as sensitized nerves are easily aggravated by stretching.

Changing Nociception in Persistent Conditions

When we look at persistent conditions from a physical perspective, one question is whether we can influence the amount of nociception arising from affected tissues. Let's look at using movement and exercise for this purpose. Exercise can be very effective in reducing pain and disability across many pain conditions.[34–38] While some effects are systemic, e.g. on nervous system sensitivity[39] and inflammation[40] (more in Chapter 8), other effects relate to optimizing muscle function, improving tissue composition (e.g. cartilage thickness)[41] and managing tissue load,[42,43] thus reducing nociceptive input.

Managing load (the amount of stress placed on the tissue) can be done in two main ways: 1) reduce the load through the painful area; and 2) increase load tolerance. Optimal management usually combines both until increased load tolerance is achieved.[43,44]

Reducing the load through the painful area: A long-distance runner with Achilles tendinopathy may have to reduce frequency or total amount of running, and maybe include cross-training as part of their rehabilitation. A manual laborer with back pain might reduce load by relaxing as they move or altering their lifting mechanics to reduce unnecessary muscle tension. Sometimes moderating load is about changing *how* a person performs a task. Technique or coordination training can be important here, e.g. reducing excessive muscle activity or adjusting alignment during movement.

During asana practice, load management might involve modifying a position by reducing the load, e.g. supported malasana (squat). Playing 'the intelligent edge' during asana practice is wise, i.e. moving to the edge or onset of discomfort. This fits nicely with optimizing tissue loading and with the principle of ahimsa or non-violence to the body. Being willing to adjust physical practices in the presence of pain and dysfunction is fundamental to ensuring the physical load we put on our bodies is appropriate and not harmful.

Building load tolerance: This is about building strength and endurance so we can tolerate loads required during activities (see Chapter 8). A runner may need to do strength and conditioning exercises to improve the Achilles tendon, calf muscle and other lower limb muscle function to build load tolerance for endurance running. The manual laborer may need to build the strength of all leg muscles to increase load tolerance for lifting, squatting and climbing ladders. Asana practice can be adapted to involve progressive load to encourage strengthening and load tolerance. Again, playing the intelligent edge and practicing ahimsa are key here, where people with pain are encouraged to increase load gradually.

Pathology and Pain

The link between pain and pathology is tenuous and one does not necessarily indicate the other. So far, we've discussed injuries and pathology and how to manage them, but how much do tissue inputs really contribute to pain? Have you worked with people who have healthy joints on scans but lots of pain, while others have advanced arthritis on X-rays but little pain? This is common clinically and growing research shows that pain and tissue damage don't always correlate. Let's explore what is *real* and what is *not true* in the following clinical scenarios, according to contemporary data.

- *I woke up this morning with severe neck pain… I can't move properly…Something must be 'out of place' in my neck.*

- Or: *My back is out.*

  Real but not true: Spinal pain can be intense and can make movement difficult. It can give the impression that the spine feels twisted or stuck. However, except in cases of severe trauma, the spinal segments and the pelvis don't 'go out of place'; they're actually much more robust than people tend to think.[45-49] Treatments like spinal manipulation (also known as adjustments) are now known to relieve pain by activating our brain's pharmacy and changing muscle tone rather than changing spinal alignment.[50,51]

- *The scan shows a cartilage tear and some wear and tear in my knee – that must be what's causing my pain.*

  Real but not (always) true: Cartilage changes can contribute to pain but it's not a given. Data from over 4,000 people without pain show cartilage changes such as tears are common, particularly in those over 40 years old.[52]

- *I have degenerative discs – I guess that will only get worse as I get older, so I can expect more pain.*

  Real but not true: Again, the 'pathology' might relate to pain, but so many people without pain have these changes that it's hard to say.[8] Back pain doesn't automatically get worse as you get older: the degenerative changes tend to increase but rates of back pain actually plateau from around age 40.[53]

Let's delve a little deeper and look at low back pain and MRI scans. While greater numbers of findings on MRI scans and some specific pathologies do show greater associations with pain and poor recovery,[54] these are not always consistent.[9] MRI scans from over 3,000 people *without* back pain show that so-called 'pathologies' such as disc degeneration and disc protrusion are very common.[8] For example, 80% of 50-year-olds have signs of degeneration. Thirty percent of 20-year-olds, 50% of 40-year-olds and 69% of 60-year-olds have disc bulges. Yet, these people didn't report pain. These findings don't necessarily predict future pain either, and other factors like depression and previous episodes of pain appear at least as, if not more, relevant.[55,56] Spines that are imperfect don't have to be painful, and vice versa: if someone has back pain, that does not mean they have pathology. If we integrate the idea of *and this too,* we can respect the potential place for considering the contribution of pathology to a person's pain without allowing pathology to be the sole focus.

It's the same story for other pathologies like shoulder rotator cuff tears, hip labral tears[57–59] and osteoarthritis[52,60]: they are commonly found in people without symptoms. Again, the degree of pathology found on scans does not always correlate with the pain people experience.[61] Recently, there have been efforts to examine different profiles in osteoarthritis.[62] While in some people the amount of degeneration seemed to correlate with pain, some profiles are more characterized by pain sensitivity and low mood,[63] and others still by broader health issues like diabetes and cardiovascular disease.[62]

The Pathology Message

The link between pathology and pain isn't linear. It certainly may be relevant for some people; however, we should consider the bigger picture of pain and its various contributors: *and this too*. Perhaps we, as clinicians and teachers, can consider how we present information about pathology, and how it relates to pain. Language deserves our attention, and in practicing ahimsa, we could use language that is less likely to be harmful. For example, if you believe people with disc bulges shouldn't bend, you may say something like: 'If you have back pain, keep your back straight.' What's the basis for this instruction? This could be a harmful thing to say. Considering the data above, many of us will have these changes naturally and don't have pain or problems with bending. You may be thinking: isn't it sensible to avoid or limit potentially painful movements? Of course, there isn't a black or white answer here. But beware: being overly cautious and advising people to *always* avoid certain movements because you consider them potentially damaging may set them up for more protection and therefore more pain later. Moreover, advising against certain movements for broad conditions like back pain or knee pain may cause people to think that particular movements are bad in general, and so fails to acknowledge that people with pain present with varied patterns of comfortable and uncomfortable movements. Recognizing the overlap between inputs to the pain experience, these thoughts and beliefs (inputs) can cause avoidance or overprotection, which may lead to unhelpful movement patterns. In turn, these inputs may all delay recovery and potentially contribute to pain persisting.

Part 2: How We Move – Does It Matter?

To recap, tissue inputs such as inflammation from injury *may* cause nociception but not in every case. Pathology can contribute too, but so-called 'pathology' is also common in people without pain. What about how we move? This is a key focus in many yoga practices, so let's examine the science.

Alignment Is Not Strongly Related to Injury or Pain

Again, let's start with a couple of common misunderstandings about pain and alignment: *real but not true.*

- *My doctor said no more bending, lifting or sitting – this is just making my back worse.*

  Real: While some people experience pain when they sit or bend, others experience pain when they stand up or move in different directions. Sometimes limiting bending, lifting or sitting for a period of time to allow healing may be recommended, but this advice should depend on the individual's presentation and should not be prescribed en masse.

  Not true: The evidence that bending while lifting or sitting actually *causes* or worsens spinal/back pain is weak.[64–67]

- *My knee has been hurting while I run. I think my alignment is off. Maybe I need some insoles to correct it.*

  Real: Knees, ankles and hips can become sore while running and altered biomechanics (how you move) may contribute to nociception.

  Not true: While biomechanics may contribute to pain for some, there isn't a direct relationship between alignment and pain or injury.[68–71] Have a look at elite athletes running a race: alignment and biomechanics vary.

This might be a challenging topic, particularly if you have spent years learning 'correct' techniques for teaching movement. Current evidence challenges a rigid focus on alignment in regard to risk of pain and injury or changing pain. We're not saying alignment never matters, but a balanced understanding of relative contributors to injury and pain allows a more realistic perspective about the risks or importance associated with so-called 'suboptimal' alignment. Importantly, we need to consider whether our traditional focus on alignment may actually cause unnecessary fear, entrenching unhelpful beliefs and ultimately contributing to more pain. That said, if a person has pain and their movement quality or

alignment looks 'suboptimal,' it *may* be contributing to their symptoms. It is justified to modify how they move and assess the response. If symptoms reduce, that's great. However, if there is no change, continued focus on specific alignment may be questionable. Worsening symptoms suggest their previous strategy was more appropriate. The crux is that we should apply this assessment and treatment approach as appropriate to the individual and not to entire groups. Keeping alignment cues as gentle suggestions may be beneficial during group classes, especially if some students mention or demonstrate struggles with pain.

Lifting and back injuries: Who among us hasn't been told to keep our back straight when lifting, or even warned, 'Watch your back'? My small stature means I get this a lot. It's amusing to me that I'll lift heavy weights at the gym but lifting a suitcase can provide cause for concern to onlookers. We must acknowledge that risk of injury for back pain includes mechanical factors like repetitive lifting; however, research highlights that these factors carry no greater risk than psychosocial factors, for example, and that traditional approaches to 'correct' lifting don't reduce back pain.[65,72,73] When comparing people who stoop while lifting to those who don't move their backs, results demonstrate no differences in back injuries or incidence of pain.[65,66] Moreover, generally, many people with back pain move with less spinal flexion,[74] which might suggest that restoring spinal movement for them, rather than avoiding it, would be helpful. Put simply, optimal techniques will vary across individuals.

Posture and back/neck pain: As for lifting techniques, we've all been told to sit up straight, and warned of the perils of slouching. Many of us will have been drilled on the benefits of good posture and its apparent ability to prevent or treat pain. However, the relationship between posture and pain is as tenuous as the relationship between pathology and pain. To say that there is an ideal posture ignores normal variation among people, including pain-free individuals.[75] While potentially relevant to some individuals, when large groups of people are examined, spinal posture is not consistently associated with pain. Recently analyses of the posture of over 1,000 adolescents found no association between posture and neck pain and headaches.[67] Further, postural retraining approaches like the Alexander Technique show inconclusive results for relieving spinal pain[76] while approaches such as Pilates show similar results to other forms of exercise.[77] If posture were the Holy Grail, surely these approaches would demonstrate better effects. There might be postures that help some individuals' symptoms; however, there is no single 'optimal' posture. This, considered alongside data that people with spinal pain move with greater stiffness,[74,78–80] challenges the merit of advocating upright postures, which can create more stiffness.

Alignment and sports injuries: The next time you watch an athletics championship, notice the variation in alignment and movement patterns across athletes. In the early 2000s I remember watching Paula Radcliffe, holder of the London marathon record for many years, who ran with a funny head nod, thinking that it couldn't be efficient. While she *looked* inefficient when she ran, she was anything but! Watch Priscah Jeptoo, another elite marathon runner– she has marked genu valgum (knocked knees) when she runs. You would think an elite athlete wouldn't run like this, but does it matter? Does this mean she's at greater risk of injury? Research examining risk factors for running injuries shows limited associations between runners' biomechanics and risk of injury. Only small associations have been found between overpronation (flat feet) and genu valgum with pain or injury.[69,81] If we look at lower limb biomechanics and patellofemoral pain syndrome (pain around the kneecap), a recent systematic review examining whether various lower limb factors *predicted the onset* of patellofemoral pain syndrome found the only factor that consistently predicted pain

was quadriceps strength,[70,71] not knee or foot angles.[71] This is echoed in studies on alignment and other lower limb injuries.[82] In tandem, recent data highlight the importance of other factors such as sleep, stress and nutrition in predicting sports injuries – back to the layers of the Pain Mandala![83–85]

Integration Into Yoga Practice

Does how you think about alignment influence how you instruct asana or teach exercise? Are there aspects of the research presented above that challenge how you instruct? In yoga classes (and many exercise situations), suggestions about alignment and posture are common. Let's consider the common instruction not to let your knee travel in front of your ankle (a restricted squat), the idea being to reduce knee loading 'to protect the knees'. While it is correct that this 'restricted squat' reduces anterior knee loading compared to an unrestricted squat (knees allowed to travel),[86] one could question what the advantage is. Our knees routinely move in front of our ankles: watch how your knee moves when you walk downstairs, or play tennis or any dynamic sport. Studies examining squats and load conclude that if the aim is to strengthen the quadriceps, then unrestricted squats may better achieve this.[86,87]

Further, while restricted squats reduce the load on knees, they increase load through the hips and spine.[86,87] Why is taking the load off the knees but placing it elsewhere better? Perhaps for some individuals with knee pain this suggestion might be helpful; for others with knee pain, gradually building tolerance to this load is appropriate, even desirable. For those without knee pain it could just be an option offered.

In summary, when drawing conclusions about whether an asana is contributing to someone's pain, injury or risk of injury, we need to hold space for the variability in alignment and postures seen across individuals as well as broader contributions to pain and injury. Perhaps we can integrate this into the concept of *and this too*, holding space for pathology or different alignment without necessarily judging it as problematic in everyone. In doing so, we can teach in a way that is likely to promote optimal healing and healthy attitudes towards the body in pain and recovery.

Movement Strategies and Pain

Movement changes in a highly variable manner when pain is present. To explore this topic, let's journey through a little of the research on 'core stability'. In the late 1990s and early 2000s research emerged that deep muscles around the spine were weaker in people with spinal pain.[88–90] This was supported with evidence of changes to the composition of these muscles.[91–93] These studies are cited frequently as the basis for 'improving core stability' in people with spinal pain. However, subsequent research has shown that muscle responses are more varied than these early studies indicated. Groups of people with back pain who demonstrate excessive muscle activation have been identified.[94–96] In those with neck pain, evidence of greater neck and trunk stiffness with higher muscle activation patterns has also recently emerged.[78,80]

This means that as we work with people with pain, assessing individual movement strategies and muscle patterning to evaluate their contribution to their pain seems wise. Some will be overactive, some underactive, some stiff, some more mobile. Advising everyone to 'activate their core' seems no longer justifiable. As with alignment, people move with variable movement and muscle strategies, particularly when pain is in the picture. Maybe this cues us to take pause before suggesting a movement strategy or muscle pattern is 'right' or 'wrong' without exploring it further. To this end we'll discuss adaptive and maladaptive movement strategies.

Are Our Adapted Movements Helpful or Not?

When we change our movement because of pain, injury or beliefs or habits, we 'adapt' our movement. The next question is whether this is helpful or not. *Adaptive movement strategies are protective altered motor behaviors in response to pain that are usually* **helpful** *at reducing pain.*[97] For example, with a recently sprained ankle, limping is an adaptive strategy – it's helpful. Initially, attempts to 'normalize' (i.e. change the pattern to something that looks more normal) this movement adaptation may provoke more symptoms and may not be helpful. However, gradually encouraging normal walking within pain limits over the week following the injury may be appropriate. Another example of an adaptive (helpful) movement strategy is an individual with spinal stenosis (narrowing of the spinal canal associated with nerve compression) who experiences back and leg pain when they try to straighten. To reduce their symptoms, they hold a more flexed spine: this is helpful to reduce symptoms associated with nerve compression.

Maladaptive movement strategies are altered motor behaviors that result in abnormal tissue loading and are usually **unhelpful** *at reducing pain.*[97] Attempts to 'normalize' movement or posture improves symptoms. For these individuals it is still important to explore why they have adopted this movement strategy. It may be unconscious – they are not aware of it. It may be associated with beliefs that this strategy is helpful or the body is weak or needs protection, and that tensing muscles is effective to protect it. For example, the person with a sprained ankle might continue to limp for weeks post injury because they thought they would do more damage if they walked normally. Returning to the case study of Phillip (see p. 51), as his pain persisted, he began to hold his right hand and arm in a 'protective pattern', with his arm across his chest as though in a sling. This provided him with some comfort and sense of safety. However, for his musculoskeletal system this was maladaptive, contributing to stiffness and potentially nervous system sensitivity.

Excessively guarded or protective movements are common when we have pain. Strategies include tensing muscles and breath holding. These strategies, if held for longer than needed, can increase nociceptive inputs and further contribute to pain. The response or *output* of muscle tension and breath holding can now become *inputs.* Commonly held beliefs can foster this too, including advice from clinicians (see Chapter 4). A good example is keeping the spine straight, with the trunk muscles engaged after an episode of back pain. While this movement strategy can be appropriate initially, it can become maladaptive (unhelpful) if the person avoids bending their spine. I encountered this with John, who had had back pain for several years before he came to see me with a recent recurrence. As I observed him move, he avoided bending his spine and was continually bracing and holding his breath. This limited his movement and seemed to increase his pain. He reported tensing his trunk muscles constantly to prevent 'going back to square one' again. He recognized much of this was psychological and protective. Moving him past this involved retraining some of his maladaptive movement and breath-holding patterns in a gradual way. As clinicians and teachers our instructions can be very helpful, but if they reinforce unhelpful beliefs about weakness and vulnerability in the body, they can contribute to maladaptive behaviors and potentially feed pain.

> Take home message: Finding balance in instructing effectively without adding to vulnerability and protective or fearful movement may promote courage and curiosity of movement, and in many cases ease discomfort.

Using Yoga to Explore Movement Patterns

While there is little research investigating using yoga in this way, for someone like John, yoga may hold benefits. Practicing asana with pratyahara (control or restraint of the senses) and dharana (concentration) may allow gentle exploration of whether movements are helpful or unhelpful. If unhelpful, this awareness can facilitate transition from protective movement patterns with excessive muscle tension to more comfortable, relaxed movement. Integrating pranayama (breath control) through asana may reinforce this and reduce associated stress responses. Moving mindfully with awareness and self-compassion also means practicing ahimsa or non-violence by removing unhelpful movement strategies. Because asana practice incorporates these elements and is a balanced and comprehensive movement system, it may provide a valuable support for rehabilitation (Figure 6.3).

Conclusion

Let's return to Phillip, and think of his scenario as a summary of what we have presented thus far. He began with a simple injury leading to inflammation and pain. Unfortunately, his immune system response became dysregulated with recurrent inflammation (among other factors). He then began moving in protective ways out of fear and sensitivity. His swollen, sore, stiff hand began to be held in a closed fist drawn up to rest on his chest: an unhelpful posture when maintained for a prolonged time, further contributing to loss of function and changes at the tissue level. As his Pain Mandala layered, outputs of protection became inputs contributing to his overall pain experience.

To begin to alter this posturing he first used a combination of breath awareness and relaxation responses (see Chapter 5) together with gentle exercises to increase his repertoire of movement. His protection tendencies turned to curiosity and he learned how to facilitate the feeling of safety, using education and breath awareness to reduce the unhelpful guarding patterns. Together, this slowly re-established freedom of movement. He explored releasing this pattern further with a controlled asana practice and then graded it into daily activities such as walking with a fluid arm swing.

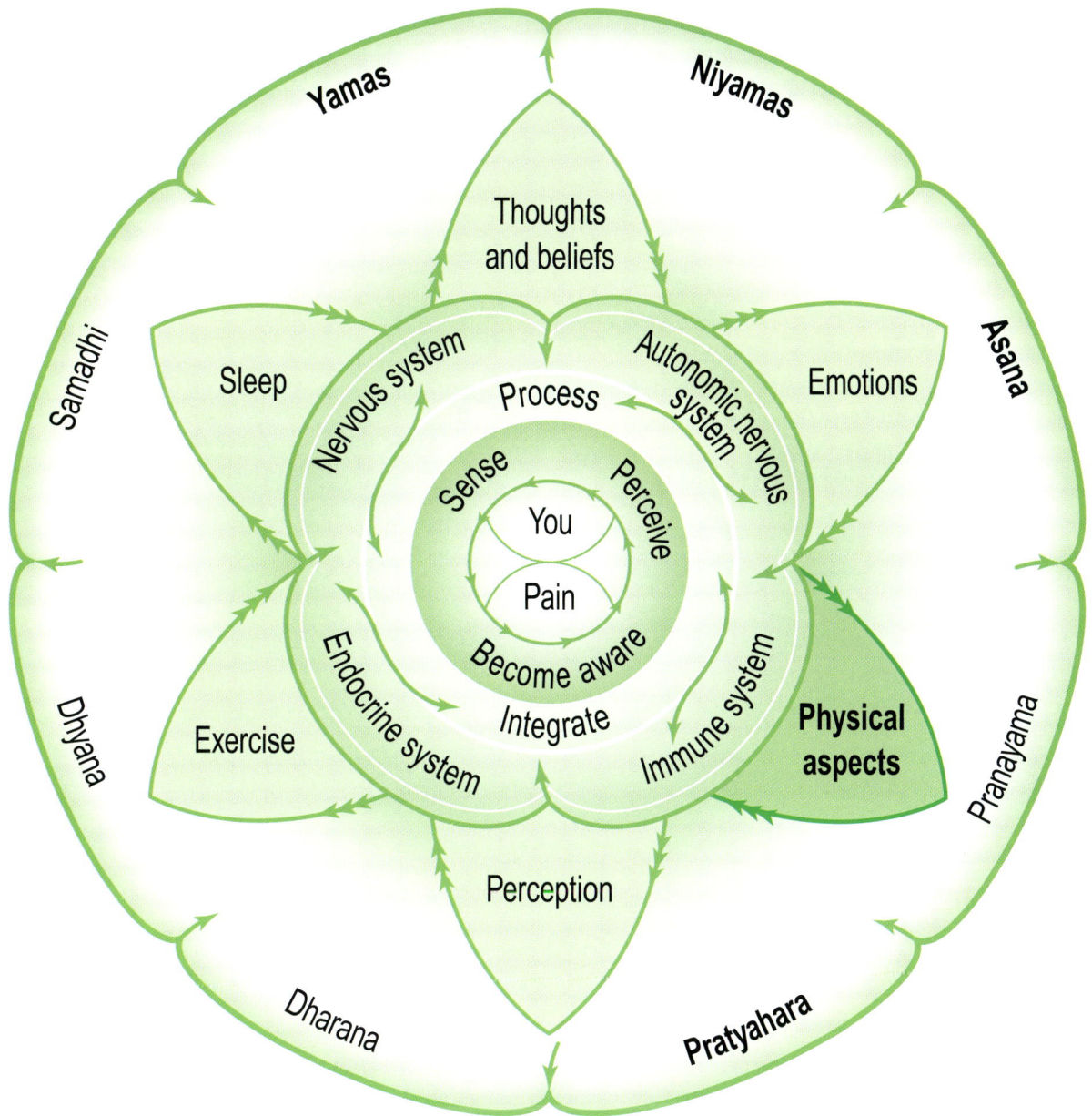

Figure 6.3

Pain and Yoga Mandala – Physical Aspects. The yoga practices of Asana (mindful movement), Pratyahara (withdrawal of the senses), Yamas–Ahimsa (non-harming), Satya (truthfulness), Niyamas–Santosha (contentment), Tapas (discipline) and Svadhyaya (self-study), combined with pain science, may offer a means to explore tissue inputs and movement patterns and to make sense of their role in the pain experience. This holds the potential for adopting helpful movement patterns, letting go of unhelpful or protective strategies and ultimately softening the sensitivity of pain.

We've covered four main themes of the physical aspects of pain: inflammatory responses and consideration of stages of healing for rehabilitation; how pathology matters but doesn't always correlate with pain; and how most of us will have some pathologies even if we don't have pain. We then considered how alignment can be relevant for some people, but that movement is so varied among individuals that 'right' or 'wrong' ways of movement are not applicable to everyone. Finally, we explored how we move in pain, whether movement is adaptive (helpful) or maladaptive (unhelpful). With these two latter points in mind, let's explore how we would put this into practice.

Out of the Head and Onto the Mat

> Transition to practice: These practice sections are not designed to be recipes for practices to give directly to a person participating in pain care. They are meant for you, the reader, to engage in experiential learning – to take the information from 'Headspace' onto your own mat and into life. As the subject, you can first explore the ideas presented, then consider how these might translate into practices for those with whom you work.

Let's explore adaptive and maladaptive movement patterns for ourselves. We've all had injuries, aches, pains, and areas that feel restricted or limited. Select four or five postures from your own practice or use Appendix 2: Asana that challenge you in ways of feeling vulnerable, restricted or uncomfortable, for any reason (physical or emotional). Generally, when discomfort is noticed, we suggest you practice gentle curiosity: moving to the point of increased tension or discomfort, pause to check in; if you feel anxious or unsafe or that you might increase soreness later, back off a little. In other words, be curious but don't bully yourself. Keep your breath soft and release resistance or straining – physical, mental or emotional.

Grab your mat, select your postures and let's practice using the following to guide this mindfulness of the body experience.

- Perform your series of postures.
  - Note your physical sensations.
  - Become aware of ingrained adjustments: alignment, bracing or guarding, etc.
  - Do these strategies cause rigidity, tension, apprehension?
  - What is your breathing pattern like?
  - Is the flow of movement or steadiness interrupted?
  - Are you aware each time that you make these adjustments or has it become automatic?
- Repeat the postures a couple of times to sense adjustments you use, then tune into your thoughts and beliefs about these postures and adjustments.
  - Do these thoughts shape your adjustments?
  - Do they reflect beliefs about tissue injury or pathology?
  - Do you have preconceived ideas about how certain movements 'should' be performed or look?
  - Are there elements of your thoughts or beliefs about your body's alignment or performance that are *real but not true*?
- Next consider whether the movement strategies you've adopted are adaptive (helpful) or maladaptive (unhelpful). Set aside any preconceived ideas you have about how the body 'should' move and allow yourself to be open to exploring variations of movement and experiencing different responses. This is important because if you have fixed beliefs that a particular movement strategy is 'bad' for you, you may still feel discomfort as

your thoughts may drive protective responses of pain or just resistance.

- Repeat the sequence of postures, taking one or two of the adjustments you made for your body and exploring them more.

- Challenge the adjustments: try to change how you move and observe your responses, physically and mentally. Move gently at first and allow your breath to be soft as you do so.

  ○ If you consciously correct your alignment, try not correcting and allowing it to flow more naturally.

  ○ If you consciously tense muscles to protect, pause and allow them time to gently let go.

  ○ If you restrict movement, try allowing yourself to move into a greater range of motion.

  ○ Are there movements or positions you have placed on the 'avoid' list? Can you explore these with gentle curiosity?

- Remember, new movements often feel vulnerable, unnatural and uncomfortable. All of these sensations are OK. This is simply an exploration to learn more about your own practice.

- Repeat this a few times and see what you experience.

  ○ Does the movement feel easier or harder?

  ○ Do you move with more or less discomfort?

  ○ When is muscle tone helpful and when does it restrict you?

  ○ What thoughts arise for you? Does this experience challenge any of your previous thoughts or beliefs?

  ○ Are there aspects of your movement that reflect beliefs that may be *real but not true*?

  ○ Try to avoid drawing hard and fast conclusions from this initial practice. It may take some time and repeated practice to explore the ideas fully.

As you explore, bear in mind that this will need time with some experimentation. Broadly, if the previous adjustment was 'maladaptive', the new movement strategy should feel more comfortable, and less painful, especially as you repeat it. It is worth training the new movement strategy and letting go of your previous adjustment.

If, however, your previous adjustment was 'adaptive', as you try to change it, the new movement may be less comfortable and more painful. At least for now, using the original movement may be helpful. You have some options here; you may want to explore this again another time, work with a clinician to see if you can identify and alter an underlying cause, or accept this adjustment as part of your current movement strategies, knowing these can change from day to day. You may find that what feels best for your body is somewhere between what you have been traditionally doing and these explorations. The goal is to find what is best for right now.

Off the Mat and Into Life
Movement Strategies in Normal Daily Life

- Do you avoid activities or movements because of conditioned responses, fear of pain, or beliefs that they are harmful? Is the concept of *real but not true* relevant here? If so, try exploring these activities gently in a similar way as the strategies identified during the asana practice. Let gentle curiosity lead your way.

- Ask yourself if your adjustments to movements in daily life are helpful or unhelpful. You may have adapted a movement strategy to cope with pain at some stage, but is it still needed now? Encourage yourself to explore whether this is still useful or it has become a limiting factor in life that no longer needs to be present.

Chapter 6

Drivers for Adaptations to Movement and Activity

We have explored this in Chapter 4; however, when in pain, it can be hard to navigate the barrage of well-meaning advice from other people that may not be so helpful. Advice can range from encouragement to take it easy to pushing through pain regardless.

- Encourage yourself and others to explore '*what's best for me?*' both on the mat and in life. Be curious and kind, finding confidence with practice.

- Acknowledge advice received as well-meaning but not always appropriate for each of us. This all might take time to balance, and it may require assistance from qualified observers to fully understand how body tissue inputs are presently contributing to limitations in activities as well as pain, and how best to move beyond them.

Bonus for Teachers

Guidance for Instructing Asanas (Movement) in an Evidence-Based Way

We teach movement based on a variety of information gained from teacher training, personal experiences, research evidence, social media, etc. The way we instruct is as important as what we instruct. We might want to consider the end goal. Is it about activating a particular muscle group, encouraging a fuller range of motion, learning a specific posture or skill, or finding comfort in our own bodies? As the science around movement, injury and pain evolves, consider whether your teaching reflects a contemporary understanding of movement. This, of course, will shift and change, depending on the goal and as knowledge grows.

The following is presented as a gentle guide based on the information presented in 'Headspace':

- Consider avoiding rigid alignment instructions that suggest a 'right' or 'wrong' way to move, as the evidence doesn't really support this. Rather, offer options.

- Encourage people to explore variations of movements to explore what feels right or comfortable for them, without the need to splint or brace.

- If providing manual adjustments, consider approaching the person and their peri-personal space gently, adjusting with softness. Take time to check how the adjustment feels for the individual. Bear in mind that what you see as 'wrong' may be an optimal or adaptive movement for that individual. Ask the individual 'What happens if I do this?' 'Does that feel OK, any better?' If not, allow them to revert to their original position.

- If working on a one-to-one basis, check responses to any suggested modifications in posture or alignment in relation to the individual's symptoms. Adjustments should feel more comfortable, not less. They should allow greater efficiency of movement or improved control of movement, not less.

- Avoid implying negative consequences of moving a certain way, e.g. 'To protect your knees, don't allow your knees to travel forwards of your ankle'; 'Keep your core engaged to avoid back pain'; 'To avoid shoulder impingement, pull your shoulder blades back.' These instructions imply that allowing your knees to travel forwards, your core to be relaxed or your shoulders to round is potentially harmful. As highlighted above, the basis for many of these instructions is not supported by research evidence and risks causing unnecessary fear or unhelpful beliefs about the body. More guidance is available in Appendix 2: Asana (Table A.1).

References

1. Woolf, C.J. and Q. Ma. Nociceptors: Noxious Stimulus Detectors. Neuron, 2007. 55(3): 353–64.

2. Choo Lee, A., W. Quillen, D. Magee, and J. Zachazweski. Injury, Inflammation, and Repair: Tissue Mechanics, the Healing Process and Their Impact on the Musculoskeletal System, in: Scientific Foundations and Principles of Practice in Musculoskeletal Rehabilitation,

D. Magee, J. Zachazweski, and W. Quillen, Editors. 2007, St Louis, MO: Saunders Elsevier. pp. 1–22.

3. Dubois, B. and J.F. Esculier. Soft-Tissue Injuries Simply Need PEACE and LOVE. British Journal of Sports Medicine, 2020. 54(2): 72-3.

4. Vuurberg, G., A. Hoorntje, L.M. Wink, et al. Diagnosis, Treatment and Prevention of Ankle Sprains: Update of an Evidence-Based Clinical Guideline. British Journal of Sports Medicine, 2018. 52(15): 956.

5. Oliveira, C.B., C.G. Maher, R.Z. Pinto, et al. Clinical Practice Guidelines for the Management of Non-Specific Low Back Pain in Primary Care: An Updated Overview. European Spine Journal, 2018. 27(11): 2791–803.

6. Blanch, P. and T.J. Gabbett. Has the Athlete Trained Enough to Return to Play Safely? The Acute:Chronic Workload Ratio Permits Clinicians to Quantify a Player's Risk of Subsequent Injury. British Journal of Sports Medicine, 2016. 50(8): 471–5.

7. Maher, C., M. Underwood, and R. Buchbinder. Non-Specific Low Back Pain. Lancet, 2017. 389(10070): 736–47.

8. Brinjikji, W., P.H. Luetmer, B. Comstock, et al. Systematic Literature Review of Imaging Features of Spinal Degeneration in Asymptomatic Populations. American Journal of Neuroradiology, 2015. 36(4): 811–16.

9. Steffens, D., M.J. Hancock, C.G. Maher, et al. Does Magnetic Resonance Imaging Predict Future Low Back Pain? A Systematic Review. European Journal of Pain, 2014. 18(6): 755–65.

10. Benson, R.T., S.P. Tavares, S.C. Robertson, et al. Conservatively Treated Massive Prolapsed Discs: A 7-Year Follow-Up. Annals of the Royal College of Surgeons England, 2010. 92(2): 147–53.

11. Zhong, M., J.T. Liu, H. Jiang, et al. Incidence of Spontaneous Resorption of Lumbar Disc Herniation: A Meta-Analysis. Pain Physician, 2017. 20(1): E45–E52.

12. Miyagi, M., T. Ishikawa, H. Kamoda, et al. ISSLS Prize Winner: Disc Dynamic Compression in Rats Produces Long-Lasting Increases in Inflammatory Mediators in Discs and Induces Long-Lasting Nerve Injury and Regeneration of the Afferent Fibers Innervating Discs: A Pathomechanism for Chronic Discogenic Low Back Pain. Spine (Phila Pa 1976), 2012. 37(21): 1810–18.

13. van den Bosch, M.H.J. Inflammation in Osteoarthritis: Is It Time to Dampen the Alarm(in) In This Debilitating Disease? Clinical and Experimental Immunology, 2018. 195(2):153–66.

14. Hanaoka, B.Y., M.P. Ithurburn, C.A. Rigsbee, et al. Chronic Inflammation in RA: Mediator of Skeletal Muscle Pathology and Physical Impairment. Arthritis Care and Research (Hoboken), 2019. 71(2): 173–7.

15. Woolf, C.J. Central Sensitization: Implications for the Diagnosis and Treatment of Pain. Pain, 2011. 15(3): S2–15.

16. Cook, J.L., E. Rio, C.R. Purdam, and S.I. Docking. Revisiting the Continuum Model of Tendon Pathology: What Is Its Merit in Clinical Practice and Research? British Journal of Sports Medicine, 2016. 50(19): 1187–91.

17. Rio, E., L. Moseley, C. Purdam, et al. The Pain of Tendinopathy: Physiological or Pathophysiological? Sports Medicine, 2014. 44(1): 9–23.

18. Barbe, M.F. and A.E. Barr. Inflammation and the Pathophysiology of Work-Related Musculoskeletal Disorders. Brain, Behaviour and Immunity, 2006. 20: 423–9.

19. Barbe, M.F., M.B. Elliott, S.M. Abdelmagid, et al. Serum and Tissue Cytokines and

Chemokines Increase with Repetitive Upper Extremity Tasks. Journal of Orthopaedic Research, 2008. 26: 1320–6.

20. Elliott, M.B., A.E. Barr, B.D. Clark, et al. High Force Reaching Task Induces Widespread Inflammation, Increased Spinal Cord Neurochemical and Neuropathic Pain. Neuroscience, 2009. 158: 922–31.

21. Elliott, M.B., A.E. Barr, B.D. Clark, et al. Performance of a Repetitive Task by Aged Rats Leads to Median Neuropathy and Spinal Cord Inflammation with Associated Sensorimotor Declines. Neuroscience, 2010. 170: 929–41.

22. Ruiz-Nunez, B., L. Pruimboom, D.A. Dijck-Brouwer, and F.A. Muskiet. Lifestyle and Nutritional Imbalances Associated with Western Diseases: Causes and Consequences of Chronic Systemic Low-Grade Inflammation in an Evolutionary Context. Journal of Nutritional Biochemistry, 2013. 24(7): 1183–201.

23. Mullington, J.M. Immune Function During Sleep and Sleep Deprivation, in: Neuroscience of Sleep, R. Stickgold and M. Walker, Editors. 2009, San Diego: Academic Press.

24. Irwin, M.R. Why Sleep Is Important for Health: A Psychoneuroimmunology Perspective. Annual Review of Psychology, 2015. 66: 143–72.

25. O'Toole, M.S., D.H. Bovbjerg, M.E. Renna, et al. Effects of Psychological Interventions on Systemic Levels of Inflammatory Biomarkers in Humans: A Systematic Review and Meta-Analysis. Brain Behavior and Immunity, 2018. 74: 68–78.

26. Rohleder, N. Stimulation of Systemic Low-Grade Inflammation by Psychosocial Stress. Psychosomatic Medicine, 2014. 76(3): 181–9.

27. Haanpää, M., N. Attal, M. Backonja, et al. NEUPSIG Guidelines on Neuropathic Pain Assessment. Pain, 2011. 152(1): 14–27.

28. Ellis, A. and D.L. Bennett. Neuroinflammation and the Generation of Neuropathic Pain. British Journal of Anaesthesia, 2013. 111(1): 26–37.

29. Woolf, C.J. Dissecting out Mechanisms Responsible for Peripheral Neuropathic Pain: Implications for Diagnosis and Therapy. Life Sciences, 2004. 74: 2605–10.

30. Chaparro, L.E., P.J. Wiffen, R.A. Moore, and I. Gilron. Combination Pharmacotherapy for the Treatment of Neuropathic Pain in Adults. Cochrane Database Systematic Reviews, 2012. 7: CD008943.

31. Basson, A., B. Olivier, R. Ellis, et al. The Effectiveness of Neural Mobilization for Neuromusculoskeletal Conditions: A Systematic Review and Meta-Analysis. Journal of Orthopaedic Sports Physical and Therapy, 2017. 47(9): 593–615.

32. Cooper, M.A., P.M. Kluding, and D.E. Wright. Emerging Relationships between Exercise, Sensory Nerves, and Neuropathic Pain. Frontiers in Neuroscience, 2016. 10: 372.

33. Eccleston, C., L. Hearn, and A.C. Williams. Psychological Therapies for the Management of Chronic Neuropathic Pain in Adults. Cochrane Database Systematic Reviews, 2015. 10: CD011259.

34. Choi, B.K., J.H. Verbeek, W.W. Tam, and J.Y. Jiang. Exercises for Prevention of Recurrences of Low-Back Pain. Cochrane Database Systematic Reviews, 2010. 1: CD006555.

35. Kay, T.M., A. Gross, C.H. Goldsmith, et al. Exercises for Mechanical Neck Disorders. Cochrane Database Systematic Reviews, 2012. 15(8): CD004250.

36. Saragiotto, B.T., C.G. Maher, T.P. Yamato, et al. Motor Control Exercise for Nonspecific Low Back Pain: A Cochrane Review. Spine (Phila Pa 1976), 2016. 41(16): 1284–95.

37. Steffens, D., C.G. Maher, L.S. Pereira, et al. Prevention of Low Back Pain: A Systematic Review and Meta-Analysis. JAMA Internal Medicine, 2016. 176(2): 199–208.

38. Fransen, M., S. McConnell, A.R. Harmer, et al. Exercise for Osteoarthritis of the Knee: A Cochrane Systematic Review. British Journal of Sports Medicine, 2015. 49(24): 1554–7.

39. Sluka, K.A., L. Frey-Law, and M. Hoeger Bement. Exercise-Induced Pain and Analgesia? Underlying Mechanisms and Clinical Translation. Pain, 2018. 159 Suppl 1: S91–S97.

40. Gleeson, M., N.C. Bishop, D.J. Stensel, et al. The Anti-Inflammatory Effects of Exercise: Mechanisms and Implications for the Prevention and Treatment of Disease. Nature Reviews Immunology, 2011. 11(9): 607–15.

41. Bricca, A., C.B. Juhl, A.J. Grodzinsky, and E.M. Roos. Impact of a Daily Exercise Dose on Knee Joint Cartilage - A Systematic Review and Meta-Analysis of Randomized Controlled Trials in Healthy Animals. Osteoarthritis Cartilage, 2017. 25(8): 1223–37.

42. Merkle, S.L., K.A. Sluka, and L.A. Frey-Law. The Interaction between Pain and Movement. Journal of Hand Therapy, 2018. pii: S0894-1130(18)30043-7.

43. Glasgow, P., N. Phillips, and C. Bleakley. Optimal Loading: Key Variables and Mechanisms. British Journal of Sports Medicine, 2015. 49(5): 278–9.

44. Cook, J.L. and C. Purdam. Is Compressive Load a Factor in the Development of Tendinopathy? British Journal of Sports Medicine, 2012. 46(3): 163–8.

45. Kibsgard, T.J. Radiostereometric Analysis of Sacroiliac Joint Movement and Outcomes of Pelvic Joint Fusion. Acta Orthopaedica Supplement, 2015. 86(359): 1–43.

46. Kibsgard, T.J., S.M. Rohrl, O. Roise, et al. Movement of the Sacroiliac Joint During the Active Straight Leg Raise Test in Patients with Long-Lasting Severe Sacroiliac Joint Pain. Clinical Biomechanics (Bristol, Avon), 2017. 47: 40–5.

47. Kibsgard, T.J., O. Roise, B. Stuge, and S.M. Rohrl. Precision and Accuracy Measurement of Radiostereometric Analysis Applied to Movement of the Sacroiliac Joint. Clinical Orthopaedics and Related Research, 2012. 470(11): 3187–94.

48. Sturesson, B., A. Uden, and A. Vleeming. A Radiostereometric Analysis of the Movements of the Sacroiliac Joints in the Reciprocal Straddle Position. Spine (Phila Pa 1976), 2000. 25(2): 214–17.

49. Palsson, T.S., W. Gibson, B. Darlow, et al. Changing the Narrative in Diagnosis and Management of Pain in the Sacroiliac Joint Area. Physical Therapy, 2019. 99(11): 1511–19.

50. Bialosky, J.E., M.D. Bishop, D.D. Price, et al. The Mechanisms of Manual Therapy in the Treatment of Musculoskeletal Pain: A Comprehensive Model. Manual Therapy, 2009. 14(5): 531–8.

51. Rabey, M., T. Hall, C. Hebron, et al. Reconceptualising Manual Therapy Skills in Contemporary Practice. Musculoskeletal Science and Practice, 2017. 29: 28–32.

52. Culvenor, A.G., B.E. Oiestad, H.F. Hart, et al. Prevalence of Knee Osteoarthritis Features on Magnetic Resonance Imaging in Asymptomatic Uninjured Adults: A Systematic Review and Meta-Analysis. British Journal of Sports Medicine, 2018. 53(20): 1268–78.

53. Hoy, D., C. Bain, G. Williams, et al. A Systematic Review of the Global Prevalence of Low Back Pain. Arthritis and Rheumatology, 2012. 64(6): 2028–37.

54. Hancock, M.J., C.M. Maher, P. Petocz, et al. Risk Factors for a Recurrence of Low Back Pain. Spine Journal, 2015. 15(11): 2360–8.

55. da Silva, T., P. Macaskill, K. Mills, et al. Predicting Recovery in Patients with Acute Low Back Pain: A Clinical Prediction Model. European Journal of Pain, 2017. 21(4): 716–26.

56. da Silva, T., K. Mills, B.T. Brown, et al. Risk of Recurrence of Low Back Pain: A Systematic Review. Journal of Orthopaedic and Sports Physical Therapy, 2017. 47(5): 305–13.

57. Minagawa, H., N. Yamamoto, H. Abe, et al. Prevalence of Symptomatic and Asymptomatic Rotator Cuff Tears in the General Population: From Mass-Screening in One Village. Journal of Orthopaedics, 2013. 10(1): 8–12.

58. Schwartzberg, R., B.L. Reuss, B.G. Burkhart, et al. High Prevalence of Superior Labral Tears Diagnosed by MRI in Middle-Aged Patients with Asymptomatic Shoulders. Orthopaedic Journal of Sports Medicine, 2016. 4(1): 2325967115623212.

59. Teunis, T., B. Lubberts, B.T. Reilly, and D. Ring. A Systematic Review and Pooled Analysis of the Prevalence of Rotator Cuff Disease with Increasing Age. Journal of Shoulder and Elbow Surgery, 2014. 23(12): 1913–21.

60. Englund, M., A. Guermazi, D. Gale, et al. Incidental Meniscal Findings on Knee MRI in Middle-Aged and Elderly Persons. New England Journal of Medicine, 2008. 359(11): 1108–15.

61. Dunn, W.R., J.E. Kuhn, R. Sanders, et al. Symptoms of Pain Do Not Correlate with Rotator Cuff Tear Severity: A Cross-Sectional Study of 393 Patients with a Symptomatic Atraumatic Full-Thickness Rotator Cuff Tear. Journal of Bone and Joint Surgery America, 2014. 96(10): 793–800.

62. Dell'Isola, A. and M. Steultjens. Classification of Patients with Knee Osteoarthritis in Clinical Phenotypes: Data from the Osteoarthritis Initiative. PLoS One, 2018. 13(1): e0191045.

63. Finan, P.H., L.F. Buenaver, S.C. Bounds, et al. Discordance between Pain and Radiographic Severity in Knee Osteoarthritis: Findings from Quantitative Sensory Testing of Central Sensitization. Arthritis and Rheumatology, 2013. 65(2): 363–72.

64. Dreischarf, M., A. Rohlmann, F. Graichen, et al. In Vivo Loads on a Vertebral Body Replacement During Different Lifting Techniques. Journal of Biomechanics, 2016. 49(6): 890–5.

65. Verbeek, J.H., K.P. Martimo, P.P. Kuijer, et al. Proper Manual Handling Techniques to Prevent Low Back Pain, a Cochrane Systematic Review. Work, 2012. 41 Suppl 1: 2299–301.

66. Wrigley, A.T., W.J. Albert, K.J. Deluzio, and J.M. Stevenson. Differentiating Lifting Technique between Those Who Develop Low Back Pain and Those Who Do Not. Clinical Biomechanics (Bristol, Avon), 2005. 20(3): 254–63.

67. Richards, K.V., D.J. Beales, A.J. Smith, et al. Neck Posture Clusters and Their Association with Biopsychosocial Factors and Neck Pain in Australian Adolescents. Physical Therapy, 2016. 96(10): 1576–87.

68. Neal, B.S., C.J. Barton, R. Gallie, et al. Runners with Patellofemoral Pain Have Altered Biomechanics Which Targeted Interventions Can Modify: A Systematic Review and Meta-Analysis. Gait Posture, 2016. 45: 69–82.

69. Neal, B.S., I.B. Griffiths, G.J. Dowling, et al. Foot Posture as a Risk Factor for Lower Limb Overuse Injury: A Systematic Review and Meta-Analysis. Journal of Foot and Ankle Research, 2014. 7(1): 55.

70. Neal, B.S., S.D. Lack, N.E. Lankhorst, et al. Risk Factors for Patellofemoral Pain: A Systematic Review and Meta-Analysis. British Journal of Sports Medicine, 2019. 53: 270–81.

71. Pappas, E. and W.M. Wong-Tom. Prospective Predictors of Patellofemoral Pain Syndrome: A Systematic Review with Meta-Analysis. Sports Health, 2012. 4(2): 115–20.

72. Sterud, T. and T. Tynes. Work-Related Psycho-social and Mechanical Risk Factors for Low Back Pain: A 3-Year Follow-up Study of the General Working Population in Norway. Occupational and Environmental Medicine, 2013. 70(5): 296–302.

73. Haukka, E., A. Ojajarvi, L. Kaila-Kangas, and P. Leino-Arjas. Protective Determinants of Sickness Absence among Employees with Multisite Pain-A 7-Year Follow-Up. Pain, 2017. 158(2): 220–9.

74. Laird, R.A., J. Gilbert, P. Kent, and J.L. Keating. Comparing Lumbo-Pelvic Kinematics in People With and Without Back Pain: A Systematic Review and Meta-Analysis. BMC Musculoskeletal Disorders, 2014. 15: 229.

75. Roussouly, P., S. Gollogly, E. Berthonnaud, and J. Dimnet. Classification of the Normal Variation in the Sagittal Alignment of the Human Lumbar Spine and Pelvis in the Standing Position. Spine (Phila Pa 1976), 2005. 30(3): 346–53.

76. Klein, S.D., C. Bayard, and U. Wolf. The Alexander Technique and Musicians: A Systematic Review of Controlled Trials. BMC Complementary and Alternative Medicine, 2014. 14: 414.

77. Saragiotto, B.T., C.G. Maher, T.P. Yamato, et al. Motor Control Exercise for Chronic Non-Specific Low-Back Pain. Cochrane Database Systematic Reviews, 2016. 1: CD012004.

78. Tsang, S.M., G.P. Szeto, and R.Y. Lee. Relationship between Neck Acceleration and Muscle Activation in People with Chronic Neck Pain: Implications for Functional Disability. Clinical Biomechanics (Bristol, Avon), 2016. 35: 27–36.

79. Heneghan, N.R., R. Smith, I. Tyros, et al. Thoracic Dysfunction in Whiplash Associated Disorders: A Systematic Review. PLoS One, 2018. 13(3): e0194235.

80. Falla, D., L. Gizzi, H. Parsa, et al. People with Chronic Neck Pain Walk with a Stiffer Spine. Journal of Orthopaedic and Sports Physical Therapy, 2017. 47(4): 268–77.

81. Buldt, A.K., G.S. Murley, P. Butterworth, et al. The Relationship between Foot Posture and Lower Limb Kinematics During Walking: A Systematic Review. Gait Posture, 2013. 38(3): 363–72.

82. Dowling, G.J., G.S. Murley, S.E. Munteanu, et al. Dynamic Foot Function as a Risk Factor for Lower Limb Overuse Injury: A Systematic Review. Journal of Foot and Ankle Research, 2014. 7(1): 53.

83. von Rosen, P., A. Frohm, A. Kottorp, et al. Too Little Sleep and an Unhealthy Diet Could Increase the Risk of Sustaining a New Injury in Adolescent Elite Athletes. Scandinavian Journal of Medicine and Science in Sports, 2017. 27(11): 1364–71.

84. von Rosen, P., A. Frohm, A. Kottorp, et al. Multiple Factors Explain Injury Risk in Adolescent Elite Athletes: Applying a Biopsychosocial Perspective. Scandinavian Journal of Medicine and Science in Sports, 2017. 27(12): 2059–69.

85. Ivarsson, A. and U. Johnson. Psychological Factors as Predictors of Injuries among Senior Soccer Players. A Prospective Study. Journal of Sports Science Medicine, 2010. 9(2): 347–52.

86. Lorenzetti, S., T. Gulay, M. Stoop, et al. Comparison of the Angles and Corresponding Moments in the Knee and Hip During Restricted and Unrestricted Squats. Journal of Strength and Conditioning Research, 2012. 26(10): 2829–36.

87. List, R., T. Gulay, M. Stoop, and S. Lorenzetti. Kinematics of the Trunk and the Lower Extremities During Restricted and Unrestricted Squats. Journal of Strength and Conditioning Research, 2013. 27(6): 1529–38.

88. Hodges, P.W. and C.A. Richardson. Inefficient Muscular Stabilization of the Lumbar Spine Associated with Low Back Pain. A Motor Control Evaluation of Transversus Abdominis. Spine (Phila Pa 1976), 1996. 21(22): 2640–50.

89. Hodges, P.W. and C.A. Richardson. Delayed Postural Contraction of Transversus Abdominis in Low Back Pain Associated with Movement of the Lower Limb. Journal of Spinal Disorders, 1998. 11(1): 46–56.

90. Hodges, P.W. and C.A. Richardson. Altered Trunk Muscle Recruitment in People with Low Back Pain with Upper Limb Movement at Different Speeds. Archives of Physical Medicine and Rehabilitation, 1999. 80(9): 1005–12.

91. Kalichman, L., E. Carmeli, and E. Been. The Association between Imaging Parameters of the Paraspinal Muscles, Spinal Degeneration, and Low Back Pain. BioMed Research International, 2017. 2017: 2562957.

92. Owers, D.S., D.M. Perriman, P.N. Smith, et al. Evidence for Cervical Muscle Morphometric Changes on Magnetic Resonance Images after Whiplash: A Systematic Review and Meta-Analysis. Injury, 2018. 49(2): 165–76.

93. Wan, Q., C. Lin, X. Li, et al. MRI Assessment of Paraspinal Muscles in Patients with Acute and Chronic Unilateral Low Back Pain. British Journal of Radiology, 2015. 88(1053): 20140546.

94. Dankaerts, W., P. O'Sullivan, A. Burnett, et al. Discriminating Healthy Controls and Two Clinical Subgroups of Nonspecific Chronic Low Back Pain Patients Using Trunk Muscle Activation and Lumbosacral Kinematics of Postures and Movements: A Statistical Classification Model. Spine (Phila Pa 1976), 2009. 34(15): 1610–18.

95. Hodges, P., W. van den Hoorn, A. Dawson, and J. Cholewicki. Changes in the Mechanical Properties of the Trunk in Low Back Pain May Be Associated with Recurrence. Journal of Biomechanics, 2009. 42(1): 61–6.

96. van Dieen, J.H., L.P. Selen, and J. Cholewicki. Trunk Muscle Activation in Low-Back Pain Patients, an Analysis of the Literature. Journal of Electromyography and Kinesiology, 2003. 13(4): 333–51.

97. O'Sullivan, P. Diagnosis and Classification of Chronic Low Back Pain Disorders: Maladaptive Movement and Motor Control Impairments as Underlying Mechanism. Manual Therapy, 2005. 10(4): 242–55.

Between stimulus and response there is a space. In that space is our power to choose our response. In our response lies our growth and our freedom.

Viktor Frankl

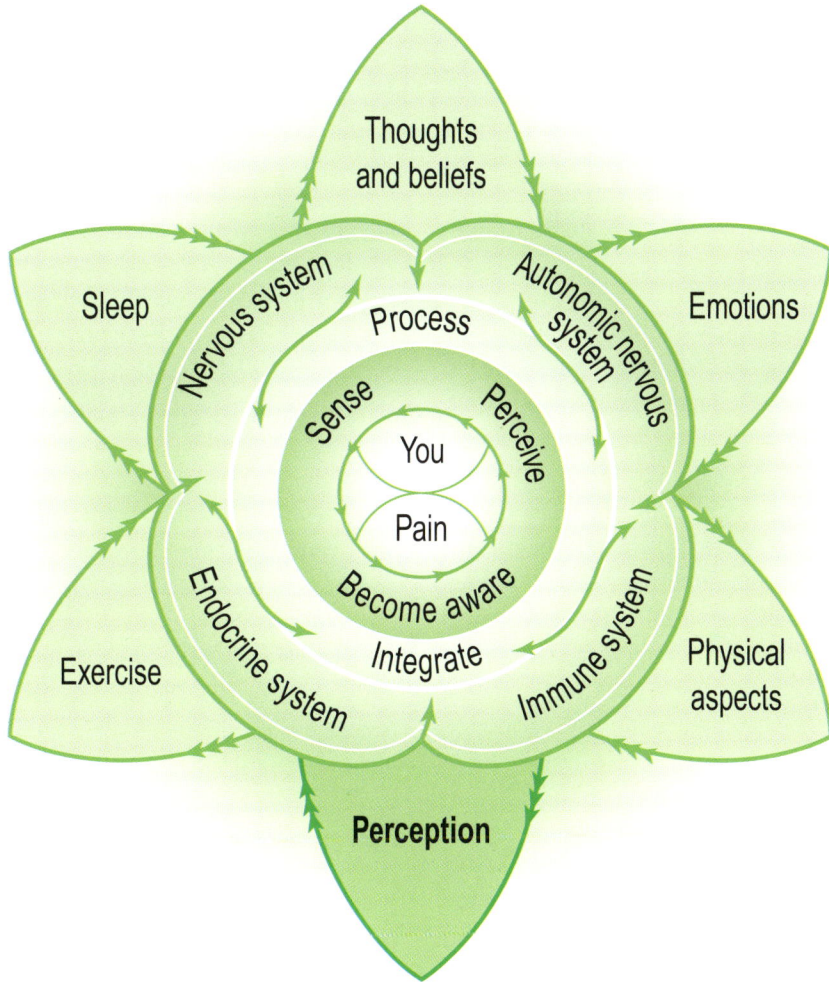

Figure 7.1
Pain Mandala – Perception. The perception of our body is an integration of inputs and awareness. The way we sense, process and integrate our physical body with our emotions, cognitions and environment feeds a dynamic loop that can increase or decrease our pain experience.
Note: This mandala depicts aspects of the human experience of pain covered in Pain Science Yoga Life. Other inputs, dimensions and body systems can contribute to pain than those noted here.

Headspace
Becoming Aware

Perception is our ability to see, hear and become aware of something through the senses. It is the way in which something is regarded or understood. Perception is also our intuitive understanding and insight. In this chapter we explore how we become aware, understand and use our senses to define our self. We focus on the physical self/body, acknowledging that the physical, psychological and emotional are integrated and cannot be separated.

How do we come to know our physical body? This is a complex question, but broadly, our physical form becomes known to us through various 'inputs' from both internal and external environments. This collection of information is processed by the brain, resulting in our own body perception and the space around us – our peri-personal space.[1] Just like the perception of all our experiences, our body perception is unique and ever-changing. Acknowledging this uniqueness and pliability is important to pain care. Pain, especially persistent pain, can impact the perception of our body,[2–6] and intriguingly, our body perception may impact the pain we experience.[3,7] However, these relationships vary across painful conditions.[2–4]

We all have dynamic representational maps* of our bodies stored in areas of our brains. These cortical maps communicate with each other and with other brain areas to form neural networks. These networks are known as neuromatrices, the brain 'orchestra' (introduced in Chapter 1). Neuromatrices are visualized using fMRI, through which we can see trends in activity in brain areas such as shifting of body maps and even how the areas interact with each other during certain experi-

---

*Use of the term 'map' to describe the awareness of the body or the perception of the body in the individual brain areas is a topic of debate currently but we use it here for ease of understanding.

ences, like pain. As we explore how we feel the physical self, we will look at these brain maps and neuromatrices with regard to the development of physical perception (body neuromatrix), including pain (pain neuromatrix). Arguably, the body neuromatrix represents an experience of our body that exists with and without pain.

Have you ever heard someone say that their knee is 'so swollen', but it appears normal? Have you worked with someone who reports stiffness of one side and yet has equal range of movement on both sides? Maybe you have heard complaints that one side or limb feels foreign? It could be easy to conclude that these individuals are exaggerating symptoms. They may have been given the impression by others that they are crazy or lying. The more likely truth is these sensations are very real.[8,9] To understand how this altered perception occurs, we need to understand how we 'feel' the body and how plastic body representations are – ever-changing. No doubt, if you've practiced yoga asanas, you've experienced moving through multiple postures directed at the right leg. Prior to doing the left side you paused in savasana. While lying flat, did you notice how the right leg felt different, like it occupied space differently than the left? Maybe it felt longer, flatter or fuller? Did the right leg really change shape, or did you just change the right leg's cortical representation – its map in areas of the brain?

Let's review a few pain specifics covered previously that might prove helpful as we increase our understanding of our body perception, and then body perception and pain. Remember we have different types of peripheral nerves (see Chapter 1) sending information to the brain. Some of these are directly involved in sensing touch, body position and movement, which we'll explain shortly. Nerves involved in nociception (warning signals) also participate in perception of other sensations (temperature, chemical and pressure changes).[10] In other words, they are polymodal[11]: they send messages warning of potential threat as well as inputs regarding other body states. These messages travel from our tissues up through the spinal cord to the brain. Signals can be turned up or down en route. But remember, the output of pain is a complex process that extends beyond the inputs detected by the peripheral nervous system.

Looking again at the neuromatrix of pain schematic (see Figure 1.9), like pain, the body-self or one's conscious awareness of the self, is influenced by the integration of inputs and unconscious activities in brain areas, producing 'the body-self neuromatrix'. The idea of the 'orchestra' in the brain is used to illustrate how development of this awareness of self arises from peripheral inputs and processing across multiple brain areas.[11–16] Contributing players in this orchestra include peripheral sensory inputs but also thoughts, beliefs, emotions, the environment and memories. All of these factors, peripheral and central, influence our sense of self, and ultimately our body's responses. This integration is also illustrated within the Pain Mandala (Figure 7.1).

Body Perception Beyond Body Inputs

As it is defined, perception is not simply about a realization of sensory inputs; it also encompasses our perspective and intuition. Can we take this idea of sensory inputs combining with intuition a step further? Conceptually, perception could be described as integrating sensory inputs with a pre-existing 'template' in the brain. This is similar to the idea of processing and scrutinizing inputs as we have seen in other chapters, and as illustrated in the Pain Mandala. This 'template' may carry expectations of a predicted pattern based on information previously learned or established – an established neuromatrix. This integration may lean our perceptions towards those of our expectations and filter out information that is incongruent with our 'template'.[17] In other words, our past and current mindsets, judgments, awareness, beliefs, etc. may influence our perception and thus our experiences.

As a teaser, can we think about our perceptions, body or otherwise, in terms of yoga and self-regulation?

Can you build a bridge between this idea of a template or scrutiny and the practice of santosha (contentment)? Let's consider first if you are well practiced in this act of choosing contentment and learning to include (*and this too*) instead of problem-seeking. This then starts to set a foundation for your 'template' and potentially your perception. Wouldn't that be great? But what about the other side of the coin? What if, instead, the template trends toward problem-seeking, sensitivity to threat and hypervigilance? How would the result of the scrutiny change the output of perception? See if you can hold on to those two scenarios as we progress forward into the science of pain and perception.

Studies have begun exploring how perception influences pain and how pain influences perception.[3–7,17–23] For example, expectations can influence sensory cortex activation, and other regions utilized in processing sensory inputs.[17,24] Even the expectation of location of pain can alter the amount of descending modulation of nociception.[25] Biased thinking may then directly influence one's perception and physical experience of pain.[6,17] Therefore, body perception should be described from multiple aspects – inclusive of sensory inputs and identifiable neural and cortical processing (maps and neuromatrices), but also inclusive of interactions with our experiences, expectations and outlook. In other words, we can't neglect the unique aspects that make us individual: potentially, the combination of these interactions creates our unique perception – body and experience. Each person in persistent pain is on a distinctive journey of their own perception. With understanding and observation, we may help those in pain to explore the root of sensations and potentially shift perception and, in turn, pain experiences.

Body Perception: Peripheral Inputs

The sense of one's physical self comprises three interrelated physiological systems: 1) proprioception and kinesthetic awareness; 2) exteroceptive senses; and 3) interoception.[26]

1. Proprioception and Kinesthetic Awareness

Proprioception is our position sense: knowing where our body is in relation to our environment based on the sensations generated by its own actions.[27] Proprioceptive inputs include trunk and limb sense of: 1) position and movement; 2) effort; 3) force; and 4) balance.[26-29] This information is communicated to the brain via particular afferent nerve fibers (called Aα fibers), linked to receptors known as proprioceptors. Proprioceptors are located in skin, muscle and joints.[27]

Kinesthetic awareness is awareness of both position and movement: what the body is doing. This awareness arises from sensory inputs plus conscious and unconscious processes. Conscious recognition of motion results from inputs from proprioceptors and other mechanoreceptors (located in muscle and joints) as well as visual and vestibular information.[26] Most of us can relate to the experience of standing on a stationary train and watching another go past: there is a split second where you may think your train is moving. The correction of awareness that confirms you are not the one moving is an example of kinesthetic awareness. Proprioception and kinesthetic awareness come together to help create a perception of how our body moves in our environment.

2. Exteroceptive Senses

Exteroceptive senses pertain to all sensory inputs from outside the body including tactile (e.g. touch, textures on the skin), visual, auditory, olfactory (smell) and gustatory (taste) inputs. The primary role of these environmental inputs is to help define the physical boundaries of the body with respect to its external environment. In other words, exteroceptive senses help us define how the external environment interacts with our physical body or how we start to define our personal space. Therefore, disrupted exteroceptive senses may compromise the way we perceive our physical self.[26]

3. Interoception

We now know where the limbs and trunk are and what they are doing, but what about the internal organs or input from the viscera? *Interoception* is the body–brain axis of sensation concerning the state of the internal body.[30] Similar to proprioception, there are receptors in our viscera that transmit messages from the periphery into the central nervous system (CNS). This is a little difficult to assess but one common measure used to represent this is heart rate awareness.[30,31]

Like all sensory experiences, interoception, proprioception and kinesthesia do not stop with inputs; the perception of sensations involves processing in the CNS. So, what happens with this information once it hits the brain, and how does this begin to create perception of the 'body-self'?

From Body Perception to Ownership

Sensory Inputs: Integration in the Brain

"If you close your eyes and take your right index finger to touch your left one, how do you know where that finger is and that it is your own?", my friend Steve asked his nine-year-old. "Because I have a brain," she quickly replied with a tone of 'duh!' in her voice. She is totally right.

A fundamental aspect of self-awareness is the acknowledgment of body ownership: the ability to know our body belongs to us and other bodies do not.[29] *Body ownership* is the discernment of our physical body, making our sensations unique.[32] But how does our brain develop this perception, and if it is compared to a pre-existing template, is it always accurate?

Enter the rubber hand illusion (Figure 7.2). The rubber hand illusion provides a controlled manipulation of body ownership and can be used to help answer such questions as: how do we identify our body as our own? The illusion works like this: a participant sits with their hands resting on a table in front of

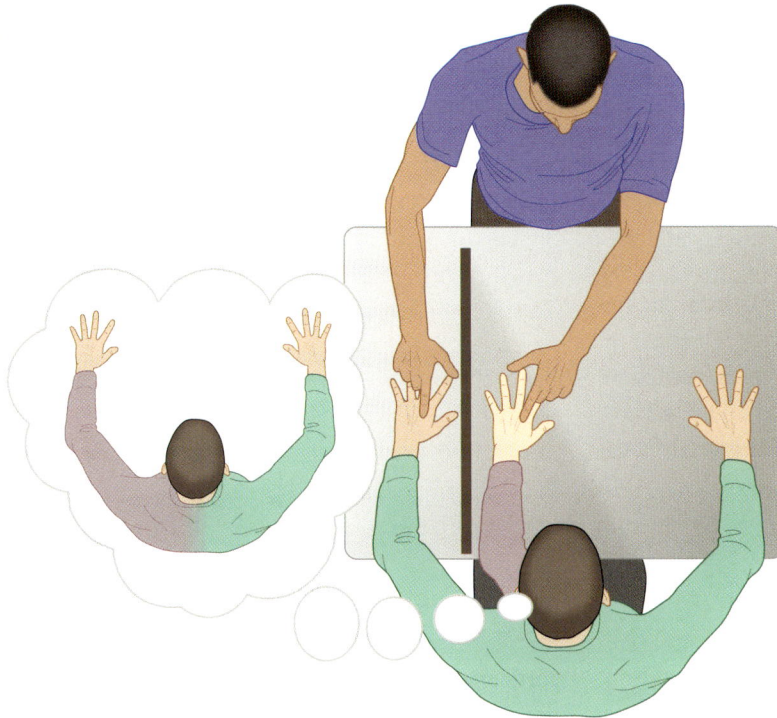

Figure 7.2
Rubber hand illusion. Subjects begin to identify a rubber hand as their own when a rubber hand is placed (in this example) where the left hand would normally be and stroked, while the actual left hand remains out of view.

them. One hand (e.g. the left as shown in Figure 7.2) is draped or blocked from view and a rubber hand is placed on the table to appear as if it is the participant's left hand. The actual hand (out of view) and the rubber hand (in view) are stroked simultaneously. Within minutes the participant begins to feel as if the rubber hand belongs to them: they develop 'ownership' or embodiment of a fake hand.[28,29,33] The rubber hand illusion demonstrates we can manipulate the *sense* of our limbs, without changing the actual limb.

> Take home message: Body perception is not a fixed entity, nor is it based strictly on peripheral sensory inputs.

Through illusions like the rubber hand, it has been shown that the brain develops a map of the body by gathering sensory information from the body and environment[28,29] and integrating this with the brain's 'template', as described earlier. This facilitates a rational representation of bodily experiences.[28] In effect, peripheral inputs are filtered through our previously developed body maps as well as our thoughts and beliefs regarding shape, position, function and integration of the body with the external environment. Potentially, the goal of this filtering is to produce an experience that provides meaning for us. Cognitive processes that change the awareness of the physical self may in turn change physiological regulation.[34] That is, the way we think impacts our physical perception and in turn our bodily responses.

Let's look at the multiple areas of the brain involved in processing afferent or incoming sensory information: the maps.

Body Perception and Mapping in the Brain

The brain areas involved in producing body awareness have been explored using fMRI. This knowledge, combined with experiments like the rubber hand illusion, highlight the brain areas most likely involved in the development of body awareness via 'map' production and communication between areas in the brain. It has been suggested that these maps and the communication between areas are available to us consciously, as well as stored in our memories,[27,35,36] which may influence our body awareness without our conscious realization. These maps and interactions continuously update based on incoming information (inputs), like a time-lapse image, with representation of each individual neuron shifting in organization over days and maybe even hours.[37] Let's look specifically at important brain areas and their roles in body perception.

Primary Brain Areas Involved in Perception

Thalamus

The thalamus acts a bit like a reception desk for the communication of multisensory information including various peripheral inputs, like nociception. Activity within the thalamus may play a role in direct integration of multisensory information, as well as in relaying it to higher brain areas that

contribute to resulting experiences and behavioral responses.[38,39]

Primary and Secondary Sensory Cortices (SI/SII)

The internal and external body surfaces are spatially mapped within SI/SII,[40] known as the sensory homunculus (from the Latin translation of 'little man'; Figure 7.3). The homunculus maintains a 'plastic' representation of the body, anatomical and positional, available for comparison to sensory inputs. These sensory inputs lead to updates of the map and/ or confirmation of the stimulation, based on the information previously stored.[28] An example here is the ability to deduce the sensation of a wool sweater versus a silk shirt on the skin.

Primary Motor and Premotor Cortices

Motor inputs are organized functionally in the motor cortices and, similar to SI/SII, a motor homunculus is described. This 'little man' represents the information used to organize inputs such as proprioception and kinesthetic awareness, and potentially guide motor response outputs.[40,41]

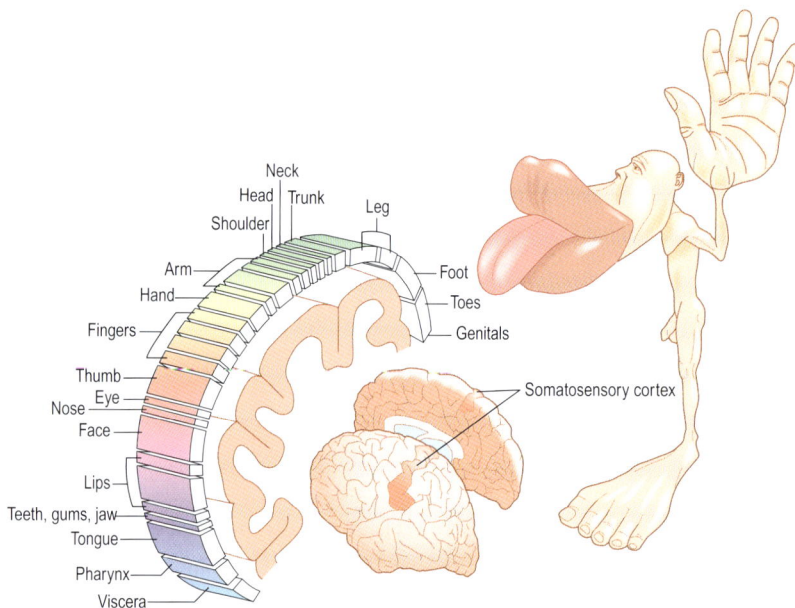

Figure 7.3
The homunculus or 'little man' is a dynamic representational 'map' of the body in the somatosensory cortices I and II, and the motor cortex.

Neck
Head | Trunk
Shoulder | Leg
Arm — — Foot
Hand — — Toes
Fingers — — Genitals
Thumb
Eye
Nose — — Somatosensory cortex
Face
Lips
Teeth, gums, jaw
Tongue
Pharynx
Viscera

Insula and Anterior Cingulate Cortex (ACC)

The insula is important for interoceptive awareness and acting as an interface between feelings, cognitions and action.[42] It is considered to be responsible for integrating both inputs that are similar and multisensory information[43,44] to help create meaning.[45] It appears the insula also connects with the brain stem, thus influencing autonomic regulation, e.g. stress responses.[1,28,43,46] Ultimately, the insula, due to its ability to integrate sensory inputs with emotions, is thought to be a primary player in the subjective experience of body ownership[28] and conscious perception.[27,47] The ACC, along with the insula, participates in processing interoceptive inputs.[26] Its role in learning, memory and emotion may also influence body perception.

Parietal Cortex

The parietal cortex is responsible for processing and integration of spatial information,[1,28] and potentially responsible for guiding initial physical responses based on this information.[27,47]

Hopefully, an understanding is developing that our sense of the physical self is ingrained (stored) and impressionable (plastic). It's not necessary to memorize the name or role of each brain area. You could, however, note that our body awareness is ever-changing, based on constant gathering, filtering and storing of information. The information comes from multiple inputs, travels through various brain areas and is correlated with the 'template' of past experiences, thoughts and beliefs. All of this occurs to produce the most meaningful representation of the individual to help determine who we physically are and how our bodies relate to the space around us.

Body Perception and Body Neuromatrix

Imagine that all of these brain regions are tags on a map: each tag is a map on its own, and lines drawn between them create a route. This becomes the neuromatrix of pain in the brain. It has been proposed that the maps come together as a dynamic entity to form a body neuromatrix.[28,40]

Does this idea of a dynamic representation of the body in the brain – a body neuromatrix – that is influenced by multiple internal and external inputs help change the understanding of what has shifted in that limb? The immediate changes in the limb itself (flexibility, strength, etc.) may be minuscule, but the changes in the brain are enough to cause a shift in perception of the physical and spatial aspects of the limb. If we look back at the example of lying in savasana after several postures focusing on the right lower limb, the right leg often feels fuller, longer and more spacious.

Physical perception is not limited to our body but extends to our peri-personal space: the space we occupy.[1] Maybe it is helpful to think about connecting this body neuromatrix with the idea of a comfort zone. Let's say you have a recent, painful injury to your right shoulder. Can you imagine your physical and emotional protective responses if someone were to suddenly reach toward that shoulder? The awareness or even assumption of an object coming anywhere near the 'space' that the shoulder occupies creates a scenario of protecting the space, not just the shoulder.

Perception and the Pain Mandala

So, if body perception goes beyond the physical and reaches toward the space the body occupies, what else is involved? Do other factors, such as what the body 'means' to us, and safety or survival, also play a role? If the maps or body neuromatrix as a whole alter due to the interpretation of what a body part means to us, that body area may be more sensitive or reactive to inputs, especially if those inputs carry a message of potential threat. Let's revisit the Pain Mandala to illustrate (see Figure 7.1). If we think of our perception as integration of internal and external inputs to create a meaningful picture of our body, and we know pain is our innate system for physical protection, then can we see that it is the synthesis of these dynamic entities (inputs, maps, emotions, cognitions, memories, beliefs, etc.) that helps us to sense, perceive and become aware of possible threat, and therefore activate the need to protect and ultimately experience pain? Let's explore the neuromatrix of pain more specifically.

Pain Neuromatrix

Hopefully, it is already clear that no one single region of the brain triggers the pain response but rather an entire neuromatrix of activity[48,49] (see Figure 4.4). It is interesting to note the common brain areas involved in both pain processing and body perception. The pain neuromatrix involves the sensory brain areas, including SI and SII, as well as cognitive–affective regions (insula and ACC).[17,48] This widespread involvement confirms that the pain neuromatrix cannot be considered solely nociception-specific, and thus the experience of pain is produced through both multisensory input and cognitive and emotional processing of that input.[17,48,50,51] This is the 'orchestra' at play. The individuality of these experiences means that for each of us, the activity in the individual brain areas will be subtly different. We all have our own body tune and our own pain tune, and the tune varies a little for each of our pain experiences.

Brain Centers Reorganize with Pain and Persistence

As pain persists the neuromatrix can change. If we continue this orchestra metaphor, the way in which the individual players are being directed will change the pain neuromatrix, and more players may join the orchestra. As highlighted in previous chapters, greater activity in brain areas responsible for emotional and cognitive processing is increasingly evident with persistent pain.[11,17,52]

When pain persists, the body neuromatrix also changes: the actual representation of the body and the space it occupies may shift at the level of the brain.[11,20,21,40,53] The sensory and motor cortices, ACC and insula all demonstrate substantial reorganization in persistent neuropathic and musculoskeletal pain.[40,54] In some specific conditions, such as fibromyalgia, persistent low back pain, phantom limb pain and neuropathic pain, the degree of reorganization has been shown to correlate directly with aspects of pain, such as intensity and duration.[3,6,40,55,56] However, this relationship is not consistent across conditions, e.g. knee osteoarthritis and complex regional pain syndrome show more variable correlations.[2,22,57–60]

Therefore, the evidence that body neuromatrix reorganization leads to pain or pain sensitivity remains uncertain.[19,20,61,62] Nonetheless, the trend seems to indicate that changes in the brain occur with pain, and people with pain demonstrate sensory and motor deficits. So, perhaps the most we can say currently is that persistence of pain may drive reorganization, and that reorganization may in turn drive persistence, for some people.[21,40,56]

The Brain: Finely Tuned, Well Practiced, Sensitive

Have you ever practiced a scale on a musical instrument or repeated a physical task to the point that you can feel it has become ingrained? Suddenly, you can hear that scale within the complexity of an entire song without any intention of listening for it. Or you can close your eyes and imagine your body performing a physical task to the point where you can feel the movement. For example, I used to be a competitive gymnast, and to this day, I can close my eyes and imagine my bar routine. I don't just see it, but I feel it and sense it in my body, down to the skin ripping from the palms of my hands, blur of the gym lights and smell of chalk. It's all there. This finely trained system is not completely different to what can occur when pain persists. Once we have experienced pain, our nervous system can learn to be more sensitive or protective even without the presence of nociception.[63,64]

Sensitization, introduced in Chapter 1, is the increase in neuronal excitability, which we described in the context of enhancing nociceptive signaling. Sensitization of central neurons within the neuromatrix means that individual neurons are more easily activated and thus the entire matrix is as well.[37,65,66] It doesn't take much to re-ignite my gym experience – the smell of a gym or chalk is enough to do it. Similarly, for pain, a sensitized neuromatrix can mean that pain and other symptoms may be elicited by various triggers.

As some brain areas of the pain neuromatrix become more sensitized and easily activated, others will be forced to the back of the orchestra pit. Some of the areas forced to the back of the orchestra relate to inhibition of brain activity. Normally, something called cortical inhibition controls brain activity and prevents over-facilitation of brain areas. The loss of this ('disinhibition') contributes to sensitization, but it also results in a loss of precision which can disrupt movement commands, sensory discrimination, and perception of the body part.[37] Together, sensitization and disinhibition change the configuration and response of neurons whose duties include body representation.[40]

What does this brain reorganization and sensitization mean for pain? Remember the fascinating things learned about body perception using the rubber hand illusion? Similarly, mental imagery, mirrors and illusions have been used to demonstrate these cortical adaptations in pain experiences. It has been reported that imagined movements[67,68] and tactile stimulation of the mirrored image[69] can elicit pain and swelling of affected or even missing limbs: without any physical input, just imagining a movement (mental imagery), or seeing a mirror image of a painful limb being stroked (but not the limb itself) can cause a person to experience pain and swelling. Many examples of such sensitization come from studies on phantom limb pain and complex regional pain syndrome (CRPS) (see Moseley & Flor[40] for review).

Stories of *'Real but Not True'*

As you read through the following, can you see how these research stories play into the idea of *real but not true*?

- Perception of body position influences tissue changes: CRPS typically involves changes in skin temperature and color. In one experiment, Moseley and team asked ten people with CRPS to cross their arms so that the affected side was placed in the space of the unaffected and vice versa. What the observers saw gave them pause: the skin temperature and color of the involved hand began to demonstrate changes that brought it closer to normal. And, incredibly, the uninvolved, previously healthy, hand began to take on the CRPS presentation. This led researchers to conclude that the body neuromatrix, inclusive of the peri-personal space, is important in influencing tissue changes.[70]

- Perception of the size of the limb can cause a shift in physiological responses: Individuals with CRPS were asked to look at their hands using binoculars both in a magnified and a minimized appearance. Swelling and pain evoked by movement of the affected limb was more severe when participants' views were magnified. Decreased swelling and pain occurred when the hand appeared smaller.[71]

- Pain perception influences motor control and vice versa: In a small sample of individuals with recurrent low back pain, impaired activation of abdominal muscles was demonstrated along with concurrent changes to the map of the trunk in the motor cortex.[55]

- Decreased tactile acuity and disrupted body perception can correlate with the location of pain: In a study of people with low back pain, participants were asked to draw their own back, not as they thought it would look but as they actually felt it. Five of six participants were unable to fully delineate the outline of the trunk, and those with unilateral back pain shifted the vertebrae toward the side of pain.[34]

- The perception of amount of movement can alter pain: Individuals with chronic neck pain were given virtual reality goggles and asked to perform a simple task of head turning. The goggles allowed the perception of movement to be manipulated, e.g. exaggerating or shrinking the actual movement. Individuals were directed to indicate at what degree of movement they experienced pain in three scenarios: 1) without visual manipulation; 2) manipulating the visual input to make the movement appear greater than actually performed; and 3) manipulating the visual input to make the movement appear less than actually performed. This allowed the point of pain to be assessed based on the *perception* of movement rather than actual movement. When the perception of motion was less than actually performed, pain was reported later in the range of motion and vice versa. This suggests the perception of movement based on visual inputs, and not solely inputs from neck tissues, influenced pain.[72]

Think about Phillip (Case Study, p.51): he reported his hand no longer felt like it belonged to him, and how, as the pain progressed, it began to feel as if pain was spreading up the arm, into the side of the face and even drifting into his trunk. Could these reports indicate a shift in body perception rather than further injury, or worsening peripheral pathology? Could the above understanding of brain changes help to create recognition of the potential changes in his body perception and pain experience, but soften the need to chase a specific cause of the drifting reports of pain?

If we recognize that these multimodal perceptual changes are potentially part of pain's persistence, then it seems reasonable to incorporate interventions in retraining body perception. Early investigation into using illusions and body perception correction to treat pain emerged from the hypothesis that incongruent inputs may be a driver of persistent pain.[17] Perceptual 'inputs' that fall outside of our brain's 'template', as we discussed earlier, may ignite a risk assessment and need to protect outcome, increasing the possibility of pain.

Perception Interventions

Can the brain be retrained? Or, indeed, can perception be retrained? Adjusting cognitive and emotional perceptions combined with movement and changing behaviors can positively influence pain (discussed in Chapters 4 and 5). These are important aspects of adjusting perception. But what about treatments specifically targeting our body perception – treatments that target the integration of sensory inputs and the body neuromatrix? This is an area where much more research is needed, especially larger randomized controlled trials, but early evidence suggests significant and clinically meaningful effects on pain and function are possible, at least in some pain conditions.[73–80] The rationale for such treatments goes something like this: altered body perception can cause the brain to conclude there is a threat to the body and so it can produce protective responses, including pain. By retraining body perception in a non-threatening way, potentially these inputs could be received and scrutinized without the conclusion of threat, and then the perception could slowly change. This might shift the need to protect and ultimately reduce the pain response. That's the theory. Let's explore these concepts further.

Interventions Targeting Body Perception

Sensory Discrimination

Did you ever write with your finger on your friend's back and have them tell you what they felt? This is called *graphesthesia* and is actually a form of assessment and treatment. Just like the game, it involves identifying drawings or letters on affected body parts to assess sensory discrimination, which requires cognitive recognition and perception of the stimulus. Some studies show this intervention increases the ability to detect tactile inputs, decrease pain and improve function.[9,40,81–83] Randomized controlled trials in phantom limb pain, chronic limb pain and CRPS have shown that sensory discrimination training can normalize the SI representation, which was coupled with improved function and decreased pain.[79,81,82] This normalization of SI and associated decrease in pain has also been demonstrated in people with chronic low back pain; however, study limitations prevent firm conclusions about its effectiveness.[84] What does this mean? Retraining sensory perception may improve body perception, which may also decrease pain.

Laterality: Do You Know Your Right From Left?

Potentially, the most reproducible example of disrupted body perception is the altered ability to determine right from left. This task, known as *laterality*, used both as a test and as a treatment to improve body perception, can be performed by showing an individual a series of pictures of a right or left body part and asking them to identify which side it is.[37] Increased time required to determine the side, as well as inaccuracies in left/right identifications, are evident in multiple pain populations.[5] Studies assessing the effectiveness of laterality training as a stand-alone treatment are limited in number and show limited effects. It is likely the potential for greater effects occurs with integration of treatments (see GMI below).[79,85]

Sensorimotor Retraining: Visualization, Virtual Reality and Illusions

These interventions vary from being easily accessible to requiring specialized equipment to create illusions and virtual realities. (Due to lack of accessibility for most of us, these won't be explored here. See Boesch et al.,[78] Stanton et al.[86] and Matamala-Gomez et al.[87] for further discussion.) Perhaps the simplest and most applicable for our purposes is a technique employed frequently by athletes in training. Visualization or imagining the desired movements may actually help to change performance and potentially pain.[88–91] 'Mirror therapy' is another simple intervention: a mirror is used for the ability to see a region typically out of sight (e.g. the back) or to 'trick' the brain into believing an affected limb is being moved; both have shown some promise.[78–80,83]

Graded Motor Imagery (GMI)

GMI was developed to target cortical disruptions in sensory and motor areas of the brain and combines the previously outlined interventions[79]: 1) left/right discrimination (laterality); 2) motor imagery (or imagined movements); and 3) mirror therapy.[37]

Early studies indicate GMI may lead to changes in pain, particularly for phantom limb pain and CRPS.[73,76,77,79,80] While GMI seems to produce better results as a combination treatment than any of the single interventions on their own, further research is needed. A distinctive aspect of this intervention is the use of a protocol specific to the person's presentation and tolerance. The theoretical goal is to subtly and gradually normalize cortical changes without eliciting protective reactions.[37,79]

Interventions Targeting Cognitive Behavioral Perceptions

Cognitive behavioral therapy (CBT) was discussed in Chapter 4. It is noted here to connect the idea that how we perceive our experiences and the perception of our physical bodies cannot be separated, and will play a role in pain, especially when our brains have changed their representational maps. Using CBT with perception in mind, the primary target for change is the need for protection and the cognitive or emotional response to that protection. Bear in mind that any input, memory, emotion, etc. accessed by the brain and determined to be a potential threat contributes to perception, which in turn can facilitate or inhibit pain. Therefore, the goals of CBT are to reduce pain-eliciting and maintaining behaviors, thoughts, emotions and beliefs,[40] or alter our perception of the experience away from threat.

Yoga and Perception

Potentially, yoga represents a system that could incorporate elements of the interventions described above. Ultimately, if persistent pain is at least partially a result of disrupted body perception and treatment aims to enhance the body maps in the brain,[11] then theoretically, simply undertaking novel movements that integrate body awareness with non-judgmental thinking may help to alter the perception of the experience and thus change pain.

Yoga for Body Perception

Could the practice of yoga be considered a form of sensory integration? First, the proprioceptive and kinesthetic awareness aspect of body perception can be influenced by yoga asanas: for example, older individuals and visually impaired individuals with balance and perception deficits have demonstrated improvements through asana practice.[92,93] Second, body perception is also about our understandings and insights, and so, potentially through meditation as well as pratayahara (drawing back the senses and turning inward), yoga may also adjust body perception through first improving the ability to identify reactive responses and subsequently reducing protective responses.

To explain this a bit further, yoga encourages the practitioner to perceive the body from the inside rather than looking at it from the outside.[94] This tends to be paired with observing the body, thoughts and emotions without judgment, attachment or reaction. With practice, sensory inputs can be held without immediate response. For example, during meditation or asanas the practitioner is often encouraged to take note of physical sensations, such as an itch or the ache of a muscle nearing fatigue. However, any sensations are simply acknowledged: to react by scratching the itch or adjusting the posture is a response, and thus a choice. Instead of reacting to the input, the yoga practitioner will draw their attention deeper into the breath or focal point, and with time the perception of sensory input may soften or dissipate. What becomes realized through this practice is that when we choose to be mindful of our reactions, be it physical or emotional, we have a deeper sense of control over the responses to inputs and ultimately their consequences.

Bringing together ideas we have previously explored: the itch in the above example could be considered a *first dart*; thoughts about what the itch could be from, what it might be in the future, and scratching it until it is red or even bleeding – these are all *second darts*. Through the introspective side of yoga and mindfulness, potentially our perception of these inputs changes, from being something perceived as a problem requiring a behavioral response (output), to a sensation noted without the need for action. If we consider Phillip again, we can see that a protective pattern of holding his right arm against his chest was initially an output; however, the continued tone and tension of the muscles used to maintain this position may have resulted in proprioceptors and brain areas sensing the arm as part of his trunk, thus switching the output response to an input. This potentially altered his body perception, leading to a further need for protection, and therefore a growing pain experience.

One study tested this idea: yoga practitioners were recruited from a variety of disciplines ensuring an integrated practice of asanas, breath control exercises and meditation.[95] Assessing pain tolerance using a cold stimulus, the yoga practitioners were able to tolerate the stimulus for twice as long as age-matched controls. Notably, the practitioners who used a coping strategy of acknowledging the input and actively maintaining

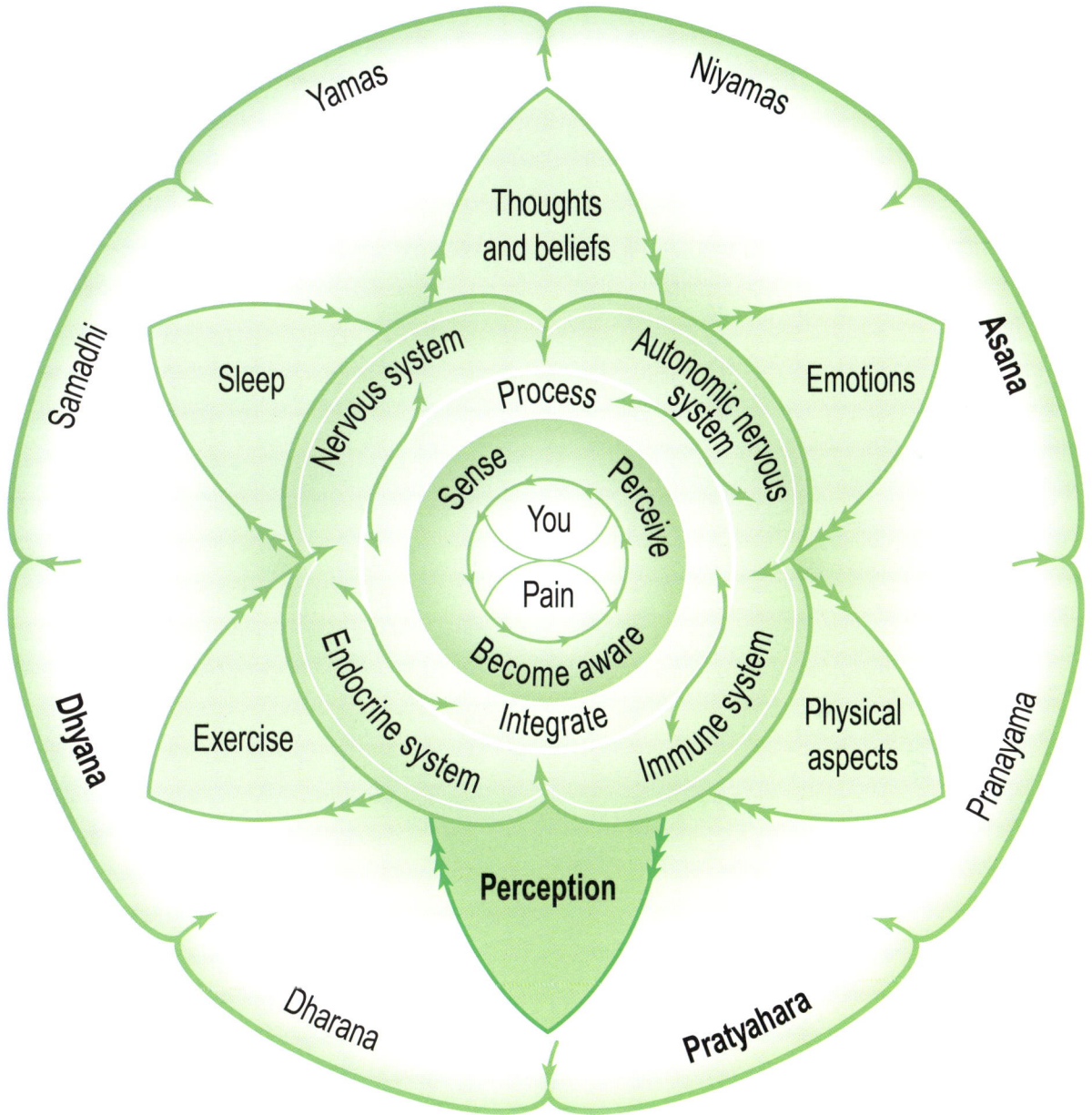

Figure 7.4
Pain and Yoga Mandala – Perception. When we combine the way we sense, process and integrate our body perception with yoga interventions such as Pratyahara (withdrawal of senses), Dhyana (meditation) and Asana (postures, movement), we potentially have the opportunity to connect more deeply with ourselves, change our body perception and soften our pain experience.

a focus on breathing or on relaxation demonstrated greater tolerance to painful stimuli as compared to controls who chose to ignore or distract from the sensation.[96] We've previously discussed how studies like this show that yoga and mindfulness can help descending modulation of nociception. What's interesting from this particular study is that the researchers also investigated brain structure using fMRI. They found structural differences in the insula in experienced yoga practitioners compared to controls, and that these differences correlated with greater pain tolerance, potentially explaining part of the effects. The insula is pivotal in perception, processing multisensory information and integrating it with cognitive–emotional processing. The techniques of relaxation and breath focus could facilitate improved interoceptive awareness: as the insula structural changes correlated with years of experience, potentially they were secondary to learned effects.[96] This was only one small study, but it is fascinating to think that experienced yoga practitioners' brains were different to those of controls in a way that adjusted their perception and, in turn, improved their pain tolerance.[96]

In another study, the ability to detect tactile inputs was superior in yoga practitioners.[94] This pilot study also examined practitioners from multiple yoga styles, but broadly consisted of physical asanas and mind–body awareness. The yoga practitioners were age-matched with a control group of regular exercisers, but who did not practice yoga. The differences observed in lumbar spine tactile precision between the groups led the researchers to conclude that yoga may help "enhance the cortical map of the back".[94] Both these studies suggest that yoga can influence the actual body perception, which may be helpful for pain.

Yoga for Cognitive Emotional Perception

As outlined in Chapter 5, large datasets on meditation practitioners have demonstrated a number of consistent changes in brain regions including the pre-frontal cortex (PFC), ACC, insula, SI and SII, inferior temporal gyrus and hippocampus.[95] It is rather encouraging to see that most of these regions are involved in body perception and pain experiences. Meditation also appears to enhance higher brain activities such as attention, memory, perceptual discrimination and compassionate behavior (see Fox et al.[95] for review).

Understanding the Pain Mandala (see Figure 7.1) and knowing how inputs of body perception, thoughts and emotions all interact and change to play a role in the persistence of pain, it might make sense to use meditation to alter one's overall perception and thus relationship with pain. Can we imagine meditation as medicine for our thinking mind? As the pain and yoga mandala (see Figure 7.4) depicts, meditation (Dhyana) and the other yoga limbs highlighted could be medicine for shifting our perception and thus the pain experience. Potentially, including an understanding of pain science could enhance the effect of meditation, to adjust the perception of threat and in turn change the pain experience. When we experience pain, our perception has shifted toward one of threat, and pain is the response produced as a means of protection. However, if we are in fact safe and can shift our perception towards feelings of safety, then our pain experience may also shift.

Conclusion

Be kind to yourself and those you work with as you wrestle with making sense of the maps, matrices in the brain, and the perception of pain: none of this is simple. As we try to understand how body perception plays a role in the experience of pain (see Figure 7.1), it may all feel rather complicated and intangible. However, perhaps body perception, the perception of experiences and the resulting perception of pain can be thought of as fascinating rather than frustrating. Maybe it is OK to not fully understand or be able to explain exactly what is happening when someone is in pain. Instead, could it be OK to consider the layers of their pain experience – their unique Pain Mandala? A starting point to pain care may be to simply choose to observe and tease out what is an input, where is it from, what information it carries and how it is processed. When we realize that some of this processing happens according to predetermined templates of expectation, we gain the opportunity to tease out how our physical perception changes with and without the involvement of the thinking mind.

Our thoughts and expectations can be altered with mindfulness – for example, the *real but not true* game could be toyed with here. What is real? The way we develop our physical sense of self, and the way it changes with repetitive inputs or practice are real. The things we add to these experiences in order to gather the meaning of what may be threatening to our sense of self are also real. However, all of this may also be combined with aspects that are not true. With gentleness and loving kindness toward ourselves and our body, we can begin to explore what is real but not actually true. We may begin to see our pain perception as a result of patterns or expectations, or attachment to experiences, beliefs or fears and a well-trained system of protection.

Phillip began to reduce his pain and symptoms with a combination of the therapeutic techniques previously discussed. Using laterality, imagined movements and mirror therapy, the perception of movement of the right hand and arm was initially facilitated, prior to performing any real movements as described in Chapter 6. While performing these therapeutic activities, he would simultaneously practice a mindfulness activity similar to the practice described below. For example, during mirror activities he would perform hand and finger motions with the left hand: watching in the mirror would give the illusion it was his right hand performing the motions, and he would notice each with conscious attention and gratitude – 'Thank you, right hand, for gripping; thank you, right hand, for opening'.

Out of the Head and Onto the Mat

Transition to practice: These practice sections are not designed to be recipes for practices to give directly to a person participating in pain care. They are meant for you, the reader, to engage in experiential learning – to take the information from 'Headspace' onto your own mat and into life. As the subject, you can first explore the ideas presented, then consider how these might translate into practices for those with whom you work.

Body Mapping Practice

In Chapter 4 we discussed practices using specific points of focus – breath, and open and focused awareness, as well as loving kindness – to act as mindfulness exercises. The practice below can be thought of as mindfulness of the body. We will use our conscious awareness to scan, notice, move and greet with gratitude our physical body. These are set in a progressive manner, beginning with a body scan and then scanning with the concept of laterality. We progress from there to noticing or scanning with a purpose of paying attention. Scanning could be thought of as a greeting of 'Hello', while noticing is a greeting with a pause to inquire, 'What is here?' After we have given attention to the body as a whole, we will come back to specific areas that were noted, this time with an intention of curious investigation without reacting or judging.

The practice goal is to use the information on body perception, body neuromatrix and the neuromatrix of pain, and combine it with these simple mindfulness practices to potentially shift the perception of threat. If we bring our attention to the region that appears to have changed, with an intention of acknowledging what is there without it being perceived as threatening, potentially our inputs can shift, and that in turn can shift body and threat perception, and maybe alter the pain experience. After you play with this experience for yourself, you can start to get creative in matching it to the specific needs of those with whom you are working. Let's practice.

- Come to your mat or choose a supportive chair. Assume a comfortable sitting posture that allows you to be relaxed yet alert. Eyes can be opened or closed.

- *Scanning:* Beginning at top of your head, slowly yet steadily scan your attention segmentally through your body until you reach your toes. No need to spend any length of time on any area; simply note the body part and move on. You can think of it like a gentle nod of hello to each body part. For example: 'This is my throat – hello, throat; this is my chest – I nod to you, chest' and so on. It may help to keep these greetings polite and gently free of any stories, questions or judgments.

- *Scanning with laterality:* Repeat the above exercise, but this time do so by separating the right from left. Start again at the top of the head and simply greet each part while identifying which side of the body it belongs to, e.g. 'Hello, right ear, right cheek, right shoulder', etc. Again, we are not spending time; we are simply noting the two sides as they are, acknowledging them politely.

- *Noticing:* For this round, repeat the body scan but let your awareness land wherever it does and allow it to linger there. Take note of the tiniest of details of this body area. It might help to open your eyes and let this be a visual focal point as well, or you can visualize the area with your eyes closed. This is done without questioning, more like a greeting, and could even take on the characteristic of wonderment. You could think of yourself as an infant discovering this area for the first time. You can also visualize how it moves with fluid strength and purpose, how it allows you to participate in a favorite activity. You could even say thank you to it. Repeat this for a few different areas of the body.

- *Noticing with intention:* Once you have completed the above activities of scanning and noticing, if at any time you noticed an area of the body that was harder to locate or that carried some sensations of sensitivity, bring your attention back to this area. Recognize that it feels or is sensed differently. This difference isn't good or bad; it just is as it is. Maybe name what you have noticed without judging. For example, the right shoulder feels sensitive, stiff, painful or foreign (difficult to find or sense).

- Once you have identified and named the sensation, try practicing the above meditation of noticing. Remember to go through the visualizations and notice, offering this body part attention with the intention of imagining, exploring and honoring what is present without judgment or scrutiny. Then start to imagine it as you would like it to be, e.g. if it feels bigger than the opposite side, imagine it feeling the same. Can you slowly and gently begin to imagine how it can shift to a perception you feel more comfortable with?

- You can also make this an asana practice. The intentions are the same: notice without judgment and bring awareness to areas that are sensitive, painful or hard to fully identify. As you move through postures, place your attention on the area that felt sensitive or different, then choose the appropriate intention as described above. For example, if it feels foreign or fuzzy, note everything else that you can about it while it moves through the posture. If it feels sensitive, painful or tender, note what else is present. So, the area may be sore but can you also feel textures or changes in muscle tone? Is it capable, stable, flexible? Is it able to function *and* be sensitive?

- *Closing the practice:* If you have time, consider repeating the whole-body scan presented first as a way of completing the practice. Either way, as you close this practice, return to your comfortable seat and encourage your attention back to your breath for a few moments before returning to life off the mat.

Off the Mat and Into Life
Noticing with Intention During Daily Life

After you have practiced the above mindfulness exercises and feel comfortable with noticing, you may like to choose a specific activity during your daily life and incorporate this practice with it (we did something similar to this in Chapter 4). Maybe you want to review the activity that you chose at that time and repeat it here, or you can select something different. Previously, we used the idea of going down the stairs with a tender knee. Let's look at that again, as an example, so imagine you have knee pain and stairs are a challenge. This time, first notice the physical tendency of turning sideways to avoid pain in the knee, recognizing the physical perception that goes along with this reaction. The perception might be that the knee is weak or unstable or feels like it can't bend. Whatever the perception is, recognize it, bring your attention to it and name it. Naming it allows us to include it just for what it is, not for what it might mean or be caused by. Then choose to notice everything else that is also present – for the knee example, this might include the contraction of the thigh muscle, the strength in the hips, the mobility in the ankle, the feel of the jeans on the skin around the knee, etc. You might even perform a marching motion or pull the heel toward the hip to feel the knee bend. You could close your eyes and imagine yourself walking down the stairs with ease. Maybe go through the movement with the contralateral limb. Then greet the knee for what it is, 'Hello, strong yet tender knee', and finally choose the appropriate response of potentially descending the stairs in a forward pattern, even if it is just a step or two first. And don't worry if initially you still don't feel ready to go down any differently than you previously did: the goal here is to first start to shift the reaction into a conscious awareness, and to respond with an intention rather than an automatic reaction.

Using this example, consider trying it with a physical struggle you can identify for yourself, then think about adapting it for use in pain care. These bullet points can be cues to help set this practice for any activity.

- Goal: shifting from reaction to response.

- Pause: name what is in your awareness.

- Make room for it and include by noticing 'What else is here?'

- Potentially bow to it, greet it and hold it for what it is.

- Then choose to respond with a conscious action or mindful intention.

References

1. Moseley, G.L., A. Gallace, and C. Spence. Bodily Illusions in Health and Disease: Physiological and Clinical Perspectives and the Concept of a Cortical 'Body Matrix'. Neuroscience and Biobehavioral Reviews, 2012. 36(1): 34–46.

2. Stanton, T.R., C.W. Lin, H. Bray, et al. Tactile Acuity Is Disrupted in Osteoarthritis but Is Unrelated to Disruptions in Motor Imagery Performance. Rheumatology (Oxford), 2013. 52(8): 1509–19.

3. Wand, B.M., M.J. Catley, M.I. Rabey, et al. Disrupted Self-Perception in People with Chronic Low Back Pain. Further Evaluation of the Fremantle Back Awareness Questionnaire. Journal of Pain, 2016. 17(9): 1001–12.

4. Nishigami, T., A. Mibu, K. Tanaka, et al. Development and Psychometric Properties of Knee-Specific Body-Perception Questionnaire in People with Knee Osteoarthritis: The Fremantle Knee Awareness Questionnaire. PLoS One, 2017. 12(6): e0179225.

5. Reinersmann, A., G.S. Haarmeyer, M. Blankenburg, et al. Left Is Where the L Is Right. Significantly Delayed Reaction Time in Limb Laterality Recognition in Both CRPS and Phantom Limb Pain Patients. Neuroscience Letters, 2010. 486(3): 240–5.

6. Martinez, E., Z. Aira, I. Buesa, et al. Embodied Pain in Fibromyalgia: Disturbed Somatorepresentations and Increased Plasticity of the Body Schema. PLoS One, 2018. 13(4): e0194534.

7. Lewis, J.S. and P. Schweinhardt. Perceptions of the Painful Body: The Relationship between Body Perception Disturbance, Pain and Tactile Discrimination in Complex Regional Pain Syndrome. European Journal of Pain, 2012. 16(9): 1320–30.

8. Stanton, T.R., G.L. Moseley, A.Y.L. Wong, and G.N. Kawchuk. Feeling Stiffness in the Back: A Protective Perceptual Inference in Chronic Back Pain. Scientific Reports, 2017. 7(1): 9681.

9. Moseley, G.L. I Can't Find It! Distorted Body Image and Tactile Dysfunction in Patients with Chronic Back Pain. Pain, 2008. 140(1): 239–43.

10. Kingsley, R.E. Concise Text of Neuroscience. 2nd ed. 2000, Baltimore: Lippincott, Williams & Wilkins.

11. Senkowski, D. and A. Heinz. Chronic Pain and Distorted Body Image: Implications for Multisensory Feedback Interventions. Neuroscience and Biobehavioral Reviews, 2016. 69: 252–9.

12. Butler, D. and L.G. Moseley. Explain Pain. 2003, Adelaide: Noigroup Publications.

13. Knudsen, L., G.L. Petersen, K.N. Norskov, et al. Review of Neuroimaging Studies Related to Pain Modulation. Scandinavian Journal of Pain, 2018. 2(3): 108–20.

14. Monroe, T.B., J.C. Gore, S.P. Bruehl, et al. Sex Differences in Psychophysical and Neurophysiological Responses to Pain in Older Adults: A Cross-Sectional Study. Biology of Sex Differences, 2015. 6: 25.

15. Schweinhardt, P. and M.C. Bushnell. Neuroimaging of Pain: Insights into Normal and Pathological Pain Mechanisms. Neuroscience Letters, 2012. 520(2): 129–30.

16. Tracey, I. and M.C. Bushnell. How Neuroimaging Studies Have Challenged Us to Rethink: Is Chronic Pain a Disease? Journal of Pain, 2009. 10(11): 1113–20.

17. Wiech, K. Deconstructing the Sensation of Pain: The Influence of Cognitive Processes on Pain Perception. Science, 2016. 354(6312): 584–7.

18. Summerfield, C. and F.P. de Lange. Expectation in Perceptual Decision Making: Neural and Computational Mechanisms. Nature Reviews Neuroscience, 2014. 15(11): 745–56.

19. Brun, C., N. Giorgi, A.M. Pinard, et al. Exploring the Relationships between Altered Body Perception, Limb Position Sense, and Limb Movement Sense in Complex Regional Pain Syndrome. Journal of Pain, 2019. 20(1): 17–27.

20. Gilpin, H.R., G.L. Moseley, T.R. Stanton, and R. Newport. Evidence for Distorted Mental Representation of the Hand in Osteoarthritis. Rheumatology (Oxford), 2015. 54(4): 678–82.

21. Bray, H. and G.L. Moseley. Disrupted Working Body Schema of the Trunk in People with Back Pain. British Journal of Sports Medicine, 2011. 45(3): 168–73.

22. Drummond, P.D. and P.M. Finch. A Disturbance in Sensory Processing on the Affected Side of the Body Increases Limb Pain in Complex Regional Pain Syndrome. Clinical Journal of Pain, 2014. 30(4): 301–6.

23. Trojan, J., V. Speck, D. Kleinbohl, et al. Altered Tactile Localization and Spatiotemporal Integration

in Complex Regional Pain Syndrome Patients. European Journal of Pain, 2019. 23(3): 472–82.

24. Fardo, F., R. Auksztulewicz, M. Allen, et al. Expectation Violation and Attention to Pain Jointly Modulate Neural Gain in Somatosensory Cortex. Neuroimage, 2017. 153: 109–21.

25. Stanton, T.R., H.R. Gilpin, E. Reid, et al. Modulation of Pain Via Expectation of Its Location. European Journal of Pain, 2016. 20(5): 753–66.

26. Tsay, A., T.J. Allen, U. Proske, and M.J. Giummarra. Sensing the Body in Chronic Pain: A Review of Psychophysical Studies Implicating Altered Body Representation. Neuroscience and Biobehavioral Reviews, 2015. 52: 221–32.

27. Proske, U. and S.C. Gandevia. The Proprioceptive Senses: Their Roles in Signaling Body Shape, Body Position and Movement, and Muscle Force. Physiological Reviews, 2012. 92(4): 1651–97.

28. Tsakiris, M. My Body in the Brain: A Neurocognitive Model of Body-Ownership. Neuropsychologia, 2010. 48(3): 703–12.

29. Walsh, L.D., G.L. Moseley, J.L. Taylor, and S.C. Gandevia. Proprioceptive Signals Contribute to the Sense of Body Ownership. Journal of Physiology, 2011. 589(Pt 12): 3009–21.

30. Garfinkel, S.N., A.K. Seth, A.B. Barrett, et al. Knowing Your Own Heart: Distinguishing Interoceptive Accuracy from Interoceptive Awareness. Biological Psychology, 2015. 104: 65–74.

31. Chiara Ribera d'Alcala, D.G.W., and Jorge E. Esteves. Interoception, Body Awareness and Chronic Pain: Results from a Case-Control Study. International Journal of Osteopathic Medicine, 2015. 18(1): 22–32.

32. Gallagher, I.I. Philosophical Conceptions of the Self: Implications for Cognitive Science. Trends in Cognitive Science, 2000. 4(1): 14–21.

33. Kilteni, K., A. Maselli, K.P. Kording, and M. Slater. Over My Fake Body: Body Ownership Illusions for Studying the Multisensory Basis of Own-Body Perception. Frontiers in Human Neuroscience, 2015. 9: 141.

34. Moseley, G.L., N. Olthof, A. Venema, et al. Psychologically Induced Cooling of a Specific Body Part Caused by the Illusory Ownership of an Artificial Counterpart. Proceedings of the National Academy of Sciences USA, 2008. 105(35): 13169–73.

35. Cardinali, L., F. Frassinetti, C. Brozzoli, et al. Tool-Use Induces Morphological Updating of the Body Schema. Current Biology, 2009. 19(12): R478–9.

36. Carruthers, G. Types of Body Representation and the Sense of Embodiment. Consciousness and Cognition, 2008. 17(4): 1302–16.

37. Moseley, G.L., D.S. Butler, T.B. Beames, and T.J. Giles. The Graded Motor Imagery Handbook. 2012, Adelaide: Noigroup Publications.

38. Yen, C.T. and P.L. Lu. Thalamus and Pain. Acta Anaesthesiologica Taiwanica, 2013. 51(2): 73–80.

39. Tyll, S., E. Budinger, and T. Noesselt. Thalamic Influences on Multisensory Integration. Communicative and Integrative Biology, 2011. 4(4): 378–81.

40. Moseley, G.L. and H. Flor. Targeting Cortical Representations in the Treatment of Chronic Pain: A Review. Neurorehabilitation and Neural Repair, 2012. 26(6): 646–52.

41. Graziano, M.S. and T.N. Aflalo. Mapping Behavioral Repertoire onto the Cortex. Neuron, 2007. 56(2): 239–51.

42. Chang, L.J., T. Yarkoni, M.W. Khaw, and A.G. Sanfey. Decoding the Role of the Insula in Human Cognition: Functional Parcellation and

Large-Scale Reverse Inference. Cerebral Cortex, 2013. 23(3): 739–49.

43. Ceunen, E., J.W. Vlaeyen, and I. Van Diest. On the Origin of Interoception. Frontiers in Psychology, 2016. 7: 743.

44. Craig, A.D. How Do You Feel? An Interoceptive Moment with Your Neurobiological Self. 2015, Princeton, NJ: Princeton University Press.

45. Maddox, R.K., H. Atilgan, J.K. Bizley, and A.K. Lee. Auditory Selective Attention Is Enhanced by a Task-Irrelevant Temporally Coherent Visual Stimulus in Human Listeners. Elife, 2015. 4.

46. Strigo, I.A. and A.D. Craig. Interoception, Homeostatic Emotions and Sympathovagal Balance. Philosophical Transactions of the Royal Society London B: Biological Sciences, 2016. 371(1708).

47. Dijkerman, H.C. and E.H. de Haan. Somatosensory Processes Subserving Perception and Action. Behavioral and Brain Sciences, 2007. 30(2): 189–201; discussion 201–39.

48. Wager, T.D., L.Y. Atlas, M.A. Lindquist, et al. An fMRI-Based Neurologic Signature of Physical Pain. New England Journal of Medicine, 2013. 368(15): 1388–97.

49. Reddan, M.C. and T.D. Wager. Modeling Pain Using fMRI: From Regions to Biomarkers. Neuroscience Bulletin, 2018. 34(1): 208–15.

50. Tracey, I. and P.W. Mantyh. The Cerebral Signature for Pain Perception and Its Modulation. Neuron, 2007. 55(3): 377–91.

51. Apkarian, A.V. A Brain Signature for Acute Pain. Trends in Cognitive Science, 2013. 17(7): 309–10.

52. Wang, S., Z.Z. Ma, Y.C. Lu, et al. The Localization Research of Brain Plasticity Changes after Brachial Plexus Pain: Sensory Regions or Cognitive Regions? Neural Plasticity, 2019. 2019: 7381609.

53. Kikkert, S., M. Mezue, D. Henderson Slater, et al. Motor Correlates of Phantom Limb Pain. Cortex, 2017. 95: 29–36.

54. Stanton, T.R., C.W. Lin, R.J. Smeets, et al. Spatially Defined Disruption of Motor Imagery Performance in People with Osteoarthritis. Rheumatology (Oxford), 2012. 51(8): 1455–64.

55. Tsao, H., M.P. Galea, and P.W. Hodges. Reorganization of the Motor Cortex Is Associated with Postural Control Deficits in Recurrent Low Back Pain. Brain, 2008. 131(Pt 8): 2161–71.

56. Wand, B.M., L. Parkitny, N.E. O'Connell, et al. Cortical Changes in Chronic Low Back Pain: Current State of the Art and Implications for Clinical Practice. Manual Therapy, 2011. 16(1): 15–20.

57. Di Pietro, F., J.H. McAuley, L. Parkitny, et al. Primary Motor Cortex Function in Complex Regional Pain Syndrome: A Systematic Review and Meta-Analysis. Journal of Pain, 2013. 14(11): 1270–88.

58. Di Pietro, F., J.H. McAuley, L. Parkitny, et al. Primary Somatosensory Cortex Function in Complex Regional Pain Syndrome: A Systematic Review and Meta-Analysis. Journal of Pain, 2013. 14(10): 1001–18.

59. Di Pietro, F., T.R. Stanton, G.L. Moseley, et al. Interhemispheric Somatosensory Differences in Chronic Pain Reflect Abnormality of the Healthy Side. Human Brain Mapping, 2015. 36(2): 508–18.

60. Pleger, B., M. Tegenthoff, P. Ragert, et al. Sensorimotor Retuning [Corrected] in Complex Regional Pain Syndrome Parallels Pain Reduction. Annals of Neurology, 2005. 57(3): 425–9.

61. Jutzeler, C.R., A. Curt, and J.L. Kramer. Relationship between Chronic Pain and Brain Reorganization after Deafferentation: A Systematic Review of Functional MRI Findings. NeuroImage: Clinical, 2015. 9: 599–606.

62. Don, S., L. Voogt, M. Meeus, et al. Sensorimotor Incongruence in People with Musculoskeletal Pain: A Systematic Review. Pain Practice, 2017. 17(1): 115–28.

63. Traxler, J., V.J. Madden, G.L. Moseley, and J.W.S. Vlaeyen. Modulating Pain Thresholds through Classical Conditioning. PeerJ, 2019. 7: e6486.

64. Madden, V.J., D.S. Harvie, R. Parker, et al. Can Pain or Hyperalgesia Be a Classically Conditioned Response in Humans? A Systematic Review and Meta-Analysis. Pain Medicine, 2016. 17(6): 1094–111.

65. International Association for the Study of Pain, IASP Terminology. 2019; Available from: http://www.iasp-pain.org.

66. International Association for the Study of Pain, Taxonomy, Part IIII: Pain Terms, a Current List with Definitions and Notes on Usage, in: Classification of Chronic Pain, H. Merskey and N. Bogduk, Editors. 1994, Seattle: IASP Press. pp. 209–14.

67. Moseley, G.L. Imagined Movements Cause Pain and Swelling in a Patient with Complex Regional Pain Syndrome. Neurology, 2004. 62(9): 1644.

68. Gustin, S.M., P.J. Wrigley, S.C. Gandevia, et al. Movement Imagery Increases Pain in People with Neuropathic Pain Following Complete Thoracic Spinal Cord Injury. Pain, 2008. 137(2): 237–44.

69. Acerra, N.E. and G.L. Moseley. Dysynchiria: Watching the Mirror Image of the Unaffected Limb Elicits Pain on the Affected Side. Neurology, 2005. 65(5): 751–3.

70. Moseley, G.L., A. Gallace, and C. Spence. Space-Based, but Not Arm-Based, Shift in Tactile Processing in Complex Regional Pain Syndrome and Its Relationship to Cooling of the Affected Limb. Brain, 2009. 132(Pt 11): 3142–51.

71. Moseley, G.L., T.J. Parsons, and C. Spence. Visual Distortion of a Limb Modulates the Pain and Swelling Evoked by Movement. Current Biology, 2008. 18(22): R1047–8.

72. Harvie, D.S., M. Broecker, R.T. Smith, et al. Bogus Visual Feedback Alters Onset of Movement-Evoked Pain in People with Neck Pain. Psychological Science, 2015. 26(4): 385–92.

73. Smart, K.M., B.M. Wand, and N.E. O'Connell. Physiotherapy for Pain and Disability in Adults with Complex Regional Pain Syndrome (CRPS) Types I and II. Cochrane Database Systematic Reviews, 2016. 2: CD010853.

74. Kregel, J., I. Coppieters, R. DePauw, et al. Does Conservative Treatment Change the Brain in Patients with Chronic Musculoskeletal Pain? A Systematic Review. Pain Physician, 2017. 20(3): 139–54.

75. Daffada, P.J., N. Walsh, C.S. McCabe, and S. Palmer. The Impact of Cortical Remapping Interventions on Pain and Disability in Chronic Low Back Pain: A Systematic Review. Physiotherapy, 2015. 101(1): 25–33.

76. Thieme, H., N. Morkisch, C. Rietz, et al. The Efficacy of Movement Representation Techniques for Treatment of Limb Pain – a Systematic Review and Meta-Analysis. Journal of Pain, 2016. 17(2): 167–80.

77. Batsford, S., C.G. Ryan, and D.J. Martin. Non-Pharmacological Conservative Therapy for Phantom Limb Pain: A Systematic Review of Randomized Controlled Trials. Physiotherapy Theory and Practice, 2017. 33(3): 173–83.

78. Boesch, E., V. Bellan, G.L. Moseley, and T.R. Stanton. The Effect of Bodily Illusions on Clinical Pain: A Systematic Review and Meta-Analysis. Pain, 2016. 157(3): 516–29.

79. Bowering, K.J., N.E. O'Connell, A. Tabor, et al. The Effects of Graded Motor Imagery and Its Components on Chronic Pain: A Systematic Review and Meta-Analysis. Journal of Pain, 2013. 14(1): 3–13.

80. Mendez-Rebolledo, G., V. Gatica-Rojas, R. Torres-Cueco, et al. Update on the Effects of Graded Motor Imagery and Mirror Therapy on Complex Regional Pain Syndrome Type 1: A Systematic Review. Journal of Back Musculoskeletal Rehabilitation, 2017. 30(3): 441–9.

81. Moseley, G.L. and K. Wiech. The Effect of Tactile Discrimination Training Is Enhanced When Patients Watch the Reflected Image of Their Unaffected Limb During Training. Pain, 2009. 144(3): 314–19.

82. Moseley, G.L., N.M. Zalucki, and K. Wiech. Tactile Discrimination, but Not Tactile Stimulation Alone, Reduces Chronic Limb Pain. Pain, 2008. 137(3): 600–8.

83. Sawyer, E.E., A.W. McDevitt, A. Louw, et al. Use of Pain Neuroscience Education, Tactile Discrimination, and Graded Motor Imagery in an Individual with Frozen Shoulder. Journal of Orthopaedic and Sports Physical Therapy, 2018. 48(3): 174–84.

84. Kalin, S., A.K. Rausch-Osthoff, and C.M. Bauer. What Is the Effect of Sensory Discrimination Training on Chronic Low Back Pain? A Systematic Review. BMC Musculoskeletal Disorders, 2016. 17: 143.

85. Suso-Martí, L., J.V. Léon-Hernández, R. La Touche, et al. Motor Imagery and Action Observation of Specific Neck Therapeutic Exercises Induced Hypoalgesia in Patients with Chronic

Neck Pain: A Randomized Single-Blind Placebo Trial. Journal of Clinical Medicine, 2019. 8(7): pii:E1019.

86. Stanton, T.R., H.R. Gilpin, L. Edwards, et al. Illusory Resizing of the Painful Knee Is Analgesic in Symptomatic Knee Osteoarthritis. PeerJ, 2018. 6: e5206.

87. Matamala-Gomez, M., A.M. Diaz Gonzalez, M. Slater, and M.V. Sanchez-Vives. Decreasing Pain Ratings in Chronic Arm Pain through Changing a Virtual Body: Different Strategies for Different Pain Types. Journal of Pain, 2019. 20(6): 685–97.

88. Beinert, K., M. Sofsky, and J. Trojan. Train the Brain! Immediate Sensorimotor Effects of Mentally-Performed Flexor Exercises in Patients with Neck Pain. A Pilot Study. European Journal of Physical and Rehabilitation Medicine, 2019. 55(1): 63–70.

89. Beinert, K., S. Preiss, M. Huber, and W. Taube. Cervical Joint Position Sense in Neck Pain. Immediate Effects of Muscle Vibration Versus Mental Training Interventions: A RCT. European Journal of Physical and Rehabilitation Medicine, 2015. 51(6): 825–32.

90. Hoyek, N., F. Di Rienzo, C. Collet, et al. The Therapeutic Role of Motor Imagery on the Functional Rehabilitation of a Stage II Shoulder Impingement Syndrome. Disability and Rehabilitation, 2014. 36(13): 1113–19.

91. Taube, W., M. Lorch, S. Zeiter, and M. Keller. Non-Physical Practice Improves Task Performance in an Unstable, Perturbed Environment: Motor Imagery and Observational Balance Training. Frontiers in Human Neuroscience, 2014. 8: 972.

92. Youkhana, S., C.M. Dean, M. Wolff, et al. Yoga-Based Exercise Improves Balance and Mobility in People Aged 60 and Over: A Systematic

Review and Meta-Analysis. Age Ageing, 2016. 45(1): 21–9.

93. Fiori, F., N. David, and S.M. Aglioti. Processing of Proprioceptive and Vestibular Body Signals and Self-Transcendence in Ashtanga Yoga Practitioners. Frontiers in Human Neuroscience, 2014. 8: 734.

94. Flaherty, M. and M. Connolly. A Preliminary Investigation of Lumbar Tactile Acuity in Yoga Practitioners. International Journal of Yoga Therapy, 2014. 24: 43–50.

95. Fox, K.C., S. Nijeboer, M.L. Dixon, et al. Is Meditation Associated with Altered Brain Structure? A Systematic Review and Meta-Analysis of Morphometric Neuroimaging in Meditation Practitioners. Neuroscience and Biobehavioral Reviews, 2014. 43: 48–73.

96. Villemure, C., M. Ceko, V.A. Cotton, and M.C. Bushnell. Insular Cortex Mediates Increased Pain Tolerance in Yoga Practitioners. Cerebral Cortex, 2014. 24(10): 2732–40.

Sometimes you have to be your own medicine.

Guy Hoffman

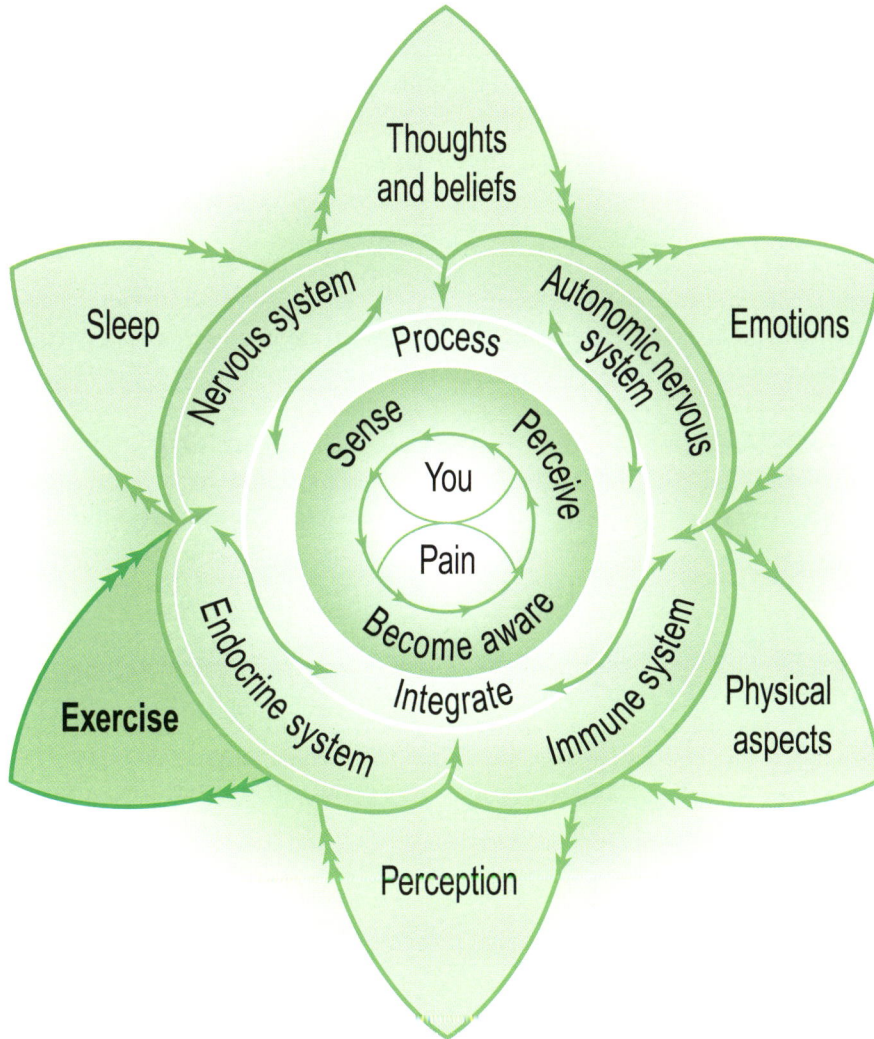

Figure 8.1

Pain Mandala – Exercise. Exercise and physical activity provide important contributions to the function of our immune, endocrine, nervous and autonomic systems. Regular exercise can improve these systems. However, in some pain states exercise can trigger negative responses, elicit the need for protection and lead to a painful flare. This, alongside our relationship with movement and exercise, creates a dynamic loop that can increase or decrease our pain experience.

Note: This mandala depicts aspects of the human experience of pain covered in Pain Science Yoga Life. *Other inputs, dimensions and body systems can contribute to pain than those noted here.*

Chapter 8

Headspace

Exercise is Medicine

If ever there was a universal action to promote health and wellbeing, it is exercise. The benefits are strongly supported by scientific evidence: exercise plays a major role in the prevention of everything from heart disease to cancer,[1,2] and future episodes of pain.[3] Its therapeutic effects are far-reaching, it being effective for pain as well as related issues like depression, anxiety and sleep disturbance.[4-6] In fact, according to the American College of Sports Medicine (ACSM), activities that promote cardiorespiratory fitness, strength, flexibility and neuromotor facilitation (coordination and balance), beyond what is performed for daily activities, are essential and outweigh the risks of participation.[7] Despite this knowledge, most adults don't reach minimum exercise recommendations of at least 150 minutes per week.[7,8]

Growing evidence supports exercise for pain relief in many persistent conditions, such as fibromyalgia,[9] chronic widespread pain,[5] osteoarthritis,[10,11] chronic neck[12] and low back pain,[13] and even neuropathic pain.[14] But sadly, levels of exercise participation and physical activity in those with persistent pain are even lower than in the general population.[15-19] It is easy to understand lower activity levels when pain is present. When it hurts even to move, or you fear damage or injury (i.e. there is an assumed risk), why would you want to exercise?

Pain is obviously one barrier but there are others. Sometimes people feel that exercise is only valuable if it is vigorous, which may deter those with low exercise tolerance. Also, for people with persistent pain, initial responses to exercise can vary, with some experiencing pain flares (see Rice et al.[20] for review). Even if this pain increase is short-term, it can be understandably discouraging, especially if individuals are unsupported in their exercise efforts. Lack of support, education and guidance is not uncommon as direction from clinicians is not always available. While attitudes of clinicians are changing, exercise and physical activity recommendations continue to take a back seat to medication prescriptions or surgery for pain,[21] in part due to lack of training or lack of knowledge regarding whom to refer to.[21-23] As yoga teachers and clinicians, we may play a valuable role in using yoga as exercise for pain care. When combined with other aspects of yoga, the asana or exercise portion may hold some unique benefits for people in pain.[24,25]

In this chapter we explore foundational principles of exercise, effects of exercise on pain, and mechanisms explaining these effects. Along the way we'll touch on exercise for mood, sleep and overall health. This subject is vast and this short chapter will not be all-inclusive. However, we aim to offer a broad understanding to support creativity and structure in the use of exercise including asanas as part of pain care.

Exercise and Physical Activity

These two terms are often used interchangeably but they are subtly different. Formally, "*Physical Activity* is any bodily movement produced by skeletal muscles, that results in energy expenditure. *Physical Exercise* is characterized as planned, structured, and repetitive physical activities with an objective to maintain or improve physical fitness."[26] It may be helpful to think of them this way: exercise should be specific and have a target goal and plan, while physical activity can be anything that gets you moving, with the focus placed more on the task or the environment rather than the physiological output. For example, hiking could be considered exercise or physical activity. Let's say I am out on a mountain trail: if I pause for photos or to take in the sounds of nature, this starts to fall into the physical activity category. However, if I keep my focus on a pre-set duration and monitor intensity, this is exercise.

Exercise Fundamentals

Let's briefly look at the building blocks of exercise relevant for pain care. These concepts are presented here in a fundamental way to ensure a basic understanding before connecting these with pain. The following American College of Sports Medicine (ACSM)[27] definitions are an important starting point as we build a strong foundation for exercise in pain care.

Cardiovascular

Aerobic means with oxygen. The ACSM defines aerobic exercise as any activity that requires the use of large muscle groups, is continuously maintained and naturally rhythmic, and increases the need for oxygen. During these activities the heart muscle pumps oxygen from the pulmonary system (lungs) via the bloodstream to the working muscles. When a consistent aerobic exercise plan is followed, the heart will gain capacity to meet the oxygen demands of the muscles with decreased effort. Regardless of weight, age, gender or medical conditions, we can all benefit from aerobic exercise.

A measure known as VO_2 max (maximum volume of oxygen) is one way that cardiovascular fitness is measured and thus intensity is often described as a percentage of this. VO_2 represents the amount of oxygen used by the tissues during physical exertion.[28] The more efficient a person is at utilizing oxygen during physical performance, the higher their VO_2 max. An alternate way to measure aerobic intensity that doesn't require special equipment is rate of perceived exertion (RPE). RPE is a subjective rating using a numeric scale. A number or intensity of performance is chosen based on how the person performing the activity perceives or feels their overall effort to be. When measured, a standard hatha yoga practice has been shown to be equivalent to low-intensity exertion, similar to slow walking.[29] There is scope for a vinyasa or repetitive sun salute style of practice to reach the level of energy expenditure considered to be moderate aerobic exercise, if it exceeds 10 minutes of continuous activity, is performed with more intensity, or in people who have lower fitness levels.[29-32]

Strength/resistance training

This type of training is simply adding resistance to build muscle strength. Depending on the individual's baseline strength, this resistance can be body weight, the weight of the working limb(s) or an external added force, e.g. dumbbells or exercise bands. The intensity of resistance training is often measured using a percentage of 1 repetition maximum. This means if the most amount of weight I can lift while performing a squat for a single repetition is 136kg, then if I am performing 15 repetitions at 50%max, I would use 68kg of added resistance.

Two common types of strength training identified as potentially useful in pain care are isometric and dynamic resistance. *Isometric* means of one length, and this type of strength training occurs when a muscle or joint is held against resistance at a consistent length or angle, e.g. utkatasana, chair pose or static half-squat position. *Dynamic resistance* training occurs when movements are performed against resistance. A push-up or yoga chaturanga could be an example of dynamic resistance training, using body weight as the resistant force.

Flexibility is the ability to move joints and lengthen muscles through a full range of motion. Flexibility training can be performed statically, where a muscle is taken to or near its end range of motion and held, or with dynamic movements throughout the entire range of motion repetitively.

Neuromuscular training can be described as training motor responses by stimulating peripheral and central mechanisms responsible for dynamic motor control. This category includes balance, proprioception, coordination, and functional activities or skills related to sport or performance.

Chapter 8

How Much Physical Activity Do We Need for Health?

The ACSM physical activity guidelines offer standards to guide individual exercise prescription.[8] If able, all adults should participate in at least 150–300 minutes per week of moderate-intensity aerobic activity, or 75–150 minutes of vigorous-intensity aerobic activity per week. Adults with and without chronic conditions should also incorporate strength training, targeting major muscle groups at least twice weekly.[33] Further, the U.S. Department of Health and Human Services advocate that any movement is better than none, and even for those with chronic conditions, inactivity should be avoided.[7] This means we should all aim for an average of 25 minutes of moderate to intense activity 6 days per week with the addition of some strength and flexibility training. That's no big deal right?

It's Not That Easy

For many of us the idea of movement for health is easy – it comes naturally. We know if we are feeling low in energy or mood, or having trouble focusing, we hop on our yoga mat or go for a jog and things will be better. However, this isn't true for all. I remember a nurse colleague asking me, "What about those of us who are not natural exercisers, how do we get moving?" If it is a struggle to just get going, trying something that makes it feel less like exercise and more like an enjoyable activity may be helpful. For example, meeting a friend to walk instead of sitting at a café, or playing music and making a game out of an indoor circuit. The best exercise is the one performed regularly. It could be helpful to have accountability, like putting it on the schedule or committing to a friend or trainer.

There is another end to this exercise spectrum that merits mention – those with super-high levels of physical activity or exercise. Too little exercise can be problematic, but so can too much, especially when it comes to pain. The overwhelming evidence is that those who don't exercise are at risk of more pain, but in contrast those who have very high levels of physical activity are also at risk of developing pain.[34–38] As a rule, being somewhere in the middle is probably a good thing. So, for some people the message may be about reducing exercise and expectations of physical activity and finding a balance that suits their current state, while others will need guided encouragement to get going.

For those in pain, barriers to exercise participation may be substantial. Even if a person was once movement-oriented, they may become hesitant because of fear of pain or fear of further injury, which could make participating in recommended exercise or physical activity more challenging. If we consider Phillip (Case Study, p.51), the pain in his hand and arm prevented him from full participation in his baseball. But, especially initially, there wasn't any physical reason why he couldn't perform other exercises such as jogging, swimming or strength training of uninvolved areas. We will come back to how he worked exercise into his pain care, but for now, simply identifying the need to educate and encourage participation, as able, is sufficient.

Teaching individuals in pain that exercise can actually help reduce pain and improve general health, mood and sleep could prove to be empowering for their recovery. The Pain Mandala (see Figure 8.1) highlights the integration of these various inputs for pain, so exercise may be one modality we can use to address multiple layers. Let's take a quick side step to overview benefits for sleep and mood, before we explore the intricacies of exercise and pain.

Exercise and Sleep

Sleep and exercise have a reciprocal relationship: good sleep facilitates increased activity and activity facilitates sleep.[4] Sleep disturbance negatively impacts both pain[39] and mood,[40] and for those struggling with persistent pain, the effects may be even greater. Thus, maintaining regular sleep and exercise habits could be highly valuable for those with pain[40–43] (more in Chapter 9).

Exercise and Mood

People who participate in regular physical activity tend to have better mental health and psychological wellbeing.[6,8,44] While the link between physical activity and psychological health in persistent pain is less clear,[5,15,45] research shows that individuals with persistent pain who are less active report greater fear of movement, fear-avoidance beliefs and pain catastrophizing, and are more likely to experience depression and anxiety than those who are more active.[15,46,47] This demonstrates again how various inputs into the pain experience converge and integrate. On the other hand, aerobic activity can improve feelings of wellbeing, cognitive function and self-efficacy, and reduce depression, even in those with persistent pain.[6,43,44]

Intensity and progression require careful consideration. An individual's personal view of exercise, as well as the intensity, can cause exercise to be stressful both physiologically and psychologically.[20] Nonetheless, the positive effects of exercise on mood tend to emerge with consistent performance.[41,47,48] Interestingly, the best outcomes for positive mood effects occur when exercise is performed at a moderate or preferred intensity – more is not always better.[44,49]

Exercise and Pain

It is encouraging to see how the data support exercise for pain care. The following are a few persuasive snippets demonstrating the medicinal effects of exercise.

Exercise as Medicine: A Circuit of Proof

- Exercise is one of the most effective treatments for persistent pain conditions, with evidence to support its use as first-line treatment in conditions ranging from back pain to arthritis and fibromyalgia.[5,10,12,13,20,50–55] Although the current level of evidence is not without limitations, and studies with longer follow-up and larger sample sizes

are still needed, we can be confident of exercise's therapeutic effects.

- Exercise can prevent recurrences. Exercise is the only modality to date effective in preventing recurrences of back pain when compared to other common treatments,[3] and can reduce recurrence of sports-related pain.[56]

- Exercise reduces the risk of developing pain in various populations: from neck pain in office workers to pregnancy-related pelvic girdle pain.[57–61] And while meeting recommended amounts of exercise is better, even small amounts seem protective,[62] e.g. people who participate in regular moderate-intensity exercise at least 1–3 times per week report less pain than those who don't.[61]

- Exercise is safe.[27] Even in conditions like osteoarthritis, where people worry about further damage, moderate levels of exercise are safe and don't worsen affected joints.[63]

- Lack of exercise and physical inactivity actually increase the risk of pain.[41,61] Further, inactivity may be an added insult for people in pain, as lifestyle diseases related to inactivity, such as obesity and type II diabetes, may actually increase sensitivity to pain.[43,64]

The Neuroscience: How Does Exercise Help with Pain?

OK, you get it: exercise has positive effects for prevention and treatment of pain, but how does this pain modulation occur? One key mechanism we will explore in some detail is exercise-induced hypoalgesia or EIH. As a brief aside, while not covered here, knowing the individual and addressing their unique limitations such as strength, flexibility and neuromuscular control specific to their impairments may hold benefits in addition to those related to EIH. Potentially, for some, beginning with general exercise participation may allow tolerance and participation in more specific or corrective exercise plans.

Exercise-Induced Hypoalgesia (EIH)

Exercise can decrease pain. But what about the cliché of exercise being all about pain and suffering – 'No pain, no gain'? Well, athletes might be able to endure pain and suffering because not only have their bodies and minds trained for the effort, but biologically they have become more tolerant to physical stress and discomfort.

If we dissect the term hypoalgesia, 'hypo' meaning low or under, and 'algesia' meaning pain, it is easy to understand the meaning: less pain. When used in this context, exercise-induced, it refers to the change in pain sensitivity following exercise. While performing exercise and shortly after completion of exercise, most individuals demonstrate increased tolerance of painful stimulation, increased pain thresholds (the amount of stimulus required to provoke a painful response) and reduced intensity of pain to that stimulus.[65-67]

> Hypoalgesia: diminished pain in response to a normally painful stimulus.
>
> Hyperalgesia: increased pain in response to a normally painful stimulus.[68,69]

It appears that three types of exercise have the greatest effect on pain sensitivity: aerobic, and dynamic and isometric strength training. (Note, most of the following findings were from healthy people.) For aerobic exercise, EIH is strongest with moderate to high-intensity.[66,70-73] Specifically, the greatest amount of hypoalgesia after aerobic exercise is demonstrated at high intensity (70–75% VO_2 max) for longer than 10 minutes, or moderate intensity (50% VO_2 max) for 30 minutes.[70] These EIH effects tend to be widespread, extending throughout the body.[74,75]

For isometric resistance exercise, research indicates EIH occurs using relatively low loads of isometric intensity, i.e. 10–30% of one repetition maximum if the duration of hold is near exhaustion, which may be 3–5 minutes.[65,74,76] Don't let the words 'relatively low' fool you as this is actually difficult to perform, especially if unaccustomed to static positions, or if getting out of a physical comfort zone feels unnatural or threatening. Interestingly, EIH effects after the performance of isometric exercises can be widespread or extend beyond the working muscle.[66,74,75,77] For example, performing a right-sided bicep isometric may reduce pain sensitivity of the left knee region. This suggests static muscle contraction facilitates central widespread inhibitory mechanisms. In other words, our natural pharmacy is activated in a broad and systemic way.

The threshold of dynamic resistance exercise required for producing EIH is not well determined, but the evidence available here demonstrates EIH is possible with performance of 2–3 sets of resistance exercise, again at high intensity.[66] To potentially mimic these effects in a yoga practice, think repeated vinyasa between warrior poses.

In general, the period of hypoalgesia carryover appears to be short, usually less than 30 minutes,[66,70,74,78] or maybe a little longer with resistance exercise.[66,74] However, what's more encouraging is that people who exercise regularly have greater tolerance to experimental pain testing than those who don't.[79-82] This might suggest, with increased consistency of performance, effects could continue with improved general tolerance to noxious inputs. One recent study looked specifically at dynamic resistance performed in a circuit class designed to target the legs, abdominals and arms. The results demonstrate the presence of EIH via improved pain tolerance, as well as participants' reports of improved tolerance to the discomfort of exercise.[83] This was only one small study, but it is an interesting investigation, given the progressive trend of circuit/interval training included in weight training, and in modern-day yoga classes.

On the whole, the research here needs to continue, since the specifics of exercise program design that are required to maximize initial and prolonged benefits for pain are still unclear. It's worth remembering that each person is different and no research can ever reproduce the exact response for individuals. The point to understand is that exercise of variable types can stimulate our natural pharmacy and improve our overall tolerance to physical discomfort. For those of us who have an affinity for exercise or work with populations of people who exercise, this is not surprising. We know first-hand the ability to sustain greater amounts of discomfort with training. But what might be surprising is the extent of these physiological changes, and how these effects may be impaired in people with persistent pain: they may have no EIH

Take home message: Exercise can activate our natural pharmacy to reduce pain.

effect, or have the opposite effect of increased pain sensitivity and/or painful flares.

Potential Mechanisms Contributing to EIH

How is it that exercise reduces pain sensitivity? Probably the most common response would be "endorphins." Though it's partially true, as with so many aspects of pain neuroscience, it's a bit more complicated. The mechanisms of EIH vary, but in a broad sense, nervous and immune system adaptations help to explain the protection that physical activity and exercise offer us in pain[15] (Figure 8.2). We will summarize a few key biological events leading to EIH; again, most studies have been performed on healthy individuals without pain and still fall short of providing exact explanations.

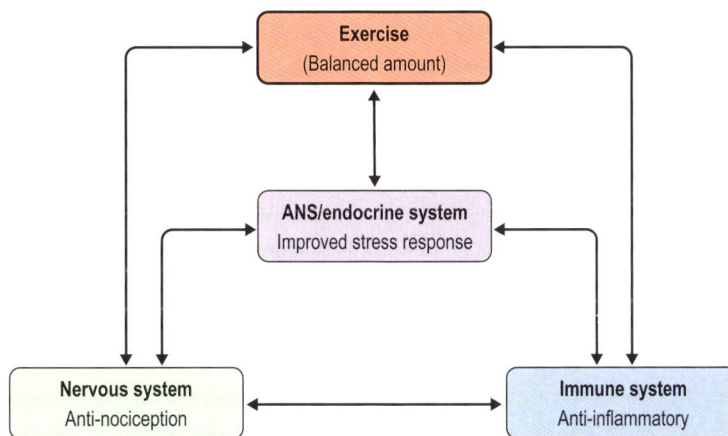

Figure 8.2
Effects of exercise on body systems. In normal circumstances, when exercise is performed at an appropriate dose it can alter our immune, nervous system and stress responses. The double arrows show that bidirectional relationships are present. 'Balanced amount' refers to the importance of exercise dose: too much or too little will not produce the desired effects. This dose will vary for different individuals and for different circumstances. *ANS*, autonomic nervous system.

Studies on persistent pain are increasing, so hopefully greater understanding is on the horizon.

Nervous System Changes and EIH: Activating Our Natural Pharmacy

Let's briefly recap some of the neurotransmitters important in modulating nociception. Opioids will be familiar to almost everyone – they are also called endorphins. The word 'endorphins' means internally produced opioids. Serotonin is another neurotransmitter we met previously. It plays a role in modulation of nociception and is an important player in controlling mood. The last group of neurotransmitters discussed here are endocannabinoids. Again, 'endo' means produced in the body; therefore these are cannabinoids our bodies naturally produce. Other neurotransmitters that have been shown to be involved in EIH are nitric oxide and noradrenaline (norepinephrine).[84]

Endorphins are released when we exercise and can modulate nociception. Long-standing evidence demonstrates they are key players in producing EIH (see Koltyn[85] for review). However, the majority of the most convincing of these studies were performed on animals. When we look at human studies, the results are a bit more ambiguous: the opioid system is activated but it doesn't fully explain the degree of EIH.[20] Subsequent research has focused on other pathways and found neurotransmitters like serotonin and endocannabinoids help produce EIH effects.[65] To highlight the complexity, it seems that *interactions* between the serotonin and opioid systems or between the endocannabinoid and opioid systems are potentially potent factors in how we gain pain relief from exercise.[76,86]

Persistent Pain and EIH: Still Not That Easy

As we have seen in other chapters, when pain becomes persistent many biological, psychological and social aspects change. When looking at the effects of exercise and specifically EIH in individuals with persistent pain, things become less clear. Instead of *hypo*algesic

effects, there have been reports of impaired EIH with *hyper*algesic effects in some populations (whiplash, chronic widespread pain, fibromyalgia) (see Rice et al.[20] for summary). *Hyper*algesic means that instead of a reduction in pain sensitivity, an increase in pain sensitivity occurs. Importantly, exercises that push individuals who struggle with persistent pain to fatigue may also produce unwanted increases in pain.[87] Perhaps recognizing the potential for exercise-induced *hyper*algesia helps us to understand the science behind the reports we hear from some individuals with persistent pain – exercise can hurt.

> Take home message: For some people with persistent pain, exercise does increase their pain.

When considering the mechanisms driving exercise-induced *hyper*algesia (or impaired EIH), even less is known about how this occurs. This may be due to factors such as central sensitization and poorer descending modulation of nociception that occur with persistent pain.[88-90] Impairment of the mechanisms responsible for descending modulation of nociception do tie in with impaired EIH seen in some people with persistent pain and arthritis.[77,91] As outlined before, descending modulation involves opioids and serotonin,[92] so it's possible that impaired EIH in persistent pain may relate to impairments in these systems.[20] Greater excitability in the central nervous system (central sensitization) may also explain impaired EIH.[87] Recently, some evidence has also emerged that decreased activation of the endocannabinoid system may explain impaired EIH in people with widespread pain, such as in fibromyalgia.[93]

Maybe all that truly needs to be understood here is that chemical shifts can happen, leaving us primed for protection. The Pain Mandala (see Figure 8.1) visually highlights integration across health dimensions, so aspects mentioned before such as fear, mood and sleep may also be inputs into or overlapping factors with impaired EIH. Therefore, typical expectations, like decreased pain and sensitivity after exercise, may not occur, and the reverse, increased pain and sensitivity, may. Preparing ourselves and those we are working with for these potential outcomes may soften the response, and help prevent people giving up on exercise prematurely.

Immune System Changes and EIH

We hear a lot about inflammation and pain. Inflammation naturally accompanies acute injuries as part of healing (see Chapter 6), but low levels of chronic inflammation, an indication of altered immune responses, are also relevant in persistent pain.[94,95] The amount of inflammation matters, as we saw in Chapter 1: pro-inflammatory chemicals (called cytokines) can trigger nociception, initiating warning signals. For most people, the effects of physical activity on the immune system are positive, with more anti-inflammatory chemicals priming for healing and protection.[96] However, inactivity and sedentary behaviors result in an increase in pro-inflammatory chemicals.[97] This makes nociception easier to trigger. Research from animal studies shows that regular physical activity causes the equilibrium to shift, with greater numbers of anti-inflammatory chemicals (for review see Sluka et al.[15]). This chemical shift potentially decreases the number of warning inputs from the tissues.

In human studies, the results are a little more complex. Some studies show a shift towards more anti-inflammatory chemicals with exercise,[96,98] but in other situations, e.g. in response to intense exercise and high training loads,[99,100] or in people with inflammatory disorders,[101] a pro-inflammatory state can occur soon after exercise. Thus, post-exercise complaints of increased pain or pain flares in people with persistent pain may be due to this initial spike of inflammation. Animal studies also show that fatiguing exercise can exacerbate this.[87] This might be relevant for some people with persistent pain, especially those with chronic fatigue as part of their clinical picture. The good news, though, is that this inflammatory profile can change. The pro-inflammatory response can actually reduce with exercise training,[101] and a shift towards an anti-inflammatory state can occur even in those with persistent pain conditions such as fibromyalgia.[15,20,96,102] Therefore, the effects of physical activity on our immune system may protect us from sensitization and inflammation that can lead to persistent pain (see Figure 8.2).

> Take home message: Physical activity and exercise can enhance our immune system.

Exercise Implementation for Persistent Pain in the Clinic and Studio

As we move into implementing exercise for people with pain, let's bear a couple of key points in mind:

- Exercise can reduce pain and inflammation but it can also increase pain sensitivity and inflammation, especially initially or if intense or fatiguing.

- While initially there is more risk of exacerbating pain with exercise, as people persist and make exercise a regular activity, they are more likely to experience pain-relieving effects, e.g. through shifting their inflammatory profile to a more anti-inflammatory state.

To help translate all of this science to a person in pain, let's meet Marie. Marie is an executive in her mid-50s, and has been struggling with widespread pain for several years, mostly affecting her trunk, shoulders and arms. She has tried various forms of exercise and rehabilitation interventions, but always ended up in more pain and feels discouraged from doing any movement above what is required for her daily tasks. However, her doctor advised her to try yoga. She is willing yet hesitant. How can we help facilitate Marie's care with what we have covered?

Marie could be told that exercise is good for her, and she'd likely sigh and tell you how she's heard that over and over, but that every time she exercises her pain worsens. This is an understandably difficult yet vicious cycle: it hurts and can feel scary to move when in pain, yet lack of movement could be making everything more sensitive and less healthy – inputs becoming outputs again.

So, how do we balance the common report of exercise increasing pain and the risk of *hyper*algesic responses, with the strong evidence that being active and participating in regular exercise is more beneficial than harmful? This is where we as clinicians and yoga teachers can help to set a scenario of safe, approachable exercise participation.

Whether we're working with an individual or in a class, setting the right tone for exercise in pain care is crucial. We can acknowledge the painful state and hold space for feelings of the important inputs of fear and apprehension, yet still encourage approaching movement with curiosity and openness. On the other end of the spectrum, we might encourage those who push too hard to ease back and explore movement with a sense of gentleness. Either way, noting initially tolerated intensity and duration of physical activity and exercise in conjunction with the consideration of other inputs – fear, past history of pain and exercise, social support systems and general tendencies toward movement – should be key parts of any pain care plan.[23,41,43,103,104] No one specific type of exercise is better than others for persistent pain.[10,105] This should be a little freeing as it means the exercise can be individualized to include personal preference and struggles, and is likely to be most beneficial when tailored this way.

So, we now have a strong foundation and sense of freedom with exercise prescription, but how do we actually start? Let's look at how we might structure an exercise prescription to optimize responses in persistent pain.

Elements of an Exercise Prescription

Aerobic exercise at a moderate intensity may be most suitable for the goal of generalized pain reduction in many pain states.[47 87,106,107] However, do tread lightly when beginning, especially with someone like Marie who has widespread pain, and those with chronic fatigue and fibromyalgia. They may be initially more prone to pain flares and increased pain sensitivity.[20] Intensity and frequency recommendations should be kept individualized and, especially initially, well supervised. Beginning at a low intensity and progressing in a slow, graded fashion may offer the most benefit[47] and reduce the risk for aggravating a sensitive system. So, for Marie, agreeing to begin at her tolerated and preferred intensity is a good place to start. This might need some adjustment during early weeks but once she's up and moving, her exercise dose can gradually be progressed until she achieves moderate intensity (50–70% of age-adjusted maximum heart rate, or 11–13 RPE, on a 6–20 scale) for at least 25 minutes, ideally six days a week. To manage expectations, allow at least six weeks for such a program to positively impact pain and function,[106,107] and it might take a long time to get to these recommendations. So, celebrate the start and recognize all the small steps along the way. Additional analgesic effects may be achieved by increasing the dose using greater frequency per week, as opposed to increased duration or intensity per exercise session.[47] In other words, small bouts every day may be more optimal than larger amounts a few days per week. For Marie, this might be 10–15 minutes of gentle, flowing asana practice focused on her legs to start with, keeping the more sensitive areas, like her arms, within aggravation-free ranges.

Generally, beginning with the insurance of success may also be helpful. For example, using a concept known as pacing,[108] if the estimated tolerance is 20 minutes of brisk walking, consider beginning with 15 minutes of moderate walking. Then increase by 1–2 minutes per day until 20 minutes every day is established. This helps build self-efficacy and reduces the risk of flares. After checking on tolerance and response, increasing the intensity can be explored.

Resistance training has also shown benefits for pain reduction and function. Again, a gradual individualized progression and avoidance of overloading is considered best practice.[41,43,61,66,103] People who struggle with pain may need a little extra reassurance and education on the safety and expectations of resistance exercise.[23] For example, knowing in advance that post-exercise muscle soreness is normal, not indicative of harm, and may actually be part of gaining strength, could be incredibly helpful for their resilience in participation. Using non- or less painful body parts[74,109] as the focus for strength training initially could achieve an EIH response, even in individuals where this response has become impaired. This indirect method may also help reassure the individual that exercise does not have to equal pain or be avoided completely, especially during times of flare-ups.[77] For Marie, adding isometric holds into warrior poses, bridge or malasana (squat) may be a way to introduce resistance training. Once her confidence, tolerance and understanding increase, then she could add in the sensitivity-prone areas like her arms.

Just like all aspects requiring practice, people need to engage in exercise programs over a sustained period to glean fuller effects, e.g. at least four weeks.[43,103] In neck pain, low back pain and knee osteoarthritis, pain relief has been found to be improved with increased exercise sessions without negative effects.[41,47,110–112]

A crucial point to note for increased adherence and positive outcomes is that, regardless of the actual activity, simply connecting with the person, increasing their confidence and understanding of movement, facilitating acknowledgment of the relationship they have with movement and their own bodies, as well as understanding how pain works, may actually be the most important part of the intervention.[103] When we recognize the level of integration between various inputs to the pain experience, and people's relationships with exercise, we can again play with *and this too*. We can be uncomfortable and hesitant, and choose to move anyway and know we are still OK. All factors get to be included when exercise is prescribed in pain care.

Asanas, Exercise or Yoga?

How does this information relate to yoga? Asanas are the physical postures of yoga and can be tailored to incorporate aspects of exercise – aerobic exercise, strength training, flexibility and neuromotor control. From a purely physical perspective, traditional yoga asanas may hold some advantages for people with pain due to the variation in body postures. A balanced yoga practice allows whole-body movement, thus improving flexibility and increasing individuals' repertoires of movement. The potential novelty of yoga asanas may create a mechanism for breaking habitual protective movement responses and offer access to improve impairments like weakness and stiffness. When we change the context of movement or exercise, we may produce a different perception – we may trick the nervous system a little, potentially altering the pain neuromatrix associated with the movement. As such, protective responses including pain may change (see Chapter 7). From a broader perspective, yoga practice, as a whole, may offer additional holistic benefits (Figure 8.3). Exercise, physical activity and asanas, when approached with intention, could be considered a mindfulness of the body practice.

The research on yoga specifically for pain remains limited. The conclusion of a Cochrane Review of yoga for chronic low back pain spells it out this way: "There is a need for additional high-quality research to truly report with confidence the long-term effects of yoga compared to other forms of exercise."[113] However, as presented previously, some investigations do show promising results for the direct use of yoga for pain reduction. Recent synthesis of research looking at yoga and mind–body approaches to exercise suggests

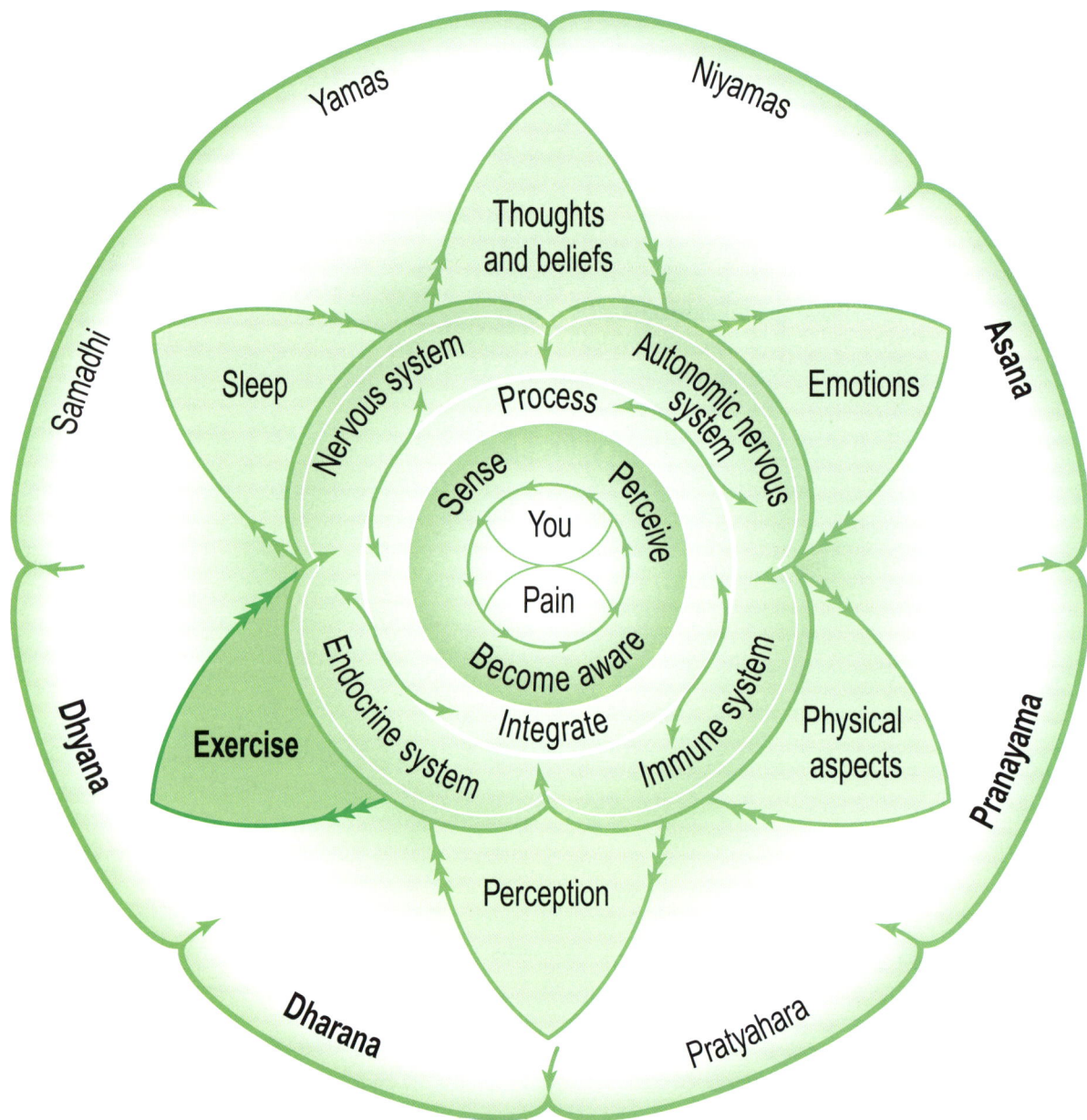

Figure 8.3

Pain and Yoga Mandala – Exercise. When we combine principles of exercise prescription and pain science with the softer side of engaging people to move from a mindful place, remaining connected to themselves, we can see how the yoga practices of Asana (postures, movement), Pranayama (breath practice), Dharana (focused attention) and Dhyana (meditation) can be used to move beyond pain. Encouraging exercise therapy to be consistent and tailored to each individual and their evolving pain journey also aligns well with many yoga principles.

yoga is a useful supportive intervention for a range of pain conditions.[24,25,114]

When approaching exercise from a yogic perspective, it should feel organic to offer a non-threatening, individualized plan, graded to fit the person's needs each time they step onto their mat. Keep in mind that yoga postures don't have to be a rigid expression of what has been demonstrated in traditional texts. So, yoga is *one* exercise option among many that may be helpful. For example, when working with someone with upper extremity pain, like Marie and Phillip, they may not tolerate a warrior stance with the arms raised. But they may gain a great deal from doing the exercise with the arms rested in a variation to allow other parts of the body to gain the benefits from the exercise, and this may actually carry over to decreased pain. The individual could even be encouraged to create the 'shape' of the posture that feels best to them initially and explore movements from there. After all, the most important aspect of providing exercise as a treatment for people in pain may well be to simply engage them, develop confidence with movement, and encourage them to become more active throughout daily life. In turn, these changes may improve function and quality of life, and reduce the impact of pain.

Conclusion

Exercise and physical activity are good for our bodies and our brains. The mechanisms behind the pain-relieving effects of exercise are complex and may take years of study and analysis to fully comprehend. Evidence-based exercise prescription for those with persistent or widespread pain varies greatly and could actually cause a person in pain to experience more discomfort if approached too aggressively. Therefore, it is imperative to be mindful, continue to monitor closely, and remember to share knowledge first and frequently. Providing the individual with an understanding of pain science may help them to embrace the value of exercise and cope with symptom

changes that may occur along the way. Exercise can span across all the following domains: aerobic and strength, land- or aquatic-based, high- and low-intensity, and specific movement-based programs (e.g. Tai Chi). Even instructions to increase activity as simple as doing one more step each day could be the exercise plan. All exercise and physical activities can be facilitated with a mindfulness of the body and connected to an awareness of breath; in this way even biking or running could be considered an asana practice. This might feel overwhelmingly unspecific but it could also be viewed as encouraging – the best exercise for people with persistent pain is movement. If one type or plan isn't quite right, lots of options exist to try something else.

Phillip required just a little encouragement and education to return to exercise. His program was initiated by doing cardiovascular activities of walking and stationary biking for at least 20–30 minutes at a comfortable pace five days per week. He slowly added isometrics for the lower extremities that were held for progressively longer periods, such as wall squats and lunges/warrior poses. Within a few weeks he was jogging and working on abdominal strengthening too. His innate drive for physical activity and challenge ignited rather quickly and he was forced to learn to slow the intensity of progression in order to prevent flares. However, this turned out to be a great opportunity because he could connect the activity with the pain flare and realize that, although he was sore, he was not under any true threat: *real but not true* again helped to manage his secondary reactions. Simultaneously, he was working through the strategies discussed in Chapter 6 to get the right hand and arm tolerating movement. Eventually, he was able to return to physical training with his baseball team. His coach agreed to vary the training schedule to allow days that included exercises most appropriate for him. This cooperative effort gave him not only the benefits of exercise but also social reconnection.

So, with a little encouragement for creativity and freedom of motion, let's get out of this headspace and start moving on and off our mats.

Out of the Head and Onto the Mat

Transition to practice: These practice sections are not designed to be recipes for practices to give directly to a person participating in pain care. They are meant for you, the reader, to engage in experiential learning – to take the information from 'Headspace' onto your own mat and into life. As the subject, you can first explore the ideas presented, then consider how these might translate into practices for those with whom you work.

This 'Onto the Mat' exercise requires a little more effort on your part to design. So first grab a pen and paper and get ready to plan yourself a practice. None of these suggestions is meant to be a rigid protocol and certainly will be too advanced for many who are in pain. Instead, they are a way to encourage you to practice incorporating exercise science into yoga asana practice and later transition to use this in pain care. As always, we recommend you experiment and experience this for yourself before designing a program for those you work with.

1. Cardiovascular Flow

Using a vinyasa style of practice, create a flow that you can move through easily with some speed in order to facilitate an aerobic state at a moderate intensity, or 'somewhat hard' (12–14 on the RPE scale).

You can use the custom flow created in Figure 8.4, or if the postures don't seem right for you, go to Appendix 2: Asana, and choose a sequence or create your own. Repeat the sequence as a flow, alternating sides for a total of 10–20 minutes. Hold each posture for 1–3 breaths, depending on comfort with rate of motion.

The goal here is to experience yoga as a form of aerobic exercise. If you are very fit aerobically, it may be more difficult for you to reach a state of moderate intensity with simple sun salutes but if you add repeated jumps or hopping for transitions you may note the elevation in heart rate and respiration. If you continue to repeat the series, you will likely experience similar benefits to walking or running.

A note to teachers: Think creatively about turning up or turning down the intensity of the poses used, creating a practice to meet the student or person in pain where they are, and then aim to offer gradual increases.

2. Strength Training, Isometrics and Neuromuscular Control

Consider the customized sequence created in Figure 8.4. Can you change the exercise focus and make this an asana practice that incorporates the principles of strength training, potentially isometrics specifically?

Here is the customized sequence (Figure 8.4) adapted for strength training, or again go to Appendix 2: Asana and create your own:

- Chair pose, hold (30 breaths').

- Forward fold, step back crescent lunge – lunge up/down 10–20 repetitions.

- Hold crescent (30 breaths).

- Step back and place hands on the floor in a plank, adding 10–12 push-ups (these can be from the knees and partial range).

- Hold plank for 30 breaths.

- Finish with downward-facing dog.

- Step forward and start again at chair and repeat for the other side.

---

* The 30-breath count hold is simply suggested to get near 1.5 minutes, in order to offer a touch of isometrics as indicated by the research presented in 'Headspace'.

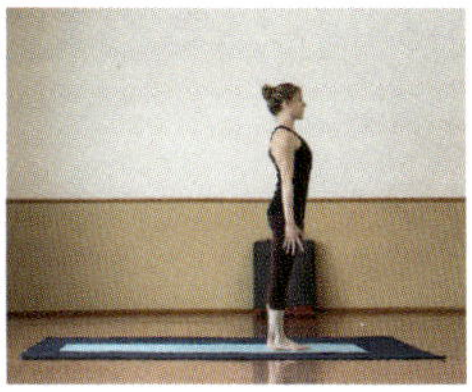 Begin in mountain pose	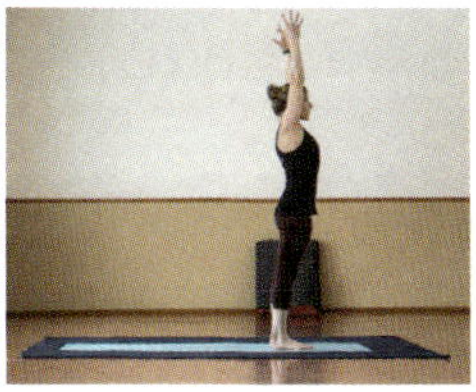 Raise arms to upward-facing mountain	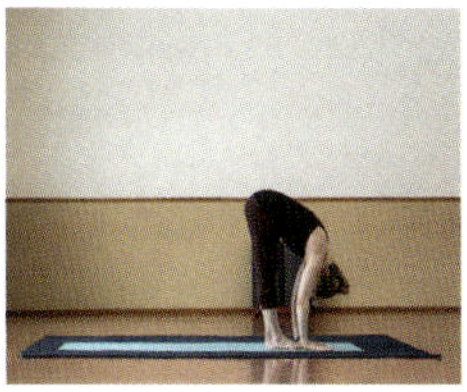 Forward fold
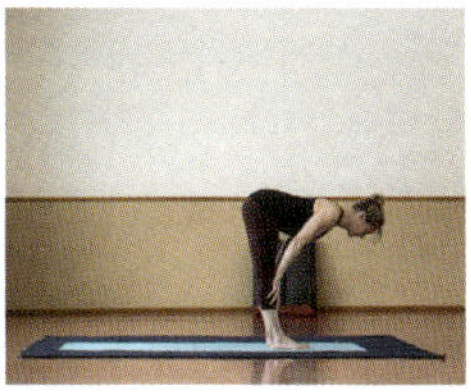 Rise halfway	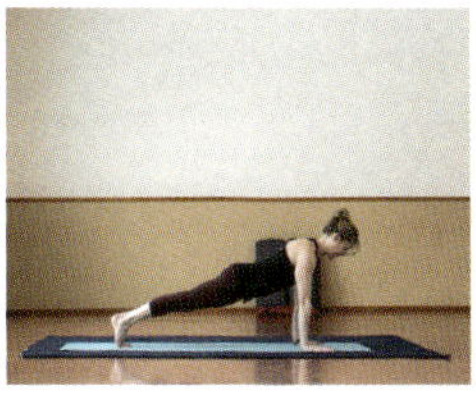 Place hands on floor; step feet back to plank	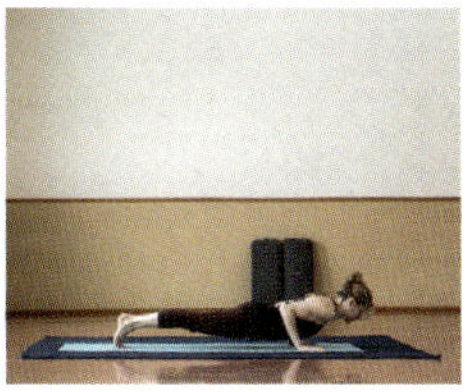 Chaturanga
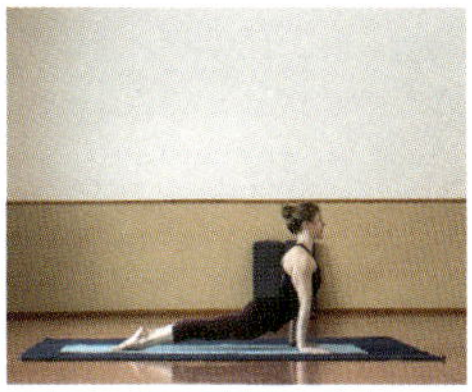 Upward-facing dog	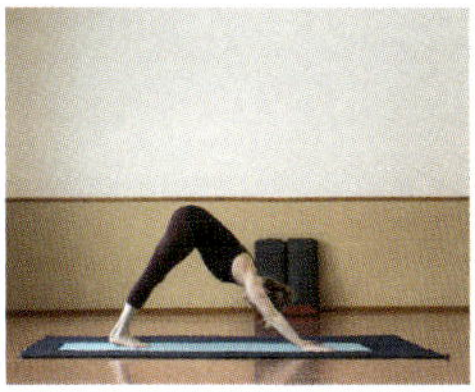 Downward-facing dog	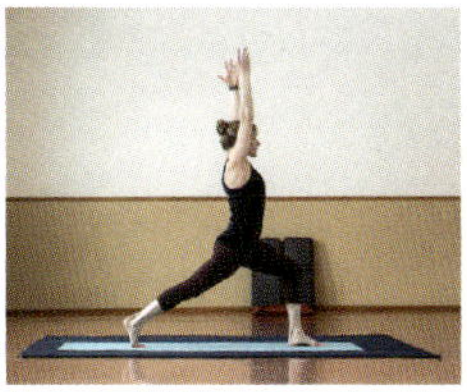 Step one foot forward to crescent lunge
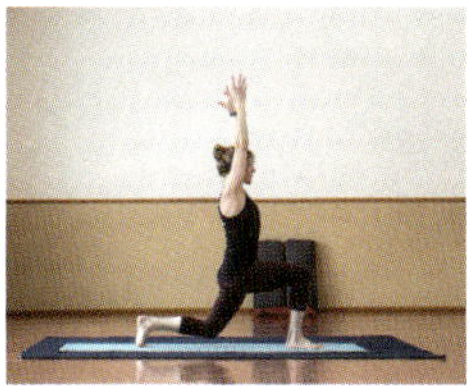 Dip back knee for dynamic lunge	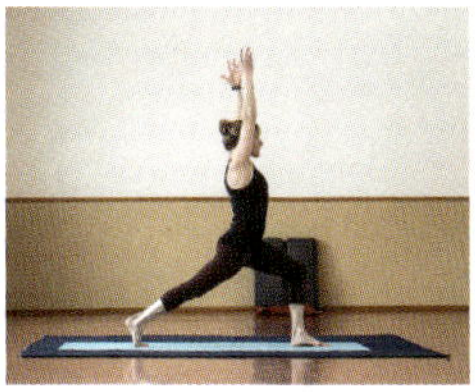 Straighten back to crescent	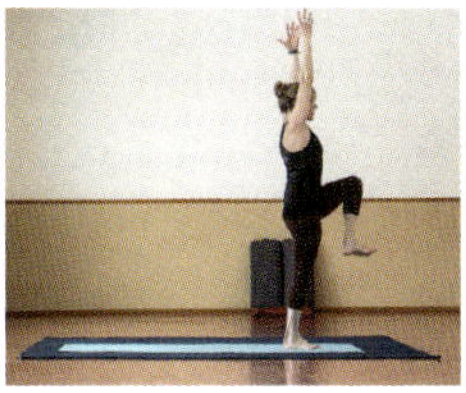 Draw back leg forward for modified tree
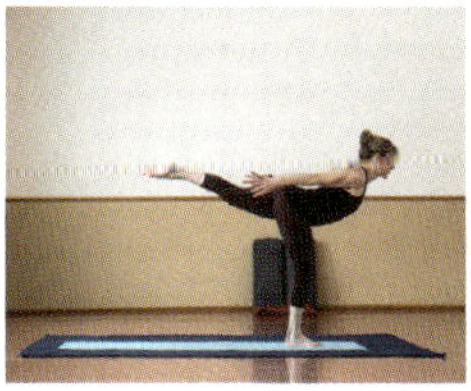 Send same leg backward for warrior 3	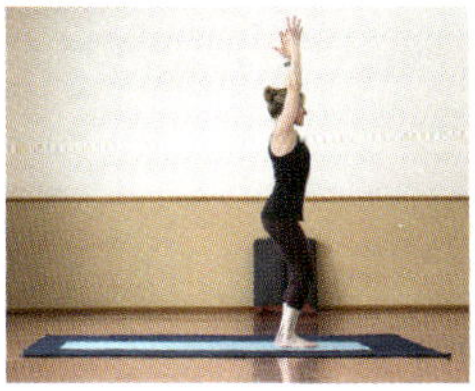 Bring back leg to meet front to find chair pose	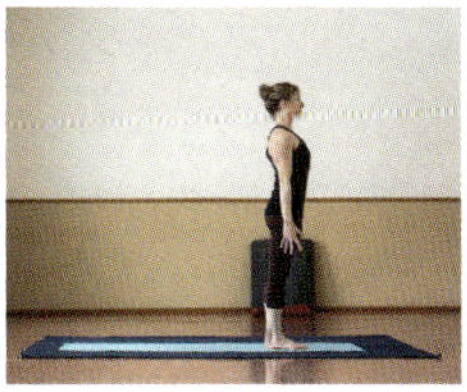 Return to mountain. Begin again to repeat on opposite side

Figure 8.4
Customized Asana Sequence. This sequence is set up so that each posture flows directly onto the next. It can also be adapted to the specifics of exercise design to reach cardiovascular, strength and neuromotor goals.
A special note on images: this is one person's body, and her individual interpretation of asanas. We encourage people to follow their own unique body shape, alignment and positions of function and comfort within these postures.

This can all be taken one step further with the addition of resistance, e.g. holding weights in your hands for curls or overhead presses, while performing an isometric exercise of the lower half.

To add an element of neuromuscular control, we can mix in some balance postures or add a creative transition that requires greater coordination to perform. Perhaps add tree pose or other standing balance between the two sides.

Now that you get the idea of it all, let's practice.

- Come onto your mat and settle into a comfortable seat.

- Place one hand on your belly and one on your heart, or both on either of those locations, whichever allows you to connect to yourself today. Stay for as many breaths as you need to feel ready to tune into yourself as an observer.

- If, at any time during the asana flow, your breath becomes labored or splinted, or your body has sensations of discomfort, lean in a little, ask, 'Am I OK?', 'Am I under threat or at risk of harm?' With clear answers, choose to continue or to back off; neither choice comes with a judgment of good or bad.

- Repeat the cardiovascular flow you've chosen as many times as feels beneficial, progressing to or adding in the strength training and neuromuscular flows when and if you are ready. Perform a simple finishing sequence of 1–2 seated postures and 1–3 supine postures (see Appendix 2) to close your practice, and then end in savasana for at least 10 breaths or as long as you have available and feels beneficial.

Off the Mat and Into Life

The following are a few potentially novel tips and tricks. Simple or creative mindfulness practices could also be incorporated with each of these suggestions. You could include focused attention on the body as you move through these playful ideas, observing how you feel or even what emotions arise (see Chapter 5) as you move. Or you could choose to move the attention away from the body by focusing on a different component altogether. For example, if with a partner, focus on the interaction with the other person, or in a scenario of playing with a child, how do they see and feel this activity? Or the attention could be on the natural environment, taking note of the temperature, breeze, bird sounds, the feeling of dirt. Each of these mindfulness strategies can serve a different purpose. Play with these for yourself and use them as guides or creative inspiration to adapt for those with whom you are working.

1. Make a playdate outside: Ask a friend or take your children or your friend's children and go outside and play (whatever that means) – crawl around in the dirt looking for bugs, swing on the swings, hang from monkey bars, play tag (this can be walking tag), play hide and seek.

2. Hallway funway: Every time you walk down your hallway at home or even at work, do it in the style of a different animal – walk like a bear, crab walk, bunny hop, frog jump, duck walk, or choose a different dance move – moonwalk, shopping cart, disco, pirouettes, etc. You might get some coworkers or family members to join in or at least you will all get a giggle.

3. Exercise of the day: Choose an exercise of the day, e.g. push-ups (these can be performed to your ability, on the floor, on the edge of a desk, at a wall or even 'air' push-ups). Then choose a number that you can already do comfortably (something that is close to 75% of your maximum): let's say that is 10. Every time you think of it or when the opportunity presents itself, stop and do 10 push-ups – if you really want a fun challenge, try doing the exercise every hour.

4. Exercise of the week: Same idea as above but each day you do the exercise you add 2–5 repetitions for a full week.

5. Take the step challenge: Get a pedometer and for one week monitor your steps without creating any change or judgments. The next week set an intention of increasing your steps by a specific but obtainable amount each day, e.g. adding 100 steps each day can get you a 1,000 step increase after just 10 days.

6. Choose to do it the hard way. Whatever 'it' is – take the stairs instead of the elevator, carry a basket at the market instead of pushing a cart, walk for your errands instead of driving, stand up out of your chair without the use of your hands three times instead of just once, stand up to put on your socks and shoes, stand on one foot to brush your teeth…

I love this stuff and could go on all day here but you get the point.

References

1. Naci, H. and J.P. Ioannidis. Comparative Effectiveness of Exercise and Drug Interventions on Mortality Outcomes: Metaepidemiological Study. British Journal of Sports Medicine, 2015. 49(21): 1414–22.

2. McTiernan, A., C.M. Friedenreich, P.T. Katzmarzyk, et al. Physical Activity in Cancer Prevention and Survival: A Systematic Review. Medicine and Science in Sports and Exercise, 2019. 51(6): 1252–61.

3. Steffens, D., C.G. Maher, L.S. Pereira, et al. Prevention of Low Back Pain: A Systematic Review and Meta-Analysis. JAMA Internal Medicine, 2016. 176(2): 199–208.

4. Dolezal, D.A., E.V. Neufeld, D.M. Boland, et al. Interrelationship between Sleep and Exercise: A Systematic Review. Advances in Preventive Medicine, 2017. 2017: 1364387.

5. Geneen, L.J., R.A. Moore, C. Clarke, et al. Physical Activity and Exercise for Chronic Pain in Adults: An Overview of Cochrane Reviews. Cochrane Database Systematic Reviews, 2017. 4: CD011279.

6. Silveira, H., H. Moraes, N. Oliveira, et al. Physical Exercise and Clinically Depressed Patients: A Systematic Review and Meta-Analysis. Neuropsychobiology, 2013. 67(2): 61–8.

7. U.S. Department of Health and Human Services. Physical Activity Guidelines for Americans, 2018. 2nd ed. U.S. Department of Health and Human Services, Washington, D.C. Available from: https://health.gov/PAGuidelines/.

8. Garber, C.E., B. Blissmer, M.R. Deschenes, et al. American College of Sports Medicine Position Stand. Quantity and Quality of Exercise for Developing and Maintaining Cardiorespiratory, Musculoskeletal, and Neuromotor Fitness in Apparently Healthy Adults: Guidance for Prescribing Exercise. Medicine and Science in Sports and Exercise, 2011. 43(7): 1334–59.

9. Bidonde, J., A.J. Busch, C.L. Schachter, et al. Aerobic Exercise Training for Adults with Fibromyalgia. Cochrane Database Systematic Reviews, 2017. 6: CD012700.

10. Fransen, M., S. McConnell, A.R. Harmer, et al. Exercise for Osteoarthritis of the Knee: A Cochrane Systematic Review. British Journal of Sports Medicine, 2015. 49(24): 1554–7.

11. Hernandez-Molina, G., S. Reichenbach, B. Zhang, et al. Effect of Therapeutic Exercise for Hip Osteoarthritis Pain: Results of a Meta-Analysis. Arthritis and Rheumatology, 2008. 59(9): 1221–8.

12. Gross, A.R., J.P. Paquin, G. Dupont, et al. Cervical Overview, Exercises for Mechanical Neck Disorders: A Cochrane Review Update. Manual Therapy, 2016. 24: 25–45.

13. Searle, A., M. Spink, A. Ho, and V. Chuter. Exercise Interventions for the Treatment of Chronic Low Back Pain: A Systematic Review and Meta-Analysis of Randomised Controlled Trials. Clinical Rehabilitation, 2015. 29(12): 1155–67.

14. Boldt, I., I. Eriks-Hoogland, M.W. Brinkhof, et al. Non-Pharmacological Interventions for Chronic Pain in People with Spinal Cord Injury. Cochrane Database Systematic Reviews, 2014. 11: CD009177.

15. Sluka, K.A., L. Frey-Law, and M. Hoeger Bement. Exercise-Induced Pain and Analgesia? Underlying Mechanisms and Clinical Translation. Pain, 2018. 159(Suppl 1): S91–S97.

16. Ellingson, L.D., M.R. Shields, A.J. Stegner, and D.B. Cook. Physical Activity, Sustained Sedentary Behavior, and Pain Modulation in Women with Fibromyalgia. Journal of Pain, 2012. 13(2): 195–206.

17. Lin, C.W., J.H. McAuley, L. Macedo, et al. Relationship between Physical Activity and Disability in Low Back Pain: A Systematic Review and Meta-Analysis. Pain, 2011. 152(3): 607–13.

18. McLoughlin, M.J., L.H. Colbert, A.J. Stegner, and D.B. Cook. Are Women with Fibromyalgia Less Physically Active Than Healthy Women? Medicine and Science in Sports and Exercise, 2011. 43(5): 905–12.

19. Mansfield, M., M. Thacker, N. Spahr, and T. Smith. Factors Associated with Physical Activity Participation in Adults with Chronic Cervical Spine Pain: A Systematic Review. Physiotherapy, 2018. 104(1): 54–60.

20. Rice, D., J. Nijs, E. Kosek, et al. Exercise-Induced Hypoalgesia in Pain-Free and Chronic Pain Populations: State of the Art and Future Directions. Journal of Pain, 2019. 20(11): 1249–66.

21. Mafi, J.N., E.P. McCarthy, R.B. Davis, and B.E. Landon. Worsening Trends in the Management and Treatment of Back Pain. JAMA Internal Medicine, 2013. 173(17): 1573–81.

22. Persson, G., A. Brorsson, E. Ekvall Hansson, et al. Physical Activity on Prescription (PAP) from the General Practitioner's Perspective - A Qualitative Study. BMC Family Practice, 2013. 14: 128.

23. Hoffmann, T.C., C.G. Maher, T. Briffa, et al. Prescribing Exercise Interventions for Patients with Chronic Conditions. Canadian Medical Association Journal, 2016. 188(7): 510–18.

24. Brosseau, L., J. Taki, B. Desjardins, et al. The Ottawa Panel Clinical Practice Guidelines for the Management of Knee Osteoarthritis. Part One: Introduction, and Mind-Body Exercise Programs. Clinical Rehabilitation, 2017. 31(5): 582–95.

25. Zou, L., Y. Zhang, L. Yang, et al. Are Mindful Exercises Safe and Beneficial for Treating Chronic Lower Back Pain? A Systematic Review and Meta-Analysis of Randomized Controlled Trials. Journal of Clinical Medicine, 2019. 8(5). pii: E628.

26. Caspersen, C.J., K.E. Powell, and G.M. Christenson. Physical Activity, Exercise, and Physical Fitness: Definitions and Distinctions for Health-Related Research. Public Health Reprorts, 1985. 100(2): 126–31.

27. American College of Sports Medicine. Guidelines for Exercise Testing and Prescription. 10th ed. 2018, Champaign, IL: Lippincott Williams & Wilkins.

28. National Strength and Conditioning Association. Essentials of Strength Training and Conditioning. 2016, 4th ed. G.G. Haff and T.N. Triplett, Editors. Champaign, IL: Human Kinetics.

29. Hagins, M., W. Moore, and A. Rundle. Does Practicing Hatha Yoga Satisfy Recommendations for Intensity of Physical Activity Which Improves and Maintains Health and Cardiovascular Fitness? BMC Complementary and Alternative Medicine, 2007. 7: 40.

30. Mody, B.S. Acute Effects of Surya Namaskar on the Cardiovascular & Metabolic System. Journal of Bodywork and Movement Therapies, 2011. 15(3): 343–7.

31. Papp, M.E., P. Lindfors, M. Nygren-Bonnier, et al. Effects of High-Intensity Hatha Yoga on Cardiovascular Fitness, Adipocytokines, and Apolipoproteins in Healthy Students: A Randomized Controlled Study. Journal of Alternative and Complementary Medicine, 2016. 22(1): 81–7.

32. Ramos-Jiménez, A., R.P. Hernández-Torres, A. Wall-Medrano, et al. Cardiovascular and Metabolic Effects of Intensive Hatha Yoga Training in Middle-Aged and Older Women from Northern Mexico. International Journal of Yoga, 2009. 2(2): 49–54.

33. Piercy, K.L., R.P. Troiano, R.M. Ballard, et al. The Physical Activity Guidelines for Americans. Journal of the American Medical Association, 2018. 320(19): 2020–8.

34. Fransen, M., M. Simic, and A.R. Harmer. Determinants of MSK Health and Disability: Lifestyle Determinants of Symptomatic Osteoarthritis. Best Practice and Research: Clinical Rheumatology, 2014. 28(3): 435–60.

35. Parekh, S.M., G.S. Fernandes, J.P. Moses, et al. Risk Factors for Knee Osteoarthritis in Retired Professional Footballers: A Cross-Sectional Study. Clinical Journal of Sports Medicine, 2019. [Epub ahead of print]

36. Heneweer, H., L. Vanhees, and H.S. Picavet. Physical Activity and Low Back Pain: A U-Shaped Relation? Pain, 2009. 143(1–2): 21–5.

37. Heuch, I., I. Heuch, K. Hagen, and J.A. Zwart. Is There a U-Shaped Relationship between Physical Activity in Leisure Time and Risk of Chronic Low Back Pain? A Follow-up in the Hunt Study. BMC Public Health, 2016. 16: 306.

38. Auvinen, J., T. Tammelin, S. Taimela, et al. Associations of Physical Activity and Inactivity with Low Back Pain in Adolescents. Scandinavian Journal of Medicine and Science in Sports, 2008. 18(2): 188–94.

39. Krause, A.J., A.A. Prather, T.D. Wager, et al. The Pain of Sleep Loss: A Brain Characterization in Humans. Journal of Neuroscience, 2019. 39(12): 2291–300.

40. Ablin, J.N., D.J. Clauw, A.K. Lyden, et al. Effects of Sleep Restriction and Exercise Deprivation on Somatic Symptoms and Mood in Healthy Adults. Clinical and Experimental Rheumatology, 2013. 31(6 Suppl 79): S53–9.

41. Ambrose, K.R. and Y.M. Golightly. Physical Exercise as Non-Pharmacological Treatment of Chronic Pain: Why and When. Best Practice and Research: Clinical Rheumatology, 2015. 29(1): 120–30.

42. Tang, N.K. and A.N. Sanborn. Better Quality Sleep Promotes Daytime Physical Activity in Patients with Chronic Pain? A Multilevel Analysis of the Within-Person Relationship. PLoS One, 2014. 9(3): e92158.

43. Hassett, A.L. and D.A. Williams. Non-Pharmacological Treatment of Chronic Widespread Musculoskeletal Pain. Best Practice and Research: Clinical Rheumatology, 2011. 25(2): 299–309.

44. Ekkekakis, P., E.E. Hall, and S.J. Petruzzello. The Relationship between Exercise Intensity and Affective Responses Demystified: To Crack the 40-Year-Old Nut, Replace the 40-Year-Old Nutcracker! Annals of Behavioral Medicine, 2008. 35(2): 136–49.

45. Carvalho, F.A., C.G. Maher, M.R. Franco, et al. Fear of Movement Is Not Associated with Objective and Subjective Physical Activity Levels in Chronic Nonspecific Low Back Pain. Archives of Physical and Medical Rehabilitation, 2017. 98(1): 96–104.

46. Elfving, B., T. Andersson, and W.J. Grooten. Low Levels of Physical Activity in Back Pain Patients Are Associated with High Levels of Fear-Avoidance Beliefs and Pain Catastrophizing. Physiotherapy Research International, 2007. 12(1): 14–24.

47. Polaski, A.M., A.L. Phelps, M.C. Kostek, et al. Exercise-Induced Hypoalgesia: A Meta-Analysis of Exercise Dosing for the Treatment of Chronic Pain. PLoS One, 2019. 14(1): e0210418.

48. Williams, D.M., S. Dunsiger, J.T. Ciccolo, et al. Acute Affective Response to a Moderate-Intensity Exercise Stimulus Predicts Physical Activity Participation 6 and 12 Months Later. Psychology of Sports and Exercise, 2008. 9(3): 231–45.

49. Ekkekakis, P. Let Them Roam Free? Physiological and Psychological Evidence for the Potential of Self-Selected Exercise Intensity in Public Health. Sports Medicine, 2009. 39(10): 857–88.

50. Bidonde, J., A.J. Busch, B. Bath, and S. Milosavljevic. Exercise for Adults with Fibromyalgia: An Umbrella Systematic Review with Synthesis of Best Evidence. Current Rheumatology Reviews, 2014. 10(1): 45–79.

51. Qaseem, A., T.J. Wilt, R.M. McLean, et al. Noninvasive Treatments for Acute, Subacute, and Chronic Low Back Pain: A Clinical Practice Guideline from the American College of Physicians. Annals of Internal Medicine, 2017. 166(7): 514–30.

52. Stochkendahl, M.J., P. Kjaer, J. Hartvigsen, et al. National Clinical Guidelines for Non-Surgical Treatment of Patients with Recent Onset Low Back Pain or Lumbar Radiculopathy. European Spine Journal, 2018. 27(1): 60–75.

53. Chen, X., B.K. Coombes, G. Sjogaard, et al. Workplace-Based Interventions for Neck Pain in Office Workers: Systematic Review and Meta-Analysis. Physical Therapy, 2018. 98(1): 40–62.

54. Juhl, C., R. Christensen, E.M. Roos, et al. Impact of Exercise Type and Dose on Pain and Disability in Knee Osteoarthritis: A Systematic Review and Meta-Regression Analysis of Randomized Controlled Trials. Arthritis and Rheumatology, 2014. 66(3): 622–36.

55. Uthman, O.A., D.A. van der Windt, J.L. Jordan, et al. Exercise for Lower Limb Osteoarthritis: Systematic Review Incorporating Trial Sequential Analysis and Network Meta-Analysis. British Medical Journal, 2013. 347: f5555.

56. Charlton, P.C., M.K. Drew, B.F. Mentiplay, et al. Exercise Interventions for the Prevention and Treatment of Groin Pain and Injury in Athletes: A Critical and Systematic Review. Sports Medicine, 2017. 47(10): 2011–26.

57. Hush, J., Z. Michaleff, C.G. Maher, and K. Refshauge. Individual Physical and Psychological Risk Factors for Neck Pain in Australian Office Workers: A 1-Year Longitudinal Study. European Spine Journal, 2009. 18: 1532–40.

58. Davenport, M.H., A.A. Marchand, M.F. Mottola, et al. Exercise for the Prevention and Treatment of Low Back, Pelvic Girdle and Lumbopelvic Pain During Pregnancy: A Systematic Review and Meta-Analysis. British Journal of Sports Medicine, 2019. 53(2): 90–8.

59. Shiri, R., D. Coggon, and K. Falah-Hassani. Exercise for the Prevention of Low Back and Pelvic Girdle Pain in Pregnancy: A Meta-Analysis of Randomized Controlled Trials. European Journal of Pain, 2018. 22(1): 19–27.

60. Munoz-Poblete, C., C. Bascour-Sandoval, J. Inostroza-Quiroz, et al. Effectiveness of Workplace-Based Muscle Resistance Training Exercise Program in Preventing Musculoskeletal Dysfunction of the Upper Limbs in Manufacturing Workers. Journal of Occupational Rehabilitation, 2019. 29(4): 810–21.

61. Landmark, T., P.R. Romundstad, P.C. Borchgrevink, et al. Longitudinal Associations between Exercise and Pain in the General Population – The Hunt Pain Study. PLoS One, 2013. 8(6): e65279.

62. Shiri, R. and K. Falah Hassani. Does Leisure Time Physical Activity Protect against Low Back Pain? Systematic Review and Meta-Analysis of 36 Prospective Cohort Studies. British Journal of Sports Medicine, 2017. 51(19): 1410–18.

63. Kraus, V.B., K. Sprow, K.E. Powell, et al. Effects of Physical Activity in Knee and Hip Osteoarthritis: A Systematic Umbrella Review. Medicine and Science in Sports and Exercise, 2019. 51(6): 1324–39.

64. Calders, P. and A. Van Ginckel. Presence of Comorbidities and Prognosis of Clinical Symptoms in Knee and/or Hip Osteoarthritis: A Systematic Review and Meta-Analysis. Seminars in Arthritis and Rheumatism, 2018. 47(6): 805–13.

65. Koltyn, K.F., A.G. Brellenthin, D.B. Cook, et al. Mechanisms of Exercise-Induced Hypoalgesia. Journal of Pain, 2014. 15(12): 1294–1304.

66. Naugle, K.M., R.B. Fillingim, and J.L. Riley, 3rd. A Meta-Analytic Review of the Hypoalgesic Effects of Exercise. Journal of Pain, 2012. 13(12): 1139–50.

67. Vaegter, H.B., G. Handberg, and T. Graven-Nielsen. Isometric Exercises Reduce Temporal Summation of Pressure Pain in Humans. European Journal of Pain, 2015. 19(7): 973–83.

68. Merskey, H. and N. Bogduk. Classification of Chronic Pain: Descriptions of Chronic Pain Syndromes and Definitions of Pain Terms. 1994, Seattle: IASP Press. p. 222.

69. International Association for the Study of Pain, IASP Terminology. 2019; Available from: http://www.iasp-pain.org.

70. Hoffman, M.D., M.A. Shepanski, S.P. Mackenzie, and P.S. Clifford. Experimentally Induced Pain Perception Is Acutely Reduced by Aerobic Exercise in People with Chronic Low Back Pain. Journal of Rehabilitation Research and Development, 2005. 42(2): 183–90.

71. Ruble, S.B., M.D. Hoffman, M.A. Shepanski, et al. Thermal Pain Perception after Aerobic Exercise. Archives of Physical Medicine and Rehabilitation, 2005. 86(5): 1019–23.

72. Meeus, M., N.A. Roussel, S. Truijen, and J. Nijs. Reduced Pressure Pain Thresholds in Response to Exercise in Chronic Fatigue Syndrome but Not in Chronic Low Back Pain: An Experimental Study. Journal of Rehabilitation Medicine, 2010. 42(9): 884–90.

73. Cook, D.B., A.J. Stegner, and L.D. Ellingson. Exercise Alters Pain Sensitivity in Gulf War Veterans with Chronic Musculoskeletal Pain. Journal of Pain, 2010. 11(8): 764–72.

74. Lannersten, L. and E. Kosek. Dysfunction of Endogenous Pain Inhibition During Exercise with Painful Muscles in Patients with Shoulder Myalgia and Fibromyalgia. Pain, 2010. 151(1): 77–86.

75. Vaegter, H.B., A.B. Madsen, G. Handberg, and T. Graven-Nielsen. Kinesiophobia Is Associated with Pain Intensity but Not Pain Sensitivity before and after Exercise: An Explorative Analysis. Physiotherapy, 2018. 104(2): 187–93.

76. Tour, J., M. Lofgren, K. Mannerkorpi, et al. Gene-to-Gene Interactions Regulate Endogenous Pain Modulation in Fibromyalgia Patients and Healthy Controls: Antagonistic Effects between Opioid and Serotonin-Related Genes. Pain, 2017. 158(7): 1194–203.

77. Vaegter, H.B., G. Handberg, and T. Graven-Nielsen. Similarities between Exercise-Induced Hypoalgesia and Conditioned Pain Modulation in Humans. Pain, 2014. 155(1): 158–67.

78. Focht, B.C. and K.F. Koltyn. Alterations in Pain Perception after Resistance Exercise Performed in the Morning and Evening. Journal of Strength and Conditioning Research, 2009. 23(3): 891–7.

79. Jones, M.D., J.L. Taylor, J. Booth, and B.K. Barry. Exploring the Mechanisms of Exercise-Induced Hypoalgesia Using Somatosensory and Laser Evoked Potentials. Frontiers in Physiology, 2016. 7: 581.

80. Ellingson, L.D., L.H. Colbert, and D.B. Cook. Physical Activity Is Related to Pain Sensitivity in Healthy Women. Medicine and Science in Sports and Exercise, 2012. 44(7): 1401–6.

81. Naugle, K.M., K.E. Naugle, R.B. Fillingim, and J.L. Riley, 3rd. Isometric Exercise as a Test of Pain Modulation: Effects of Experimental Pain Test, Psychological Variables, and Sex. Pain Medicine, 2014. 15(4): 692–701.

82. Jones, M.D., J. Booth, J.L. Taylor, and B.K. Barry. Aerobic Training Increases Pain Tolerance in Healthy Individuals. Medicine and Science in Sports and Exercise, 2014. 46(8): 1640–7.

83. Baiamonte, B.A., R.R. Kraemer, C.N. Chabreck, et al. Exercise-Induced Hypoalgesia: Pain Tolerance, Preference and Tolerance for Exercise Intensity, and Physiological Correlates Following Dynamic Circuit Resistance Exercise. Journal of Sports Science, 2017. 35(18): 1–7.

84. Da Silva Santos, R. and G. Galdino. Endogenous Systems Involved in Exercise-Induced Analgesia. J Physiol Pharmacol, 2018. 69(1): 3–13.

85. Koltyn, K.F. Analgesia Following Exercise: A Review. Sports Medicine, 2000. 29(2): 85–98.

86. Pacheco Dda, F., A. Klein, A.C. Perez, et al. Central Antinociception Induced by Mu-Opioid Receptor Agonist Morphine, but Not Delta- or Kappa-, Is Mediated by Cannabinoid CB1 Receptor. British Journal of Pharmacology, 2009. 158(1): 225–31.

87. Lima, L.V., T.S.S. Abner, and K.A. Sluka. Does Exercise Increase or Decrease Pain? Central Mechanisms Underlying These Two Phenomena. Journal of Physiology, 2017. 595(13): 4141–50.

88. Ossipov, M.H., K. Morimura, and F. Porreca. Descending Pain Modulation and Chronification of Pain. Current Opinion in Supportive and Palliative Care, 2014. 8(2): 143–51.

89. Woolf, C.J. Central Sensitization: Implications for the Diagnosis and Treatment of Pain. Pain, 2011. 152(3 Suppl): S2–15.

90. Zhuo, M. Descending Facilitation. Molecular Pain, 2017. 13: 1744806917699212.

91. Fingleton, C., K.M. Smart, and C.M. Doody. Exercise-Induced Hypoalgesia in People with Knee Osteoarthritis with Normal and Abnormal Conditioned Pain Modulation. Clinical Journal of Pain, 2017. 33(5): 395–404.

92. Sandkuhler, J. Models and Mechanisms of Hyperalgesia and Allodynia. Physiology Reviews, 2009. 89(2): 707–58.

93. Ghafouri, N., B. Ghafouri, B. Larsson, et al. Palmitoylethanolamide and Stearoylethanolamide Levels in the Interstitium of the Trapezius Muscle of Women with Chronic Widespread Pain and Chronic Neck-Shoulder Pain Correlate with Pain Intensity and Sensitivity. Pain, 2013. 154(9): 1649–58.

94. Slade, G.D., M.S. Conrad, L. Diatchenko, et al. Cytokine Biomarkers and Chronic Pain: Association of Genes, Transcription, and Circulating Proteins with Temporomandibular Disorders and Widespread Palpation Tenderness. Pain, 2011. 152(12): 2802–12.

95. Mendieta, D., D.L. De la Cruz-Aguilera, M.I. Barrera-Villalpando, et al. IL-8 and IL-6 Primarily Mediate the Inflammatory Response in Fibromyalgia Patients. Journal of Neuroimmunology, 2016. 290: 22–5.

96. Haaland, D.A., T.F. Sabljic, D.A. Baribeau, et al. Is Regular Exercise a Friend or Foe of the Aging Immune System? A Systematic Review. Clinical Journal of Sports Medicine, 2008. 18(6): 539–48.

97. Hashem, L.E., D.M. Roffey, A.M. Alfasi, et al. Exploration of the Inter-Relationships between Obesity, Physical Inactivity, Inflammation, and Low Back Pain. Spine (Phila Pa 1976), 2018. 43(17): 1218–24.

98. Ortega, E., J.J. Garcia, M.E. Bote, et al. Exercise in Fibromyalgia and Related Inflammatory Disorders: Known Effects and Unknown Chances. Exercise Immunology Reviews, 2009. 15: 42–65.

99. Greenham, G., J.D. Buckley, J. Garrett, et al. Biomarkers of Physiological Responses to Periods of Intensified, Non-Resistance-Based Exercise Training in Well-Trained Male Athletes: A Systematic Review and Meta-Analysis. Sports Medicine, 2018. 48(11): 2517–48.

100. Peake, J.M., O. Neubauer, N.P. Walsh, and R.J. Simpson. Recovery of the Immune System after Exercise. Journal of Applied Physiology (1985), 2017. 122(5): 1077–87.

101. Ploeger, H.E., T. Takken, M.H. de Greef, and B.W. Timmons. The Effects of Acute and Chronic Exercise on Inflammatory Markers in Children and Adults with a Chronic Inflammatory Disease: A Systematic Review. Exercise Immunology Reviews, 2009. 15: 6–41.

102. Bote, M.E., J.J. Garcia, M.D. Hinchado, and E. Ortega. An Exploratory Study of the Effect of Regular Aquatic Exercise on the Function of Neutrophils from Women with Fibromyalgia: Role of IL-8 and Noradrenaline. Brain, Behavior and Immunity, 2014. 39: 107–12.

103. Booth, J., G.L. Moseley, M. Schiltenwolf, et al. Exercise for Chronic Musculoskeletal Pain: A Biopsychosocial Approach. Musculoskeletal Care, 2017. 15(4): 413–21.

104. van Koulil, S., W. van Lankveld, F.W. Kraaimaat, et al. Tailored Cognitive-Behavioral Therapy and Exercise Training for High-Risk Patients with Fibromyalgia. Arthritis Care Research (Hoboken), 2010. 62(10): 1377–85.

105. Jones, K.D., D. Adams, K. Winters-Stone, and C.S. Burckhardt. A Comprehensive Review of 46 Exercise Treatment Studies in Fibromyalgia (1988–2005). Health and Quality of Life Outcomes, 2006. 4: 67.

106. Busch, A.J., S.C. Webber, M. Brachaniec, et al. Exercise Therapy for Fibromyalgia. Current Pain and Headache Reports, 2011. 15(5): 358–67.

107. O'Connor, S.R., M.A. Tully, B. Ryan, et al. Walking Exercise for Chronic Musculoskeletal Pain: Systematic Review and Meta-Analysis. Archives of Physical and Medical Rehabilitation, 2015. 96(4): 724–34 e3.

108. Guy, L., C. McKinstry, and C. Bruce. Effectiveness of Pacing as a Learned Strategy for People with Chronic Pain: A Systematic Review. American Journal of Occupational Therapy, 2019. 73(3): 7303205060p1-7303205060p10.

109. Burrows, N.J., J. Booth, D.L. Sturnieks, and B.K. Barry. Acute Resistance Exercise and Pressure Pain Sensitivity in Knee Osteoarthritis: A Randomised Crossover Trial. Osteoarthritis Cartilage, 2014. 22(3): 407–14.

110. Jones, K.D., C.A. Sherman, S.D. Mist, et al. A Randomized Controlled Trial of 8-Form Tai Chi Improves Symptoms and Functional Mobility in Fibromyalgia Patients. Clinical Rheumatology, 2012. 31(8): 1205–14.

111. Kelley, G.A., K.S. Kelley, J.M. Hootman, and D.L. Jones. Effects of Community-Deliverable Exercise on Pain and Physical Function in Adults with Arthritis and Other Rheumatic Diseases: A Meta-Analysis. Arthritis Care and Research (Hoboken), 2011. 63(1): 79–93.

112. Kaleth, A.S., C.K. Saha, M.P. Jensen, et al. Effect of Moderate to Vigorous Physical Activity on Long-Term Clinical Outcomes and Pain Severity in Fibromyalgia. Arthritis Care and Research (Hoboken), 2013. 65(8): 1211–18.

113. Wieland, L.S. and N. Santesso. A Summary of a Cochrane Review: Yoga Treatment for Chronic Non-Specific Low Back Pain. European Journal of Integrated Medicine, 2017. 11: 39–40.

114. Bussing, A., T. Ostermann, R. Ludtke, and A. Michalsen. Effects of Yoga Interventions on Pain and Pain-Associated Disability: A Meta-Analysis. Journal of Pain, 2012. 13(1): 1–9.

May this new night of rest
Repair the wear of time
And restore youth of heart
For the adventure
That awaits tomorrow

John O'Donohue

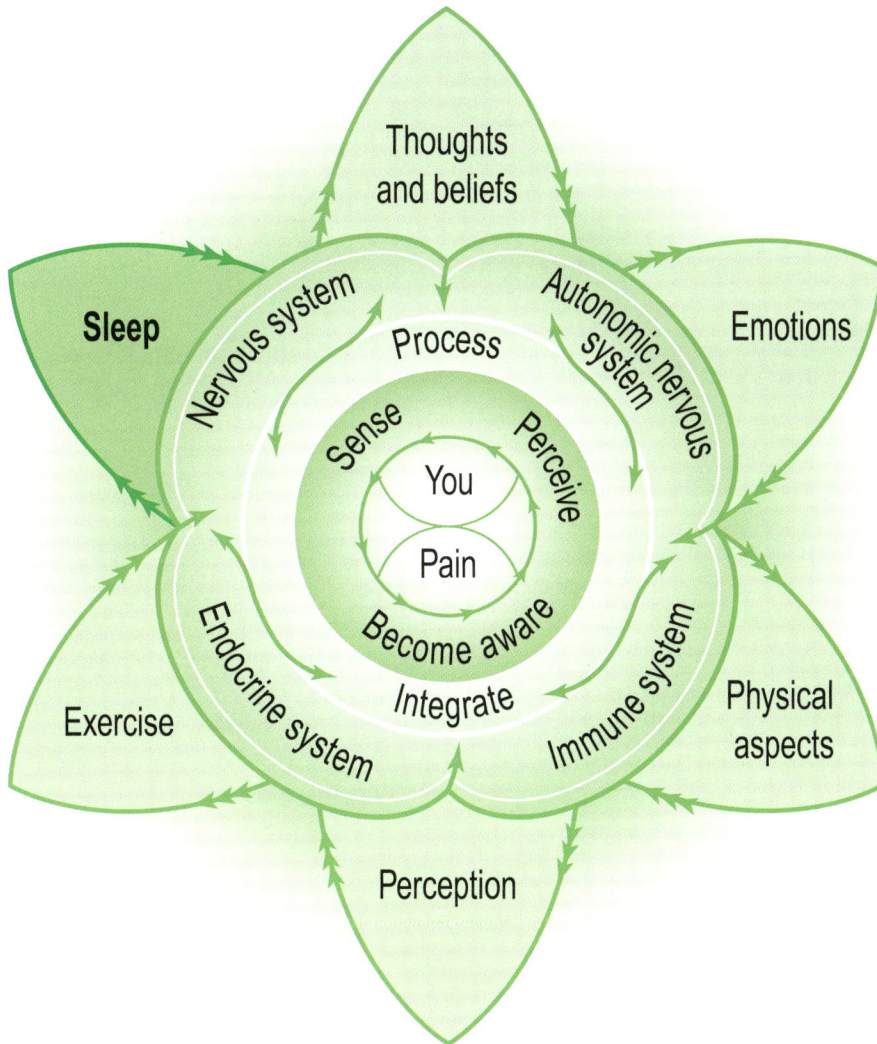

Figure 9.1

Pain Mandala – Sleep. Sleep is a powerful regulator of our immune, endocrine, nervous and autonomic systems. When sleep disturbance is part of the pain picture, as is often the case, these systems can suffer and subsequent processes can integrate to lead to more pain. The reverse can also be true: as sleep improves, so too can regulation of these systems and processes. In turn, all aspects of our health and our sense of self, including pain, may also improve.

Note: This mandala depicts aspects of the human experience of pain covered in Pain Science Yoga Life. *Other inputs, dimensions and body systems can contribute to pain than those noted here.*

Chapter 9

Headspace
Painfully Tired

Oh, those nights of tossing and turning, when you just can't find a position of comfort, be it your thoughts or your body or both that keep sleep at bay. Such was the case for Phillip (Case Study, p.51), whose mind would spin during the night with thoughts of what his life would be like if he couldn't use his hand, and with his pain being so intense that sleep just wouldn't come. Many of us have had the experience of feeling more pain or being sensitive (physically or emotionally) after a poor night's sleep. Sleep disorders are the continuation of such interruptions, which become problematic. According to the *International Classification of Diseases*, there are six main categories of sleep disorders.[1] In this chapter, we will focus on just one, insomnia, and its relationship with pain.

Insomnia is defined as: "a complaint of persistent difficulty with sleep initiation, duration, consolidation, or quality, that occurs despite adequate opportunity and circumstances for sleep, and results in some form of daytime impairment."[1] In other words, difficulty falling asleep or staying asleep frequently enough that it interrupts daily life, could be considered insomnia. Given our understanding of inputs to the pain experience, addressing sleep disturbance could positively impact pain and many aspects of a person's health and quality of life.

In the general population, approximately one-third of adults report some symptoms of insomnia including difficulty initiating or maintaining sleep, with almost 10% fulfilling criteria for insomnia syndrome.[2] But in those with persistent pain, rates are higher, with insomnia affecting over 40%.[3,4] Large community-based studies demonstrate that pain and sleep disturbance frequently co-exist and that this relationship is partly explained by depression, anxiety and stress sensitivity.[5] The Pain Mandala (Figure 9.1) highlights these interactions. We see sleep disturbance commonly in our work as clinicians and teachers, yet perhaps surprisingly, sleep receives little attention in the care of many people with pain. Let's step into this void and explore how pain and sleep interact, how sleep disturbance can be a significant input to pain, and whether improved sleep impacts pain and its effects.

> Scope of practice consideration: If a sleep disorder is present, a referral to a qualified sleep expert for full evaluation and treatment is warranted.

What Is Sleep and What Drives It?

Sleep is defined as: "a reversible condition of reduced responsiveness usually associated with immobility. The decreased ability to react to stimuli distinguishes sleep from quiet wakefulness, while its reversibility distinguishes sleep from coma."[6] Sleep serves many functions, ranging from tissue restoration and brain-metabolite clearance, to emotional regulation and learning.[7] The more sleep has been studied, the more apparent it is that sleep is critical to optimal cognitive, emotional and bodily function.[8]

With the advent of wearable activity technology (that fancy thing on your wrist that you can wear in bed too), many of us are becoming more aware of sleep and its stages. But what is this information telling us? Many people I see in clinic are concerned that only a proportion of their sleep recorded on their device is 'deep sleep'; however, when you look at sleep cycles, this is potentially completely normal. There are two major types of sleep: REM (rapid eye movement) and non-REM sleep, which alternate at regular periods 4–5 times per night. Each cycle lasts about 90–120 minutes. Non-REM sleep is made up of three stages: light sleep (called N1, N2) and deep sleep (N3). Deep sleep is referred to as slow wave sleep and considered to be the most restorative phase of sleep.[7] So, our sleep is naturally made up of light and deep phases.

In theory, loss of slow wave sleep has been thought to contribute to pain, as during slow wave sleep there is a shift towards greater parasympathetic nervous system activity and increased normal endocrine release; therefore, loss of this is important.[9] However, while sleep disturbance is common in people with pain, with evidence of macrostructure changes (e.g. difficulty falling asleep, greater wakefulness through the night and reduced total sleep time), alterations in sleep microstructure (stages of sleep) are more controversial. There is some evidence of loss of slow wave sleep in people with fibromyalgia, but overall, it's not yet clear how relevant this is or how concerned we should be about it in pain states.[9]

What Is Optimal Sleep?

Given the importance of sleep for bodily function, let's check in on what is considered optimal sleep. If we look at the definition of insomnia, then key factors in determining optimal sleep depend more on quality of sleep rather than just quantity, e.g.:

- Ease with which one goes to sleep.
- Ability to stay asleep for reasonable amounts of time.
- Waking reasonably refreshed and not feeling tired during the day.
- Able to function in a productive way the next day.
- Good overall health.

Does 'how much' matter? Like everything else in human nature, that depends on the individual. For one adult, seven hours of sleep will be sufficient, but for another nine hours will be optimal. That said, broad guidelines do exist (Table 9.1):[10] below six hours' sleep is considered deprivation and is associated with higher risk for poor health.[11] What about broken sleep? Well, we all wake slightly at the end of sleep stages. Mostly we're not aware of this but it's not abnormal to wake periodically during the night and

Table 9.1 Sleep Recommendations[10]

Age category	Recommended hours of sleep per day
Newborns (0–3 months)	14 – 17
Infants (4–11 months)	12 – 15
Toddlers (1–2 years)	11 – 14
Preschoolers (3–5)	10 – 13
School-age children (6–13)	9 – 11
Teenagers (14–17)	8–10
Younger adults (18–25)	7–9
Adults (26–64)	7–9
Older adults (65+)	7– 8

as long as this doesn't interrupt quality of sleep too much, it's not necessarily abnormal.

Drivers of Sleep

We'll discuss what influences sleep as a basis for understanding how to address it as part of pain care. Two main processes are thought to control our sleep–wake cycles: homeostatic mechanisms and circadian rhythms.[12]

Homeostatic Mechanisms

The basis for homeostatic mechanisms is that a build-up of substances in the brain occurs as a result of time spent awake. These are called endogenous somnogens (e.g. nitric oxide, cytokines, prostaglandin).[13] As these substances build up, the longer someone is awake they cause 'sleep drive'. We all know that feeling of not being able to keep our eyes open, nodding off despite our best efforts – this is our 'sleep drive'.

Circadian Rhythm: Our Body's Master Clock

Circadian rhythms are processes that are governed by our body's master clock and follow typical patterns throughout the day. This master clock is thought to reside in a part of the brain called the suprachiasmatic nucleus of the hypothalamus. The hypothalamus, as discussed previously, is central to driving many body responses like stress responses and hormonal processes. Its major role for sleep is the secretion of the hormone melatonin.[12] Under normal circumstances the body's master clock is reset daily by light inputs (daylight/artificial light) during the day, and melatonin secretion at night. Indeed, exposure to natural light early in the day helps regulate melatonin release later at night. While the master clock acts as a guide, our circadian rhythm and the processes it drives are not fixed, and demonstrate a degree of plasticity, as in our adjustment to seasonal changes in daylight.[14] People who are morning larks might recognize this as the pull from bed earlier and earlier with the rise of the sun in summer.

'Masking' of the circadian rhythm can occur. This means that non-circadian or environmental factors can affect this natural rhythm,[14] and there are many examples of these: distraction, stress, food, exposure to bright lights and screen-time, caffeine and alcohol intake, irregular sleep patterns, sleep habits and irregular work schedules. As we'll see later, many things we do to improve sleep aim to address some of these lifestyle habits in a bid to recalibrate our natural body clock. Sometimes we need to 'get out of our own way' to allow our body's natural rhythm to re-establish itself – to stop masking our body clock. In practice this is called *sleep hygiene,* referring to our sleep habits and how this influences sleep. Utilizing the yoga practices of saucha (cleanliness) and ahimsa (non-harming) may mean adjusting our daily routines and behaviors to facilitate optimal working of our master body clock to promote good sleep.

> Take home message: Our body's master clock regulates our sleep but is influenced by many factors like stress, diet, caffeine and alcohol, light exposure, screen-time, bed-time routines and exercise.

The Role of Neurotransmitters and Exercise in Sleep

Related to both circadian rhythm and homeostatic mechanisms, sleep and wakefulness are driven by complex interactions between many parts of the brain and their related neurotransmitters.[13] Importantly, inhibitory chemicals like GABA, and neuropeptides, which neurons use to communicate, influence transition into and maintenance of sleep.[13] GABA is a primary inhibitory neurotransmitter (a calming chemical messenger) of the central nervous system (or CNS), and as we learnt in earlier chapters, is important in inhibition of nociception. Its role in sleep is mostly associated with nervous system inhibition and suppression of sensory stimuli during sleep. This is one reason why you don't always wake when there's a loud noise or your partner rolls over in bed. GABA also plays a key role in influencing circadian rhythms.[15] Interestingly, studies examining GABA levels in sleep disorders show differences between healthy controls and those with insomnia but the direction (more or less GABA) is actually inconsistent.[16-18] The key message, then, is that it can become dysregulated.

While sleep studies have traditionally studied the role of CNS processes in governing sleep, increasing attention is being paid to broader contributing factors, e.g. to the role of exercise on sleep. Exercise may exert its influence on sleep in a number of ways (see Uchida et al.[19] for review). For example:

- Exercise can induce CNS fatigue and promote slow wave sleep.

- Exercise can change core body temperature, increasing blood flow to the periphery (peripheral vasodilation). Preliminary data suggest that increases in body temperature from exercise earlier in the day likely reduce body temperature during sleep and facilitate greater slow wave sleep.[20] In contrast, evening exercise may result in higher core body temperatures and greater sympathetic nervous system activity,[20] hence may impede sleep.

- Regular exercise can improve parasympathetic nervous system activity, and hence relaxation responses, reflected in improvements in measures like heart rate and heart rate variability.[20]

- Exercise improves mood and as poor mood negatively influences sleep, exercise may help indirectly by improving mood.[21,22] This may in part be due to the way exercise modulates brain chemicals like dopamine and serotonin, neurotransmitters important in stress, depression and anxiety.[23]

Further research is needed to clarify these mechanisms; however, the positive effects of exercise on sleep provide a basis for the use of physical activity, including asana practice, to improve sleep. As we will explore, this in turn may help pain.

Physiological Effects and Hormonal Function Related to Sleep

The complexity of sleep and all of its physiological and hormonal effects is vast. Let's simply look at key functions that help our understanding of pain.

The Autonomic Nervous System and Sleep

Non-REM sleep is associated with greater parasympathetic (rest and digest) nervous system activity: slowing of heart and respiratory rates and lowering of blood pressure and muscle tone. In tandem, sympathetic (fight or flight) nervous system activity decreases. This is particularly the case during slow wave sleep.[9] During REM sleep sympathetic nervous system activity increases with increases in heart and respiratory rates but muscle tone stays suppressed and parasympathetic nervous system activity remains high or dominant.[24]

Think of a time when you've been feeling stressed, particularly in the evenings – perhaps worrying over the events of the day or future plans. Was your sleep affected? Was it harder to get to sleep? Or perhaps you woke up in the middle of the night? Did you notice your heart rate or how you were breathing? When Phillip (Case Study, p.51) was asked these questions, he noted he would wake with his heart racing and an unsettled feeling. He said the day of the injury would replay like a movie over and over again in his head. For him this may be related to greater sympathetic nervous system activity late in the day, when ideally we would be settling into a more restful state. Looking at the normal function of the autonomic nervous system during sleep, it's easy to see how shifts in the balance between parasympathetic and sympathetic nervous system activity can influence sleep. In turn, both sleep and autonomic nervous system disturbance can be linked to difficulties with pain.

Hormones and Sleep

Regulation of the endocrine system and hormone levels are closely linked with sleep, so sleep disturbance can influence many different aspects of health. Let's look briefly at melatonin and cortisol, two key hormones that are altered when sleep is disturbed, which warrant our attention for regulating sleep, and relating to pain (see Mullington[25] for overview).

Melatonin is important in stimulating sleep – it helps us fall asleep. Although it's technically a nighttime hormone, with higher levels present in the pre-sleep period, regulation of melatonin is heavily influenced by exposure to light. Ideally, we should have some exposure to natural light early in the day, as this suppresses its release. Later in the day as natural light fades, melatonin levels should then increase. However, low daytime exposure to light and exposure to bright light in the pre-sleep period can both reduce melatonin and impede sleep.

Cortisol is an abundant, naturally occurring steroid hormone that, as we've seen, is involved in many bodily processes including stress and inflammatory responses. Cortisol is strongly circadian in its secretion, generally reaching its lowest levels 1–2 hours after sleep onset, and peaking shortly after waking. As discussed in Chapter 5, cortisol is also released as part of our stress response, and high levels of cortisol are associated with greater sympathetic nervous system activity. Cortisol levels are affected by many factors like first exposure to light and exposure to noxious or stressful stimuli. So, having a stressful conversation right before bedtime is likely to raise cortisol levels at a time when they should be reducing and therefore may interrupt sleep. In pain research, cortisol is one of the most commonly studied hormones, due to its role in inflammatory responses and because it is often used to quantify stress responses, which are critically linked with pain.

Let's consider Martha, who has knee osteoarthritis and experiences frequent knee pain. Sleep disturbance and low physical activity are also major issues for her. She could get to sleep quite easily but woke frequently during the night. She often felt tired, which made motivating herself to exercise difficult. A common story! She also reported watching TV late into the evening. As part of her overall care, Martha was asked to consider how sleep and exercise may be interacting with her pain, e.g. how inappropriate light exposure and low physical activity may be 'inputs' affecting her sleep, and in turn, how her sleep disturbance may be an important input for her pain – interactions between the different layers of her Pain Mandala. We discussed options of either starting with small amounts of regular exercise or changing sleep habits, e.g. turning off the TV earlier and doing a short, guided meditation before bed, explaining that this could promote both appropriate melatonin release (by reducing light exposure) and relaxation responses that promote sleep. She chose the latter with great effect. Her sleep improved, as did her motivation to exercise, and in turn, her osteoarthritis symptoms started to settle.

Sleep and Pain Interactions

How do you think sleep and pain interact? Do you think of it as unidirectional: poor sleep drives pain? Or that if poor sleep existed first, then it isn't a factor? This seems to be a common view. Interestingly, the research tells us a two-way relationship between sleep and pain exists: insomnia is a risk factor for persistent pain,[26] and persistent pain is a risk factor for insomnia.[27] Back to the Pain Mandala (see Figure 9.1): poor sleep could be an input or a response, or both. The situation is likely even more complex, with interactions between sleep, pain and other factors highly relevant. Let's explore possible mechanisms and interactions linking sleep and pain. The following is admittedly simplified, but hopefully, the interplay between different mechanisms will be evident.

Sleep and Inhibition of Nociception

In Chapter 1 we discussed inhibition of nociception and how our natural analgesic system (the brain's pharmacy) works, and why this is important in influencing pain experiences. Experimental sleep–pain studies have shown that sleep deprivation is associated with lower pain thresholds[28]: it takes less stimulation to provoke a pain response. How does this happen? One pathway may be 'inhibition of descending analgesia'.[29] In other words, when we're sleep-deprived, our natural pain-relieving system stops working so well, reducing the release of pain-relieving chemicals such as GABA, dopamine, serotonin and endorphins.[13,15,17,28,30] This also makes it easier for incoming signals from tissues to be 'turned up' within the nervous system, increasing the potential for pain. Sleep disturbance can be considered an input that negatively influences nociception, reducing the work of the brain's pharmacy and causing a pro-nociceptive state (Figure 9.2).

When individuals experience persistent pain and ongoing sleep disturbance, it is an open question as to which comes first: does pain drive poor sleep, or poor

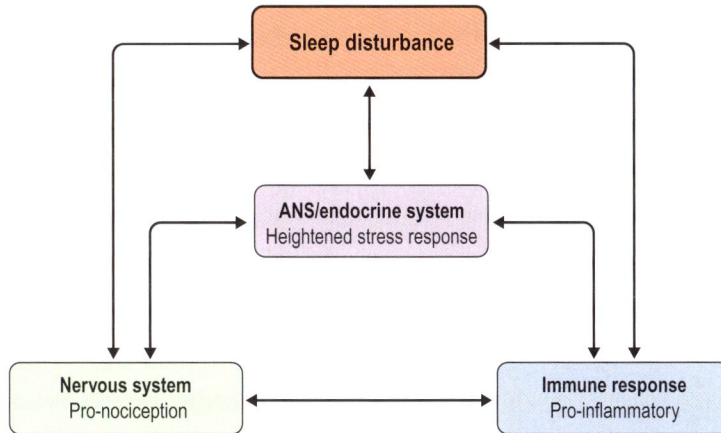

Figure 9.2

Effects of sleep disturbance on pain mechanisms. You haven't been sleeping well lately. Then last night you had an argument with your partner just before bed. You didn't sleep well at all last night and now you've got a terrible headache. How can this poor sleep affect pain?

Sleep disturbance can influence pain by effects on multiple systems. Sleep disturbance can heighten stress responses (ANS and endocrine system), meaning you were probably a little more emotionally reactive in the first place. Vice versa, stress can disrupt your sleep – the argument before you went to bed feeds a vicious circle. Sleep disturbance can influence a pro-nociceptive state (nervous system) and impair immune system responses, causing a pro-inflammatory state (immune system), both of which can increase your pain sensitivity.

The two-way arrows indicate all systems can influence one another. *ANS*, autonomic nervous system.

sleep drive pain? There is certainly evidence of both directions; interestingly, slightly more evidence demonstrates poor sleep drives persistent pain.[28] Further, there may be common mechanisms underpinning both: for example, inflammation and mood.

Sleep and Inflammation

How you ever been through a really busy period, where life was hectic and sleep in short supply, only to find yourself battling a nasty cold or flu? Most of us recognize how being run down like this hampers our immune system, leaving us open to various illnesses. We are less likely to think about this in the context of bodily pain, but actually it's highly relevant.

By now you can see that pain, from a neurophysiological perspective, is the result of many processes in our nervous, immune and hormonal systems.[30–35] This makes sense when we look at immune system functions like inflammation, which we closely associate with pain. In optimum health, immune system function is fairly robust and on the whole resilient to short-lived periods of sleep deprivation.[36] However, prolonged sleep deprivation (e.g. longer than 10 days) can profoundly affect our immune system, promoting a pro-inflammatory state,[36,37] and with greater inflammation comes increased potential for pain (see Figure 9.2). Again, the relationship between sleep and inflammation is a two-way street[30] with poor sleep driving greater inflammation, while the presence of excessive pro-inflammatory cells impedes sleep.[36] So, how does prolonged sleep disturbance influence inflammatory responses? The stress response systems are key pathways here. Remember the HPA (hypothalamic–pituitary–adrenal) axis and the sympathetic nervous systems that we discussed in Chapter 5? These are integral in the relationship between sleep and altered inflammatory responses. Let's discuss cortisol again, which not only is involved in the stress response but also regulates inflammatory responses.

Dysregulation of cortisol (either too much, too little or altered timing) is associated with pro-inflammatory responses.[34,36] As highlighted earlier, cortisol levels are strongly influenced by our circadian rhythm with peaks and troughs evident through our sleep–wake cycle. Cortisol should be at its lowest levels 1–2 hours after sleep onset and peak shortly after waking.[38] Think of cortisol as a Cinderella-like hormone – keep her up too late and her ball-gown turns to rags. Sleep studies show that sleep deprivation and disturbed sleep are associated with altered cortisol levels and in turn a more pro-inflammatory state.[30,36,39–41] A pro-inflammatory state means our tissues are more susceptible to sending warning signals even in the absence of other tissue damage, and more warning signals can mean more pain.[30] The effects of poor sleep on the immune system and in promoting pro-inflammatory responses may also impair tissue healing in acute injury states, providing a further link between sleep disturbance and pain.[30,42,43]

Sleep and Mood Disturbance

In people suffering from persistent pain, mood disorders and cognitive changes can co-exist with sleep disturbance. These relationships represent yet another vicious circle with one inputting on another[27,28,30] (Figure 9.1). Certainly, depression is established as one link between pain and insomnia.[5,15] As outlined in Chapter 5, our mood profoundly influences our natural pain-relieving system,[44–47] so low mood, anxiety and stress can all contribute to pain. In turn, low mood and anxiety co-exist with sleep disturbance,[48,49] each influencing the other.[48] Depressive symptoms and stressful or worried thoughts may explain some of the relationship between sleep disturbance and

pain.[50] For example, cognitive and emotional arousal in the pre-sleep period has been shown to prevent the transition into restful sleep in people with pain and lead to greater pain on the day following sleep disturbance.[51] These worried thoughts may relate to the effects of sleep or pain or broader concerns.

Preoccupation with pain or sleep-related anxieties have also been shown to enhance the influence between pain and insomnia.[52] And so we see a complex dance between depressive symptoms, anxiety, pre-sleep arousal, sleep disturbance and pain – our thoughts, mood, sleep and pain all interacting[30] (see Figure 9.1).

> Take home message: Common interactions between sleep, mood, inflammation and pain include[30]:
>
> - Activation of common neurobiological pathways (areas of the brain and nervous system).
> - Alterations in serotonin, GABA and other inhibitory neurotransmitters creating a pro-nociceptive state.
> - Hyperarousal and elevated sympathetic nervous system and hypothalamus–pituitary axis activity.
> - Pro-inflammatory responses.

Evidence for Sleep Therapies for Sleep and Pain

Ask most people about sleep treatments, and usually they will mention sleeping tablets. Thanks to successful marketing campaigns, most people know more about sleep medication than other sleep therapies. While prescription pharmacological interventions and melatonin have some effectiveness in improving sleep, the degree is often small,[53] and they carry the risk of adverse effects including reducing non-REM slow wave sleep, thus impairing the restorative nature of sleep.[53–55] Further, long-term use of sleep medication carries risks of rebound insomnia, depression, anxiety and addiction, particularly with high doses.[56] The most well-studied and effective *non-pharmacological* intervention is *cognitive behavioral therapy for insomnia (CBT-I)*. CBT-I is a structured psychological intervention for sleep. It is similar to CBT, described previously for mood and pain, in that it combines cognitive and behavioral elements of treatment, but it is different in that these specifically relate to sleep. Components include[57]:

1. Addressing knowledge, thoughts and beliefs about sleep, aiming to reduce stressful and counterproductive thoughts about sleep (e.g. worrying about not being asleep, fear of not sleeping and the consequences of poor sleep).

2. Addressing sleep habits and contributing lifestyle habits (e.g. exercise, diet, alcohol/caffeine intake).

3. Sleep restriction and pacing (i.e. actually reducing time spent in bed) in order to improve sleep efficiency.

4. Relaxation strategies.

CBT-I has the strongest evidence over any other non-pharmacological therapy with modest effects, and demonstrates at least comparable if not superior effects to pharmacological interventions.[57]

Next in the treatment line are *sleep hygiene* interventions – addressing sleep habits. This involves ensuring regular bedtimes, creating an environment that's conducive to sleep, minimizing screen use in the pre-sleep period and addressing lifestyle factors like exercise, diet and alcohol/caffeine consumption, particularly in the pre-sleep period. These approaches form part of CBT-I, and have some positive effects on their own, but are not as effective as the more comprehensive CBT-I.[58] For people with milder sleep disturbances, sleep hygiene practices on their own may do the trick; however, for most people with greater levels of sleep disturbance, more comprehensive treatments may be required.

So, how effective is CBT-I in changing pain and insomnia? So far, CBT-I has been shown to have large effects on insomnia but small effects on pain among people with various pain-related conditions.[59,60]

However, some results show that if people attained at least a 30% improvement in sleep, pain relief was more likely,[61] and the greatest impacts were seen in those with more severe pain and insomnia symptoms.[62]

Exercise is also a potential treatment to aid sleep, with possible underlying mechanisms outlined earlier. Exercise is associated with moderate benefits on sleep quality when performed regularly,[63] and both aerobic and resistance exercise demonstrate positive effects on sleep.[22,63–65]

Is Yoga Effective for Sleep in People with Pain?

When research is grouped together, at present there is insufficient evidence that yoga is effective for improving sleep quality, with some studies showing positive effects but others showing no or limited effects.[66,67] The studies included in these reviews all involved participants attending a yoga class at least once a week. The classes typically involved asana, pranayama and guided relaxation or meditation. In addition, one study included yoga nidra,[68] while another included lectures on yoga philosophy.[69] Further research is needed before we draw conclusions about the effects of yoga on sleep, as most studies to date have investigated specific populations or were preliminary in nature, e.g. had small sample sizes. Future work in this field may allow this evidence to change but for now it would be hard to advocate using yoga as a sole intervention for sleep, particularly in those who are more than mildly affected. So, does yoga have a role at all? Perhaps as part of an overall sleep management program, yoga may be helpful. Here are a few ways yoga may form part of sleep hygiene and/or CBT-I interventions and vice versa (Figure 9.3).

1. As exercise: Depending on the intensity of yoga performed, yoga can be tailored to gain aerobic effects and/or constitute resistance training, both of which have shown positive effects on sleep.[63,64] As some evidence suggests, exercise late

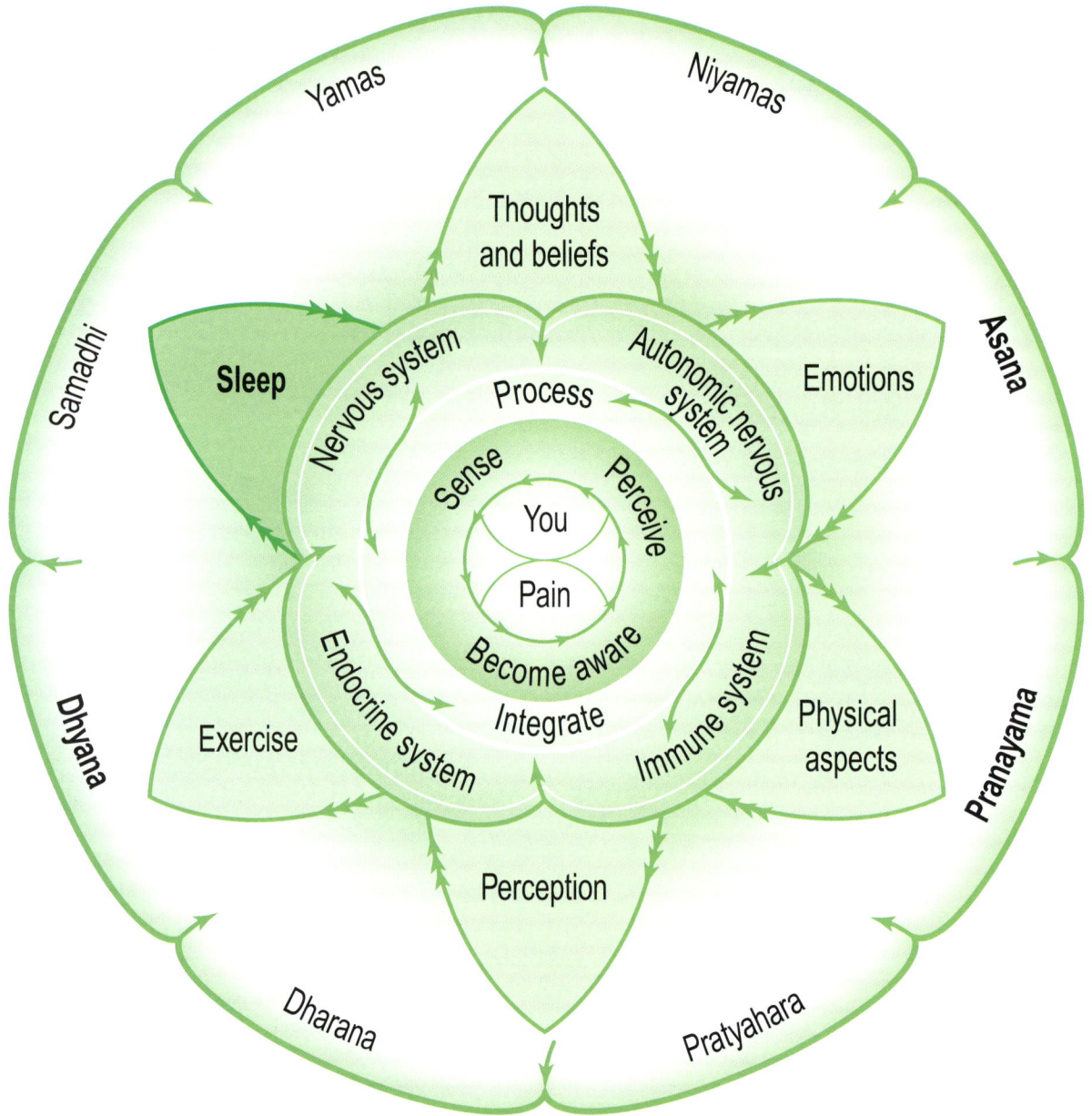

Figure 9.3
Pain and Yoga Mandala – Sleep. Harnessing the yoga limbs Dhyana (meditation), Pranayama (breath awareness) and Asana (postures, movement) may have value to support better sleep in the overall pain care plan. These approaches have the potential to facilitate a relaxation response, improve physiological regulation and help reduce our sensitivity to pain.

in the day may negatively impact sleep;[19,20] current guidelines advocate for the avoidance of intensive exercise late in the evening and advocate for this earlier in the day.[10]

2. To stimulate a relaxation response (reducing stress responses) in preparation for sleep: Gentle asana, meditation and breathing practices and/or yoga nidra could facilitate greater parasympathetic nervous system activity, which could serve as an ideal preparation for sleep. There is low- to moderate-quality evidence that yoga reduces stress responses, e.g. with large effects on lowering cortisol levels (particularly morning and evening cortisol levels),[70] as well as reductions in blood pressure and heart rate.[70,71]

3. As a mindfulness practice to improve mood and reduce the stress and anxiety that can drive poor sleep. As discussed in Chapters 4 and 5, yoga may facilitate sleep by helping to adjust emotional responses and reduce cognitive arousal in relation to both pain and life's stresses in general.

4. Breathing and meditation practices could serve as useful practices during periods of night-time wakefulness: This might serve as a practical tool to moderate stress responses to wakefulness during the night, again reduce stress responses, and promote parasympathetic nervous system activity, and thereby potentially earlier return to sleep.

Conclusion

Sleep and pain are common bedfellows for many with persistent pain. Our journey into sleep and pain has seen us revisit some familiar territory with changes in inflammation, stress responses and mood, interacting with sleep and in turn pain, as illustrated by the Pain Mandala (see Figure 9.1). We've also explored how some of our habits fundamentally disrupt our sleep–wake cycles and how these can be targets for change.

To address Phillip's sleep struggles, he began shutting his phone down and completing all schoolwork by 9:00pm and he committed to a 10:00pm bedtime. During the hour in between, he would choose one or more of the following activities to help set the scene for relaxation and sleep: 1) journaling; 2) body scan; 3) breathing; 4) gentle asanas; or 5) visualization with a sankalpa (positive intention). He liked the ability to alter the hour's activity based on how he was feeling that day. For example, if he was feeling full of worry or seeking, journaling helped him process these thoughts. If he was feeling tense or painful, breathing and asanas proved to be valuable tools to help him find a sense of physical relaxation and reconnection with his body. Some nights he would practice only one of the techniques while other nights he would go through more.

When he laid his head to rest, he was encouraged to utilize the skills of mindfulness he had already been practicing to include all that was there, using *and this too* as a mantra to include his fears and his pain. He chose to reflect with gratitude on his struggles as well as his gifts. He found sleep came more easily, and if he did happen to wake in the night with pain or worry, he would again practice these mindfulness strategies. If he did not return to sleep within 20 minutes, he would rise, turn on a dim light and go back to one of the five items previously noted for no more than 45 minutes, then return to bed. This strategy worked well for Phillip, and after about a month of consistent practice, he re-established an average of 7–8 hours of sleep per night. With these strategies and benefits in mind, let's head onto the mat and into life to see how we can influence sleep.

Out of the Head and Onto the Mat

Transition to practice: These practice sections are not designed to be recipes for practices to give directly to a person participating in pain care. They are meant for you, the reader, to engage in experiential learning – to take the information from 'Headspace' onto your own mat and into life. As the subject, you can first explore the ideas presented, then consider how these might translate into practices for those with whom you work.

Two practices are described below: progressive muscle relaxation and yoga nidra. Progressive muscle relaxation is a simple guided relaxation that can be used as a process for stimulating the relaxation response/parasympathetic nervous system activity. Yoga nidra is somewhat more complex, involving a body scan, intention setting and visualization. Both options are presented as a relaxation exercise that can be used to facilitate winding down into sleep. As you practice, note what allows you to shift to a place of calm, mindfulness and acceptance. This then becomes a place to teach from.

The following examples of scripts are just that – examples derived from multiple sources.[72,73] Feel free to change the wording to suit your personal practice, prior knowledge, style of teaching or the person you are working with. Recording these for yourself and your students may allow more complete relaxation.

Progressive Muscle Relaxation

- **Set up:** Choose to rest in a comfortable seated or lying position.

- **Breath awareness:** Bring your attention to your breath, monitoring the inhalation and exhalation without judgment for a few rounds until you feel settled and ready to proceed with the practice. (See Appendix 1: Pranayama for specific cues if needed.)

- **Muscle relaxation:** You will work your way around the body, squeezing and tensing the muscles in your body and then releasing them. If you find it hard to relax certain parts of your body, don't worry: do what you can without increasing tension and just let it be. Forcing 'relaxation' is a bit of a paradox, as sometimes the harder you try, the more tension you generate. So just let it be. Let's start at your hands:

  o Tighten your hands as much as you can, tighter, tighter…and now release.

  o Tighten your shoulders as much as you can, tighter, tighter…and release.

  o Press your shoulder blades against the floor/chair…press further…and release.

  o Press the back of your head against the floor…press harder…and release.

  o Tense your stomach muscles, pressing your lower back against the floor/chair…and release.

  o Squeeze your hips…squeeze harder…and release.

  o Tighten your thigh muscles, pressing the backs of your legs against the floor/chair…tighter, tighter…and release.

  o Point your toes away to tense your calf muscles…squeeze harder…and release.

  o Point your toes towards your face to tense your shin muscles…squeeze harder…and now release.

  o Now allow your whole body to relax and let go, softening further, allowing the floor/chair to support you fully. Let your body come to stillness. If some areas are hard to relax, just notice them and let them be; remain free from judgment or questions about your body's responses.

Yoga Nidra

- **Set up:** Choose to rest in a comfortable seated or lying position.

- **Breath awareness:** Bring your attention to your breath, monitoring the inhalation and exhalation without judgment for a few rounds until you feel settled and ready to move forward with the practice. (See Appendix 1: Pranayama for specific cues if needed.)

- **Sankalpa:** Create a sankalpa, which is an intention or affirmation based on your deepest desire or wish for yourself. State this as a positive statement in the present tense, as though it's already happening. For example, 'I am comfortable and at ease in my body.' Repeat it to yourself at least three times as though it is already happening.

- **Perform a body scan:** Begin to consciously scan your body, starting at the crown of your head or the tip of your toes. Slowly move your awareness throughout your whole body. You are simply noting, greeting, maybe acknowledging with gratitude or offering an exhalation of relaxation to each body area, without adding any judgments or questions. Take the time you need to gently scan your whole body. (See Appendix 1: Meditation and Pranayama for more specific cues if needed.)

- **Visualization:** Now bring your attention to the area behind your closed eyes. As though you are watching a movie or slides projected on a screen, allow the following images to appear for you.

    o Blue sky with white drifting clouds.

    o A forest, with trees all around you reaching up to the sky.

    o A bonfire on a beach.

    o Waves crashing on the beach.

    o A tall mountain.

    o A candle in a cave.

    o Raindrops.

    o Crescent moon at night, crescent moon shining brightly against a starlit night.

    o A candle flame.

    Note: you can use many forms of visualization, so feel free to choose options you feel comfortable with.

- Continue watching the space of the mind, and observe the thoughts that arise. For the next minute or so allow these thoughts or feelings to come up, taking the role of the witness, and simply observe without any hope or repression.

- **Return:** Repeat your intention to yourself at least three times. Allow this sankalpa to sink into your consciousness.

    o Now bring your awareness back to your body on the floor.

    o Notice your breath. Take some deep breaths, noticing the movement of your body.

    o Now bring your awareness back into the room: notice where you are, notice the sounds that are around you, reminding you of where you are. Bring your attention back to the here and now. Start to wriggle your fingers and toes.

    o When you are ready, start to gently move and stretch your body and open your eyes.

Off the Mat and Into the World

In daily life, identifying habits that contribute to poor sleep and taking positive action to improve sleep are key elements of any sleep therapy. Here are some tips for better sleep, considered key components of sleep hygiene.

- Establish a bedtime: Go to bed and get up at the same time every day, even at weekends. When possible, sleep as much as needed to feel refreshed and healthy during the following day, but not more.

- Try to make your bedroom conducive to sleep: De-clutter it, keep it at a slightly cooler temperature than other rooms, ensure it is well ventilated, and work on soundproofing where necessary. Make the bedroom device-free – this includes a TV. Spoil yourself with a comfortable bed and pillows: there are no set rules here, find the ones that feel best to you.

- Develop a wind-down routine: Spend an hour or so slowing down before you go to bed. Take a bath, read a book, practice meditation or gentle yoga – anything that allows you to relax.

- Be careful using screens, as while they might feel relaxing, a lit screen is quite stimulating for your brain and can prevent the release of sleep-inducing melatonin. For the same reasons, consider reducing exposure to any bright light in the pre-sleep period.

- Avoid stressful or highly stimulating conversations or activities late in the evening. Even highly cognitive tasks or tasks requiring a lot of concentration late in the evening can impede sleep. Meditation or yoga nidra may be a good antidote for stress, and some people find journaling a helpful way to defuse the day's activities.

- Participate in daily exercise. Alternate your exercise times during the day until you find what works well for you.

- Diet matters: Caffeine, alcohol and nicotine, particularly later in the evening, can all lead to wakeful nights. Alcohol may initially help with going to sleep but is associated with more waking during the night. And while going to bed on a full stomach may not be conducive to sleep, neither is going to bed hungry. A light bedtime snack (especially a warm drink) helps many individuals sleep better.

What to do if you wake during the night

- Avoid clock watching: Getting frustrated about being awake is usually counter-productive.

- Rather than trying harder and harder to fall asleep during a poor night, switching on a dim light and doing something else may be helpful. Some might find practicing a guided meditation or yoga nidra helpful to get back to sleep. Otherwise, activities that are relaxing and/or monotonous, such as reading, routine housework/tasks or making to-do or shopping lists, are also recommended.

References

1. World Health Organisation, International Classification of Diseases. 2018; Available from: https://icd.who.int/en.

2. Morin, C.M., M. LeBlanc, M. Daley, et al. Epidemiology of Insomnia: Prevalence, Self-Help Treatments, Consultations, and Determinants of Help-Seeking Behaviors. Sleep Medicine, 2006. 7(2): 123–30.

3. Karaman, S., T. Karaman, S. Dogru, et al. Prevalence of Sleep Disturbance in Chronic Pain. European Review for Medical and Pharmacological Sciences, 2014. 18(17): 2475–81.

4. Mathias, J.L., M.L. Cant, and A.L.J. Burke. Sleep Disturbances and Sleep Disorders in Adults Living with Chronic Pain: A Meta-Analysis. Sleep Medicine, 2018. 52: 198–210.

5. Stubbs, B., D. Vancampfort, T. Thompson, et al. Pain and Severe Sleep Disturbance in the General Population: Primary Data and Meta-Analysis from 240,820 People across 45 Low- and Middle-Income Countries. General Hospital Psychiatry, 2018. 53: 52–8.

6. Cirelli, C. and G. Tononi. Is Sleep Essential? PLoS Biol, 2008. 6(8): e216.

7. Brinkman, J.E. and S. Sharma. Physiology, Sleep, in: StatPearls. 2018, Treasure Island, FL: StatPearls Publishing LLC.

8. Stickgold, R. and M. Walker. Neuroscience of Sleep. 2009, San Diego: Academic Press.

9. Bjurstrom, M.F. and M.R. Irwin. Polysomnographic Characteristics in Nonmalignant Chronic Pain Populations: A Review of Controlled Studies. Sleep Medicine Reviews, 2016. 26: 74–86.

10. Hirshkowitz, M., K. Whiton, S.M. Albert, et al. National Sleep Foundation's Updated Sleep Duration Recommendations: Final Report. Sleep Health, 2015. 1(4): 233–43.

11. Walker, M. Why We Sleep. 2017, New York: Scribner.

12. Pace-Schott, E.F. Sleep Architecture, in: The Neuroscience of Sleep, R. Stickgold and M. Walker, Editors. 2009, San Diego: Academic Press.

13. Monti, J.M. The Neurotransmitters of Sleep and Wake, a Physiological Reviews Series. Sleep Medicine Reviews, 2013. 17(4): 313–5.

14. Minkel, J.D. and D.F. Dinges. Circadian Rhythms in Sleepiness, Alertness, and Performance, in: Neuroscience of Sleep, R. Stickgold and M. Walker, Editors. 2009, San Diego: Academic Press.

15. Ono, D., K.I. Honma, Y. Yanagawa, et al. Role of GABA in the Regulation of the Central Circadian Clock of the Suprachiasmatic Nucleus. Journal of Physiological Sciences, 2018. 68(4): 333–43.

16. Winkelman, J.W., O.M. Buxton, J.E. Jensen, et al. Reduced Brain GABA in Primary Insomnia: Preliminary Data from 4T Proton Magnetic Resonance Spectroscopy (1H-MRS). Sleep, 2008. 31(11): 1499–506.

17. Plante, D.T., J.E. Jensen, and J.W. Winkelman. The Role of GABA in Primary Insomnia. Sleep, 2012. 35(6): 741–2.

18. Morgan, P.T., E.F. Pace-Schott, G.F. Mason, et al. Cortical GABA Levels in Primary Insomnia. Sleep, 2012. 35(6): 807–14.

19. Uchida, S., K. Shioda, Y. Morita, et al. Exercise Effects on Sleep Physiology. Frontiers in Neurology, 2012. 3: 48.

20. Yamanaka, Y., S. Hashimoto, N.N. Takasu, et al. Morning and Evening Physical Exercise Differentially Regulate the Autonomic Nervous System During Nocturnal Sleep in Humans. American Journal of Physiology: Regulatory-Integrative and Comparative Physiology, 2015. 309(9): R1112–21.

21. Wegner, M., I. Helmich, S. Machado, et al. Effects of Exercise on Anxiety and Depression Disorders: Review of Meta-Analyses and Neurobiological Mechanisms. CNS and Neurological Disorders: Drug Targets, 2014. 13(6): 1002–14.

22. Banno, M., Y. Harada, M. Taniguchi, et al. Exercise Can Improve Sleep Quality: A Systematic Review and Meta-Analysis. PeerJ, 2018. 6: e5172.

23. Lin, T.W. and Y.M. Kuo. Exercise Benefits Brain Function: The Monoamine Connection. Brain Science, 2013. 3(1): 39–53.

24. Caples, S.M. and V.K. Somers. Autonomic Dysregulation During REM Sleep, in: Neuroscience of Sleep, R. Stickgold and M. Walker, Editors. 2009, San Diego: Academic Press.

25. Mullington, J.M. Endocrine Function During Sleep and Sleep Deprivation, in: Neuroscience of Sleep, R. Stickgold and M. Walker, Editors. 2009, San Diego: Academic Press.

26. Afolalu, E.F., F. Ramlee, and N.K.Y. Tang. Effects of Sleep Changes on Pain-Related Health Outcomes in the General Population: A Systematic Review of Longitudinal Studies with Exploratory Meta-Analysis. Sleep Medicine Reviews, 2018. 39: 82–97.

27. Doufas, A.G. Pain and Sleep, in: Principles and Practice of Sleep Medicine, M. Kryger, T. Roth, and W.C. Dement, Editors. 2017, Philadelphia: Elsevier.

28. Finan, P.H., B.R. Goodin, and M.T. Smith. The Association of Sleep and Pain: An Update and a Path Forward. Journal of Pain, 2013. 14(12): 1539–52.

29. Smith, M.T., R.R. Edwards, U.D. McCann, and J.A. Haythornthwaite. The Effects of Sleep Deprivation on Pain Inhibition and Spontaneous Pain in Women. Sleep, 2007. 30(4): 494–505.

30. Boakye, P.A., C. Olechowski, S. Rashiq, et al. A Critical Review of Neurobiological Factors Involved in the Interactions between Chronic Pain, Depression, and Sleep Disruption. Clinical Journal of Pain, 2016. 32(4): 327–36.

31. McEwen, B.S. Protective and Damaging Effects of Stress Mediators. New England Journal of Medicine, 1998. 338(3): 171–9.

32. McEwen, B.S. Protective and Damaging Effects of Stress Mediators: Central Role of the Brain. Dialogues in Clinical Neuroscience, 2006. 8(4): 367–81.

33. Simons, L.E., I. Elman, and D. Borsook. Psychological Processing in Chronic Pain: A Neural Systems Approach. Neuroscience and Biobehavioral Reviews, 2014. 39: 61–78.

34. Hannibal, K.E. and M.D. Bishop. Chronic Stress, Cortisol Dysfunction, and Pain: A Psychoneuroendocrine Rationale for Stress Management in Pain Rehabilitation. Physical Therapy, 2014. 94(12): 1816–25.

35. Grace, P.M., M.R. Hutchinson, S.F. Maier, and L.R. Watkins. Pathological Pain and the Neuroimmune Interface. Nature Reviews Immunology, 2014. 14(4): 217–31.

36. Mullington, J.M. Immune Function During Sleep and Sleep Deprivation, in: Neuroscience of Sleep, R. Stickgold and M. Walker, Editors. 2009, San Diego: Academic Press.

37. Irwin, M.R. Why Sleep Is Important for Health: A Psychoneuroimmunology Perspective. Annual Review of Psychology, 2015. 66: 143–72.

38. Hucklebridge, F., T. Hussain, P. Evans, and A. Clow. The Diurnal Patterns of the Adrenal Steroids Cortisol and Dehydroepiandrosterone (DHEA) in Relation to Awakening. Psychoneuroendocrinology, 2005. 30(1): 51–7.

39. Chrousos, G., A.N. Vgontzas, and I. Kritikou. HPA Axis and Sleep, in: Endotext, L.J. De Groot, G. Chrousos, K. Dungan, et al., Editors. 2000, South Dartmouth, MA: MDText.com, Inc.

40. Abell, J.G., M.J. Shipley, J.E. Ferrie, et al. Recurrent Short Sleep, Chronic Insomnia Symptoms and Salivary Cortisol: A 10-Year Follow-up in the Whitehall II Study. Psychoneuroendocrinology, 2016. 68: 91–9.

41. Morgan, E., L.P. Schumm, M. McClintock, et al. Sleep Characteristics and Daytime Cortisol Levels in Older Adults. Sleep, 2017. 40(5).

42. Smith, T.J., M.A. Wilson, J.P. Karl, et al. Impact of Sleep Restriction on Local Immune Response and Skin Barrier Restoration with and without "Multinutrient" Nutrition Intervention. Journal of Applied Physiology (1985), 2018. 124(1): 190–200.

43. Nyland, J., A. Huffstutler, J. Faridi, et al. Cruciate Ligament Healing and Injury Prevention in the Age of Regenerative Medicine and Technostress: Homeostasis Revisited. Knee Surgery Sports Traumatology Arthroscopy, 2020. 28(3): 777–89.

44. Jennings, E.M., B.N. Okine, M. Roche, and D.P. Finn. Stress-Induced Hyperalgesia. Progress in Neurobiology, 2014. 121: 1–18.

45. Lockwood, S.M., K. Bannister, and A.H. Dickenson. An Investigation into the Noradrenergic and Serotonergic Contributions of Diffuse Noxious Inhibitory Controls in a Monoiodoacetate Model of Osteoarthritis. Journal of Neurophysiology, 2019. 121(1): 96–104.

46. Nation, K.M., M. De Felice, P.I. Hernandez, et al. Lateralized Kappa Opioid Receptor Signaling from the Amygdala Central Nucleus Promotes Stress-Induced Functional Pain. Pain, 2018. 159(5): 919–28.

47. Zhuo, M. Descending Facilitation. Molecular Pain, 2017. 13: 1744806917699212.

48. Alvaro, P.K., R.M. Roberts, and J.K. Harris. A Systematic Review Assessing Bidirectionality between Sleep Disturbances, Anxiety, and Depression. Sleep, 2013. 36(7): 1059–68.

49. Lovato, N. and M. Gradisar. A Meta-Analysis and Model of the Relationship between Sleep and Depression in Adolescents: Recommendations for Future Research and Clinical Practice. Sleep Medicine Reviews, 2014. 18(6): 521–9.

50. Harrison, L., S. Wilson, J. Heron, et al. Exploring the Associations Shared by Mood, Pain-Related Attention and Pain Outcomes Related to Sleep Disturbance in a Chronic Pain Sample. Psychology and Health, 2016. 31(5): 565–77.

51. Tang, N.K., C.E. Goodchild, A.N. Sanborn, et al. Deciphering the Temporal Link between Pain and Sleep in a Heterogeneous Chronic Pain Patient Sample: A Multilevel Daily Process Study. Sleep, 2012. 35(5): 675–87a.

52. Akerstedt, T. Psychosocial Stress and Impaired Sleep. Scandinavian Journal of Work Environment and Health, 2006. 32(6): 493–501.

53. Wilt, T.J., R. MacDonald, M. Brasure, et al. Pharmacologic Treatment of Insomnia Disorder: An Evidence Report for a Clinical Practice Guideline by the American College of Physicians. Annals of Internal Medicine, 2016. 165(2): 103–12.

54. Glass, J., K.L. Lanctôt, N. Herrmann, et al. Sedative Hypnotics in Older People with Insomnia: Meta-Analysis of Risks and Benefits. British Medical Journal, 2005. 331(7526): 1169.

55. Rosner, S., C. Englbrecht, R. Wehrle, et al. Eszopiclone for Insomnia. Cochrane Database Systematic Reviews, 2018. 10: CD010703.

56. Li, C.-T., Y.-M. Bai, Y.-C. Lee, et al. High Dosage of Hypnotics Predicts Subsequent Sleep-Related Breathing Disorders and Is Associated with Worse Outcomes for Depression. Sleep, 2014. 37(4): 803–9.

57. Trauer, J.M., M.Y. Qian, J.S. Doyle, et al. Cognitive Behavioral Therapy for Chronic Insomnia: A Systematic Review and Meta-Analysis. Annals of Internal Medicine, 2015. 163(3): 191–204.

58. Chung, K.F., C.T. Lee, W.F. Yeung, et al. Sleep Hygiene Education as a Treatment of Insomnia: A Systematic Review and Meta-Analysis. Family Practice, 2017. 35(4): 365–75.

59. Tang, N.K.Y., S.T. Lereya, H. Boulton, et al. Non-pharmacological Treatments of Insomnia for Long-Term Painful Conditions: A Systematic Review and Meta-Analysis of Patient-Reported Outcomes in Randomized Controlled Trials. Sleep, 2015. 38(11): 1751–64.

60. Ho, K.K.N., P.H. Ferreira, M.B. Pinheiro, et al. Sleep Interventions for Osteoarthritis and Spinal Pain: A Systematic Review and Meta-Analysis of Randomized Controlled Trials. Osteoarthritis Cartilage, 2019. 27(2): 196–218.

61. Smith, M.T., P.H. Finan, L.F. Buenaver, et al. Cognitive-Behavioral Therapy for Insomnia in Knee Osteoarthritis: A Randomized, Double-Blind, Active Placebo-Controlled Clinical Trial. Arthritis and Rheumatology, 2015. 67(5): 1221–33.

62. McCurry, S.M., S.M. Shortreed, M. Von Korff, et al. Who Benefits from CBT for Insomnia in Primary Care? Important Patient Selection and Trial Design Lessons from Longitudinal Results of the Lifestyles Trial. Sleep, 2014. 37(2): 299–308.

63. Kredlow, M.A., M.C. Capozzoli, B.A. Hearon, et al. The Effects of Physical Activity on Sleep: A Meta-Analytic Review. Journal of Behavioral Medicine, 2015. 38(3): 427–49.

64. Kovacevic, A., Y. Mavros, J.J. Heisz, and M.A. Fiatarone Singh. The Effect of Resistance Exercise on Sleep: A Systematic Review of Randomized Controlled Trials. Sleep Medicine Reviews, 2018. 39: 52–68.

65. Singh, N.A., T.M. Stavrinos, Y. Scarbek, et al. A Randomized Controlled Trial of High Versus Low Intensity Weight Training Versus General Practitioner Care for Clinical Depression in Older Adults. Journals of Gerontology: Series A, Biological Sciences and Medical Sciences, 2005. 60(6): 768–76.

66. Rubio-Arias, J.A., E. Marin-Cascales, D.J. Ramos-Campo, et al. Effect of Exercise on Sleep Quality and Insomnia in Middle-Aged Women: A Systematic Review and Meta-Analysis of Randomized Controlled Trials. Maturitas, 2017. 100: 49–56.

67. Patel, N.K., A.H. Newstead, and R.L. Ferrer. The Effects of Yoga on Physical Functioning and Health Related Quality of Life in Older Adults: A Systematic Review and Meta-Analysis. Journal of Alternative and Complementary Medicine, 2012. 18(10): 902–17.

68. Newton, K.M., S.D. Reed, K.A. Guthrie, et al. Efficacy of Yoga for Vasomotor Symptoms: A Randomized Controlled Trial. Menopause, 2014. 21(4): 339–46.

69. Manjunath, N.K. and S. Telles. Influence of Yoga and Ayurveda on Self-Rated Sleep in a Geriatric Population. Indian Journal of Medical Research, 2005. 121(5): 683–90.

70. Pascoe, M.C., D.R. Thompson, and C.F. Ski. Yoga, Mindfulness-Based Stress Reduction and Stress-Related Physiological Measures: A Meta-Analysis. Psychoneuroendocrinology, 2017. 86: 152–68.

71. Pascoe, M.C. and I.E. Bauer. A Systematic Review of Randomised Control Trials on the Effects of Yoga on Stress Measures and Mood. Journal of Psychiatric Research, 2015. 68: 270–82.

72. Miller, R. Yoga Nidra: A Meditative Practice for Deep Relaxation and Healing. 2010, Boulder, CO: Sounds True Inc.

73. Lusk, J. Yoga Nidra for Complete Relaxation and Stress Relief. 2015, Oakland, CA: New Harbinger Publications Inc.

Namaste – I bow to you.

I bow to the divine in you.

I bow to the essence of you.

Perhaps a fitting way to bring this book to a close is to acknowledge the essence in us. Despite the presence of pain and the suffering it may cause, the essence or true self is ever present, at the heart of each and every one of us. Yoga is an experiential practice to be cultivated, with the true benefits emerging like a journey with consistent practice over time. Moving beyond pain also takes a journey, one that requires considerable strength and resilience, wisdom and hope. We started this book with the recognition that each person in pain is on a journey of their own; each person in pain has their own unique past, their unique story, their diagnosis, their own contributing factors or 'inputs' to their pain and suffering. Starting with this recognition we may create awareness and gentle shifts away from pain and the suffering it causes.

As we moved through the chapters and explored different dimensions of pain, we recognized the science of each and the interplay between them. This dimensional interplay was represented in the Pain Mandala – how the different constructs discussed have effects on our physiology, psychology and behaviors, and ultimately how these all come together to become the pain experience. We are complex. We are integrated. The pain we experience arises with this. And while we understand this complexity, we try not to take for granted the layers of integration at play – multidimensional systems, and the body, mind and spirit all dancing separately and together. Perhaps when we learn to pause, notice and become aware, we can see each of us has the ability to become our own medicine. Though the current evidence base for yoga as a stand-alone treatment is not strong, it can support pain care. Through a few relatively simple practices great health benefits can be gained. This realization may allow new opportunities for pain care.

We recognize that some of the approaches to pain care presented may appear simple, but that doesn't make them easy. For those with pain, there are skills to be learned, awareness to be created and shifts to be made. Listed below are some of the challenges and limitations facing us as teachers and clinicians, as well as our clients.

- *Thoughts and beliefs*: It can be a challenge to come to an understanding of how our pain works. It can be a challenge to let go of some things that we thought we always knew and embrace new ways of thinking. It can be a challenge to realize what is *real but not true*. It can be a challenge to know that this might change in the future too.

- *Mood*: It can be a challenge to start to notice our reactions, to notice how mood influences pain, to notice when we've moved into a stress response, or indeed, we can become so caught up in a stress cycle that we're not even aware when we're in a state of distress. It can be a challenge to start to gently shift away from patterned responses and choose a different response, to cultivate practices and carve out enough time to teach our bodies and minds how to relax and find balance. And it can be a challenge to stay patient and hopeful through this potentially long journey.

- *Physical aspects*: When we're in pain or working with people in pain, it can be easy to blame the physical body for all of the pain and suffering we experience. It may be the only explanation for pain until now. It can be a challenge to let some of this go. In the sense of *real but not true* we might see diagnoses, pathology, or alignment issues as only one part of the story and maybe not the full explanation for pain. It can be a challenge to hold space for a diagnosis as well as holding space for all that we *can* do, even with a diagnosis – *and this too.*

It can be a challenge to explore when our approach to movement is helpful or not so helpful, to become aware that what once served us may not be serving us still, and again to let go of unhelpful patterned movement strategies. It can be a challenge to acknowledge when our body has changed and we need to adjust how we see our body's capacity: to recognize when we need to pull back a little and move with gentleness – to practice kindness for ourselves through satya (truth) and ahimsa (non-violence) during movement when we're in pain or healing an injury – but to also practice self-compassion and contentment (santosha) for what we *can* do.

- *Perception:* All of these factors feed into our sense of self. This can be a sense of our physical body, our pain, our situation, or indeed a broader awareness of our purpose and sense of self. Our self-perception may be an ideal space for exploring *real but not true.* This can be a challenge, but perhaps this is the place where great opportunity arises.

With an aim of moving beyond pain, we can start to integrate these concepts to develop a deeper awareness of who we are, what pain is and how it can be helpful and unhelpful for us and for those participating in pain care. The Pain Mandala highlights this integration and development of awareness. As the center of the mandala demonstrates, the 'you', the true self, can grow stronger while pain and our suffering fade. We can see how pain science and yoga can start to offer not only an insight into pain and suffering but some of the tools needed to move beyond pain: simple tools like moving mindfully, meditating, incorporating exercise and sleep hygiene into our day, replacing our reactive patterned thoughts and emotional responses for more conscious responses. Our roles as clinicians and teachers using yoga is to help people become aware, offer guidance and encouragement but ultimately meet people where they are: it is their own journey. Hopefully, we can provide the catalyst for a step toward a life they desire.

For each of us on our unique journey of learning, and for those we work with on their journey beyond pain – *namaste.*

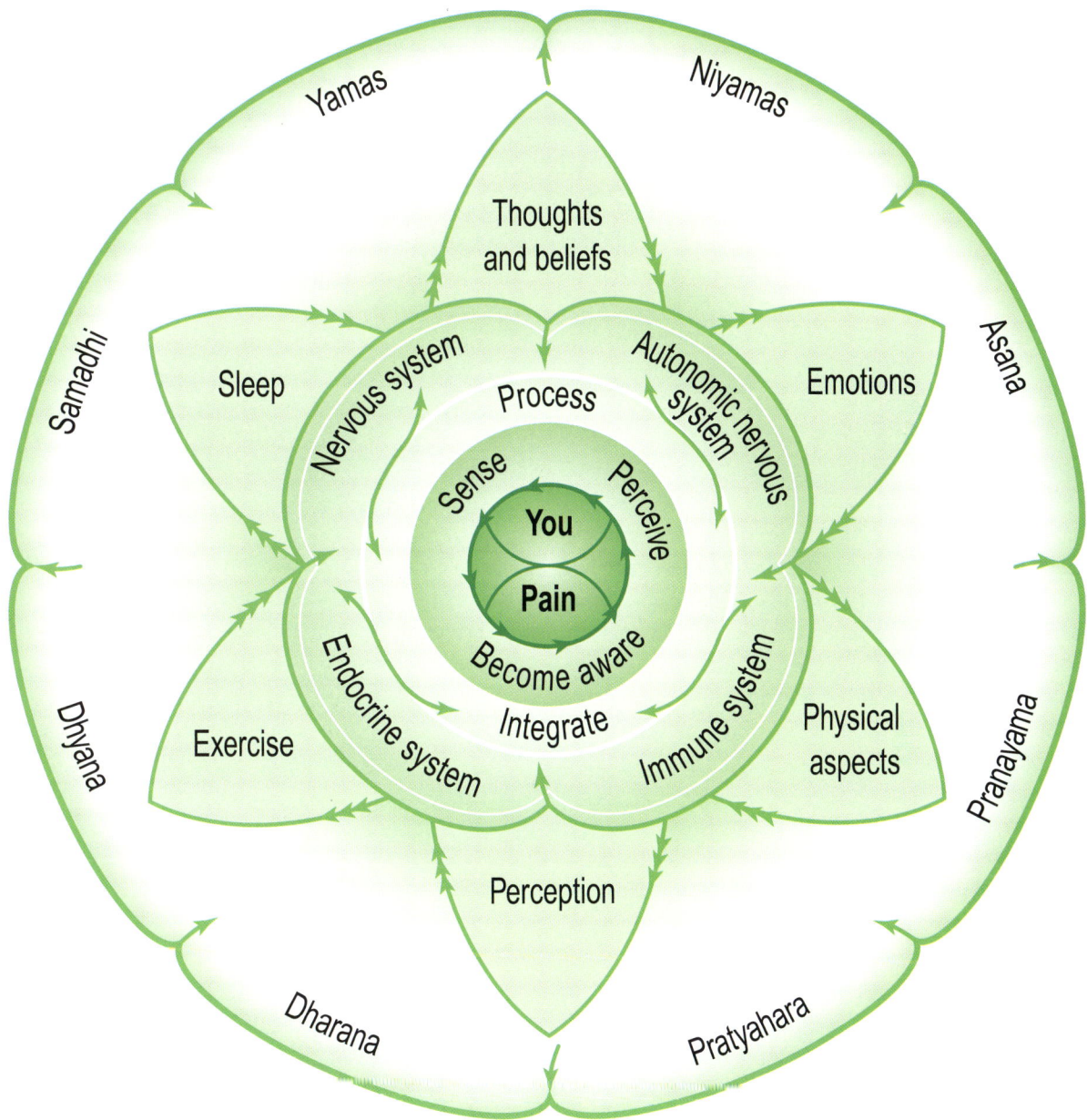

Yamas

Niyamas

Thoughts and beliefs

Sleep

Nervous system

Process

Autonomic nervous system

Emotions

Samadhi

Asana

Sense

Perceive

You

Pain

Become aware

Dhyana

Exercise

Endocrine system

Integrate

Immune system

Physical aspects

Pranayama

Perception

Dharana

Pratyahara

203

Meditation

Meditation Notes

Meditation is a practice. Becoming skilled at finding and keeping the desired focus can take a lifetime of practice. Throughout this book we have discussed the evidence that supports the use of meditation and mindfulness as an intervention for persistent pain. In the practice sections we introduced creative, therapeutic adaptations to some standard practices. Here we would like to share a few general points about meditation and share a few practices as they tend to be generally used without the specificity for pain. We hope you can see how easy adapting these for pain care can be and find courage to do this on your own. Each time you notice your focus has drifted away with thoughts, sounds, images or sensations, that's OK: simply encourage yourself back to the point of focus. This is the practice: you go away and you come back, each time finding forgiveness for yourself and your struggles – these all get to be included with kindness.

Notes on Cues

A few common cues used to encourage you to find a focal point within yourself and let go of the distractions happening around you are things like: go within, drop in, consider your internal landscape, from an inward-looking perspective, etc.

Notes on Posture

During led meditation the facilitator may open with verbal instructions on posture and alignment. These instructions can be a form of mindfulness of the body or act as an opportunity for a brief check-in. As the practitioner follows cues to settle into a purposeful position, these cues may help to set the physical scene

of an intention to focus. However, as we discussed at length in Chapter 6 on physical aspects of pain, the expectations of specific postures may not be helpful when it comes to pain care. Therefore, we have opted to simply encourage taking a comfortable position prior to beginning meditation. If you are interested in exploring the common cues given for seated meditation, they are included here. Most importantly, the posture chosen should encourage a sense of relaxation and alertness.

Posture Cues

1. Assume a comfortable sitting posture.

2. Relax your hips and legs; allow yourself to be rooted in your seat.

3. Hands rest on the knees – palms turned up or turned down or one of each.˙

4. The spine is upright yet relaxed.

5. Shoulders are relaxed away from the ears.

6. Chin is slightly dropped.

7. Allow the crown of the head to be lifted.

8. Eyes can be opened or closed.

Find a Comfortable Seat

It may be assumed that movement of any kind is not permitted during meditation; however, that is not true. Forcing and straining yourself to stay in

---

˙ The positioning of the palms can act as a reflection of intention for the practice. Palms up: the reflected intention is openness to receive. Palms down: the intention is to be internally focused without allowing distractions from external inputs. One up and one down: reflects balance of inward and outward awareness.

one position is discouraged. If you notice postural discomfort while you are meditating, you may like to first try acknowledging its presence and reassuring yourself that you are OK, and return to the focus of the meditation. This may be enough to allow the feelings to shift, and for comfort to settle back in. If the discomfort persists or is intense enough to be distracting, forcing yourself to stay is not helpful for your body or your mind. Feel free to adjust your position as needed. Seated meditations are not the only option; you could stand or lie down, or even walk. The position itself is not the focal point; that's what asanas are designed for. The use of props such as blocks, bolsters, pillows and chairs is welcomed to help you form a supported shape, allowing your body to be relatively still and your mind to focus.

Meditation Mudras

These are hand positions or gestures that may be instructed as part of a meditation practice. They encourage you to form a specific shape with the hand that has a traditional representation to support or channel the focus of the practice. For example, forming the 'OK' sign with your fingers (touching the tip of index finger to tip of the thumb with the other three fingers extended) is said to represent concentration and the 'yoking or union' of the yoga practice.

Sankalpa

A specific individualized intention. This is instructed by some meditation teachers prior to each practice. It is another point of focus for harnessing your own self-will or prana.

Guided Meditations

Open Monitoring Meditation

- Find a comfortable posture.
- Close your eyes or drop your gaze and bring your attention to your breath. Spend a few minutes on breath awareness (breath awareness practice is described in detail in Chapter 5, or you can use a technique of your own).

- Set an intention of mental focus that is all-inclusive. You are aware and open to your own inner and outer environments. Allow the mind to be calm and relaxed, not focused on anything in particular, but present and willing to include.

- When thoughts arise, notice them and simply let them pass through your mind. If you find yourself following those thoughts, engaging in an internal conversation, simply acknowledge this and encourage your focus to that of open and aware. If you need to reconnect with the breath to discourage the tracking of thoughts or images, you can do so. Once you feel focused, allow the openness to return.

- Allow the mind to be present and all-inclusive. When you notice sounds or other sensations, let them be as they are without engaging them or rejecting them. When thoughts or sensations arise, acknowledge them and permit them – tell yourself, 'It's OK to think this, it's OK to feel this,' each time gently encouraging a return to the open awareness.

- Continue this practice for several minutes. When you're ready to end, bring your attention back to your breath for a few moments, then back into the room you are in, before opening your eyes and ending the exercise.

Loving-Kindness Meditation

- Find a comfortable position.
- Close your eyes or drop your gaze and bring your attention to your breath as described above. Spend a few minutes on breath awareness. When the mind wanders, acknowledge it and bring it back to rest on your breath.

- Allow your attention to turn inward to your body. Notice what you feel, how that part of your body feels. How does this make you feel?

- When you are ready, allow these phrases to come to mind:

  May I be filled with loving kindness

  May I be free from suffering

  May I be well in body and mind

  May I be at ease and happy

- Take your time, and allow each phrase to settle, listening to any thoughts, feelings and bodily sensations as you do. There is no need to judge what arises; simply acknowledge it and allow it to be.

- Play with this meditation by:

  o Extending it to a person whom you love or have loved unconditionally, wishing them well in the same way, using the same phrases.

  o Extending it to someone you see regularly but whom you don't really know like a bus driver or shop assistant.

  o Extending it to someone with whom you have a more difficult relationship.

  o Then return to practice this extending these wishes to yourself.

- To close this practice, bring your attention back to your breath for a few moments and then drop your attention into your body once more. Finish with a few deep breaths. Bring your attention back to the room you are in and finish your practice.

Body Scan Meditation

- Allow your awareness to travel through your body, sensing your body. Simply feel each part as it is mentioned without moving. Notice all sensations and allow them to be, just as they are, without judgment. If thoughts arise or you get caught in a narrative about your body, just notice that and come back to simply sensing your body.

- Bring your attention to your right hand. Feel and sense your whole right hand: right forearm, elbow, upper arm, shoulder. Have a sense of your whole right arm and hand as one.

- Sense the right side of your trunk: your chest, upper abdomen, lower abdomen.

- Bring your attention to your right hip, thigh, knee, lower leg and foot – the top and sole of the foot. Have a sense of your whole right leg and foot.

- Now feel the whole right side of your body.

- Now move your attention to the left hand. Feel and sense the whole of your left hand: left forearm, elbow, upper arm, shoulder. Have a sense of your whole left arm and hand as one.

- Sense the left side of your trunk: your chest, upper abdomen, lower abdomen.

- Bring your attention to your left hip, thigh, knee, lower leg and foot – the top and sole of the foot. Have a sense of your whole left leg and foot.

- Now feel the whole left side of your body.

- Move to the back of your body: the backs of your legs against the floor/chair, left buttock, right buttock, lower back, middle back, upper back, back of your neck. Run your awareness along the whole spinal column, from bottom to top. Sense the back of your head against the floor.

- Now move your awareness to the front of your body. Starting at your forehead, eyebrows, space between the eyebrows, nose, left cheek, right cheek, jaw, tongue, front of your neck, chest. And back to your breath.

- Have a sense of your whole body as one: your whole body resting, supported on the floor.

Pranayama
Guidance and Reflections

As I read various texts to brush up on the more traditional forms of pranayama, I am fascinated by the number of 'should(s)' written. 'You should practice first thing in the morning, you should practice after bathing, you should practice in a specific space,' should, should, should…makes me think, "*Stop shoulding all over yourself.*" (My friends hear this from me frequently; as I recall, it, or something similar, comes from the HBO show, *Sex and the City.*) I am sure some of these should(s) may help to maximize the mechanisms of the practice as well as establish healthier rituals, but for now let's just agree the best time and place to practice is the one that works best for you in your life, right now.

Posture

Traditionally, pranayama is performed while seated with a few specific practices done standing. Ultimately, the principles discussed in meditation stand true here as well. The aim is a comfortable position that allows the body and mind to be relaxed and alert.

Nostril Breathing

Unless otherwise indicated, the pranayama practice is performed through the nostrils, both the inhalation and the exhalation. If the natural tendency is to breathe through the mouth, setting an intention for a certain number of breaths in and out through the nostrils can be a pranayama practice in itself.

Don't Strain

This includes any sensation of straining, with the breath, posture, pain or dizziness. Here we go again with the 'shoulds' and 'don'ts', but this one is important. No matter what style or duration, pranayama should not be performed with a sense of physical straining. If the recommended length of time or repetitions creates a sensation of straining, be it the inhalation, exhalation or retention, simply soften the expectation and start with a shorter breath or skip retaining the breath. Sometimes these feelings of straining occur in the beginning of a practice and a simple encouragement to the self to relax can shift it. Sometimes straining sensations occur

after minutes of performance: again, encouragement for relaxation can help or it might be necessary to stop the practice and take a few natural breaths. The practice can then be resumed or completed.

Contraindications

Individuals with some specific conditions should not practice forms of pranayama. It is always a good idea to consult someone with formal training in medicine and yoga prior to beginning a new practice. If in doubt, keeping to simple breath awareness (see Chapter 5) is beneficial and safe.

Pranayama Practices

Start each of the practices described here with breath awareness: begin to relax, breathe through the nose and take gentle note of your inhalations and exhalations. Breath awareness is outlined specifically in Chapter 5.

Ujjayi: victorious breath, psychic breath or ocean breath

Slowly draw your awareness to the back of the throat. Begin to imagine the breath is coming in and out from your throat. It becomes slightly audible like a soft snoring sound with each breath, long and deep. Ujjayi can be a stand-alone practice for 10 breaths to 5 minutes, or it can be used to accompany a meditation practice for the duration. It can also be used to lead into other pranayama practices or in conjunction with asana performance.

Nadi shodhana: alternate nostril breathing

Take one hand in front of your face, placing the second and third fingers either on the forehead or in the palm of the hand. This allows the thumb and fourth finger to be used to block the nostrils. Traditionally, the right hand is used, the thumb blocks the right nostril and the fourth finger blocks the left. If this isn't comfortable, just change it. Use either hand and any finger/thumb combination that works for you. After a few rounds of breath awareness or ujjayi, perform the following:

- Block the right nostril and inhale slowly through the left.

- Then pause to block the left, release the right, and exhale completely through the right nostril; pause; inhale through the right.

- Then pause to block the right and release the left, and exhale completely.

- Keeping the right blocked, now inhale through the left …

- Continue alternating side to side in this way.

Keep this alternating pattern going for as long as you feel comfortable. This practice can also be reversed to inhale right and exhale left. Traditionally, these are said to have different effects on the nervous system.

Kapalbhati: frontal lobe cleansing breath

This practice consists of a forced exhalation and relaxed inhalation. Exhalation is through the nose by contracting the abdominal muscles (drawing the belly back to the spine). The inhalation occurs with a relaxed passive recoil of the abdomen. The exhalation is rapid and strong and a result of only the abdomen contracting; the face, neck, shoulders and chest all remain relaxed. The rate is slowly and steadily increased. Begin with 10 consecutive breaths in this fashion. Pause to a natural inhalation and exhalation, then resume kapalbhati breathing of 10 breaths, repeating 2–5 rounds or as long as it is comfortable. This is contraindicated for anyone with heart disease, high blood pressure, vertigo, epilepsy, stroke, hernia or gastric ulcer, and in pregnancy.

APPENDIX 2: ASANA

The following images of asanas or yoga postures could be used to help set up a simple asana practice for the 'Out of the Head and Onto the Mat' sections. There are many resources available in print and on the web to offer a greater array of postures. Please use these images as a sample and reference; the model is human and lets the abilities and limitations of her own body guide her practice. This is what we advocate for others to do as well.

Scope of practice consideration: There is more to yoga asana than matching a picture or following a sequence. We encourage all who are not yoga practitioners or teachers to recognize the scope of skills and training. Please consider working with someone who is trained to help initiate an individualized practice.

Standing Sequence

Surya Namaskara A – Sun Salutation A

Surya: sun; *namaskara:* respectful greeting or salute

Tadasana	Urdva Tadasana	Uttanasana	Urdva Uttanasana
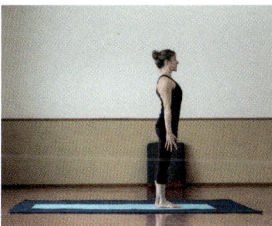	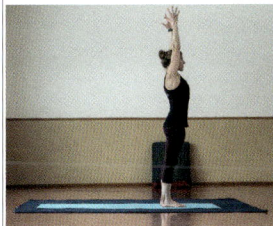	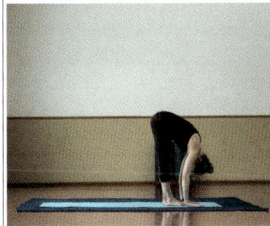	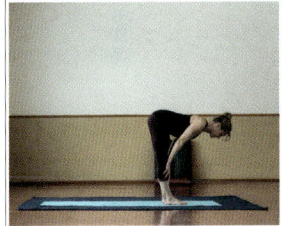
Mountaln	Upward-facing mountain	Standing forward fold	Upward-facing forward fold

Dondasana	Chaturanga Dandasana	Urdhva Mukha Svanasana	Adho Mukha Svanasana
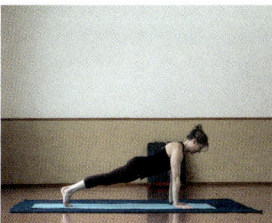	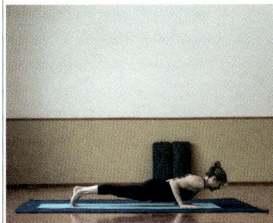	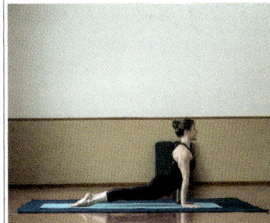	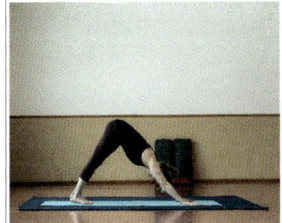
Plank	Four limbs posture: lowering aspect of push-up	Upward-facing dog	Downward-facing dog

Standing sequence posture options to add into Surya Namaskara to create a flow (see Chapter 8 for example).

Virabhadrasana I (modified)	Virabhadrasana II	Utthita Parsvakonasana	Utthita Trikonasana
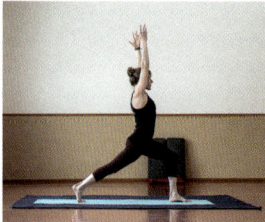	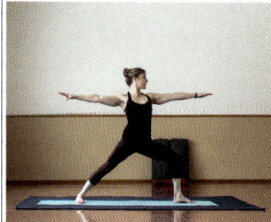	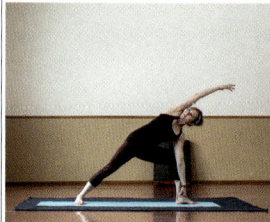	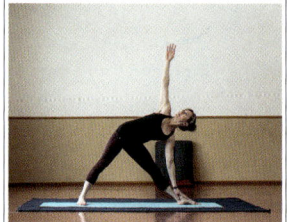
Warrior 1 (modified to crescent lunge)	Warrior 2	Extended side angle	Extended triangle

Prasarita Podottanasana	Vriksasana	Virabhadrasana III	Utkatasana
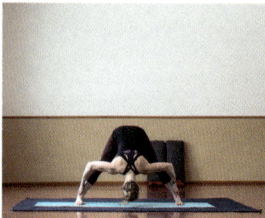	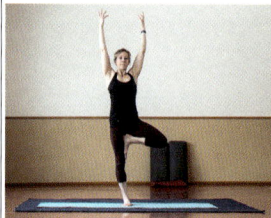	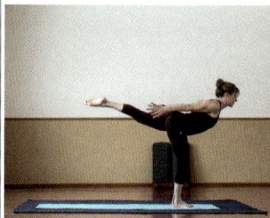	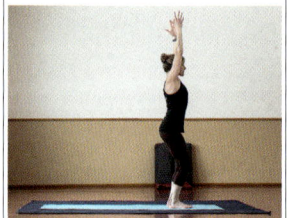
Wide leg forward fold	Tree	Warrior 3	Chair

Kneeling or Modified Sequence

Bharmanasana	Marjaryasana	Bitilasana	Balasana
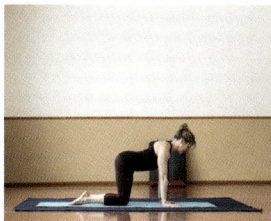	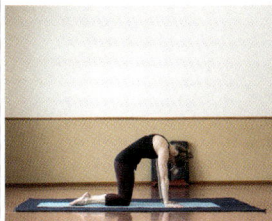	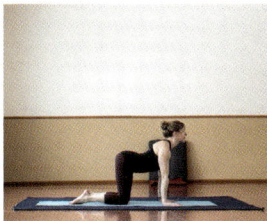	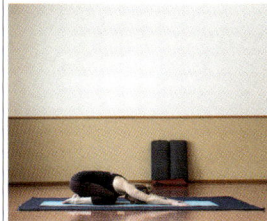
Table top	Cat	Cow	Child's pose

Uttana Shishosana	Anjaneyasana	Parsva Balasana	Modified Dandasana
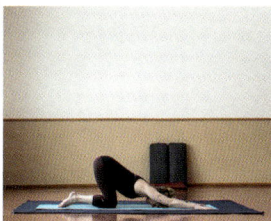	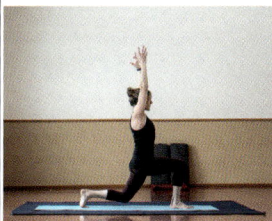	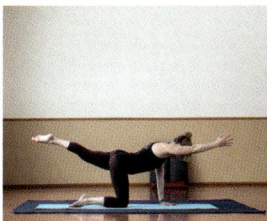	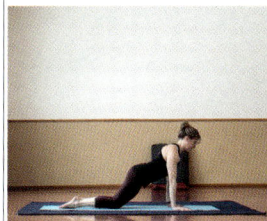
Puppy	Kneeling crescent or low lunge	Bird-dog	Modified plank

Modified Chaturanga Dandasana	Bhujangasana
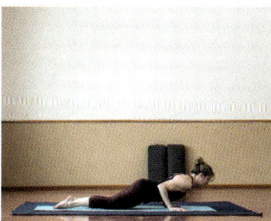	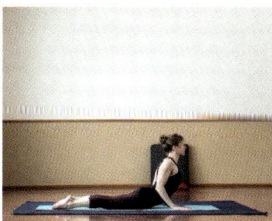
Modified four limbs posture: lowering aspect of push-up	Cobra

Seated Postures

Baddha Konasana	Matsyendrasana (modified)	Janu Sirsasana	Sukhasana
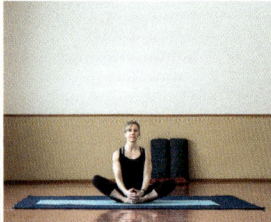	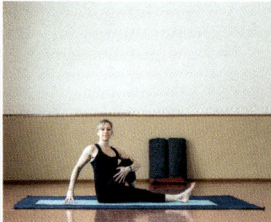	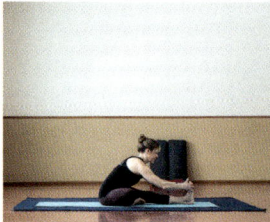	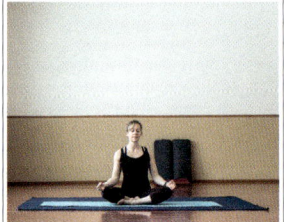
Cobbler's/Butterfly	Seated twist modified	Seated hamstring stretch	Simple cross-legged

Closing Postures

Urdhva Dhanurasana modified	Apanasana	Supta Ardha Apanasana	Supta Matsyendrasana
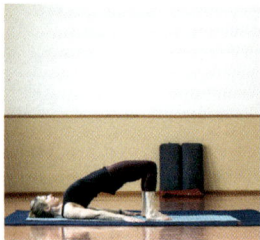	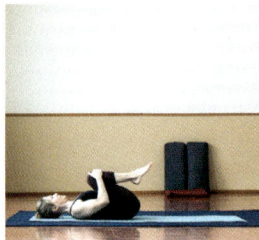	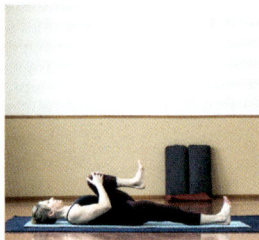	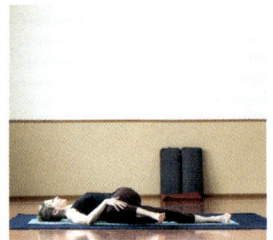
Bridge	Supine double knee to chest	Supine single knee to chest	Supine simple twist

Savasana
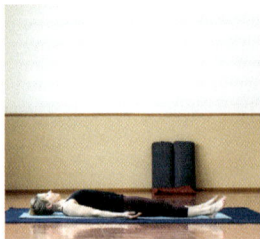
Corpse

Table A.1 Evidence-Based Hints for Asana Instruction

Asana/example of instruction to avoid	Reasons to adjust this instruction	Guidance for evidence-based and balanced instruction
Utkatasana (chair pose); Virabhadrasana (Warrior poses) '(To protect your knees) Don't let your knees travel in front of your ankle'.	1. While this instruction may lead to reductions in load on the knee and quadriceps, it increases the load through hips and spine. 2. Training to improve load tolerance of knees and quadriceps to these normal positions may be advantageous for people who find this difficult. 3. Our knees travel in front of our ankles frequently in normal life: walking downhill/downstairs, playing tennis or squash.	Alternate phrases: 'If you wish to reduce the load on your knees'. 'Sitting back more will reduce the load on your knees and increase the work around your hips and lower back'. Consider playing with each position to feel the differences in your own body and decide what works best for you, today.
'To avoid injury, make sure x body part is in line with x body part'.	1. Alignment is not nearly as important in preventing injury as we once thought. 2. Many people with supposedly 'suboptimal alignment' don't develop problems. 3. Attributing the cause of pain and injury solely to tissues and alignment fails to recognize the complexity of pain, and blames the physical body for more than it may be responsible for. This can cause unnecessary fear and fuel unhelpful beliefs about the body. 4. Programs to improve 'alignment', e.g. ergonomics, manual handling training, have not led to marked reductions in injury or pain. 5. The risk of injury is complex and involves multiple factors like sleep stress, general health and social support as well as physical factors.	Acknowledge that alignment may be relevant for some people but there are no rules for whole groups of people. Offer options and encourage people to explore moving in different ways and to find movement that feels good for them. Use neutral language that does not infer 'cause and effect'. Alternate phrases: 'If your x body part rolls in/out, try straightening it to see if that's more comfortable'. 'Roll your arm/knee/ankle in fully, then roll it out fully. Now try to find a position within that range that allows you to gain greater comfort/strength/mobility'. 'In this position, play with the tilt of your pelvis/breastbone. Now try to find a position within that range that allows you to gain greater comfort/strength/mobility'. 'If your x is not comfortable here, some different positions you could try are…'

continued

213

Table A.1 *continued*

Asana / example of instruction to avoid	Reasons to adjust this instruction	Guidance for evidence-based and balanced instruction
'To protect your back/pelvis/hip, activate mula bandha/your core/pelvic floor during this posture'	1. This instruction infers that strengthening these muscles can prevent injury, for which there is little evidence. 2. Pre-activation of pelvic floor and/or deep abdominal muscles has not been shown to consistently improve muscle activation patterns or result in better results than other exercise approaches for people with back pain. 3. While weakness may be an issue for some, for many people with back, hip and pelvic or pelvic girdle pain, these muscles are over-active and potentially contribute to pain.	Practice activating the pelvic floor or abdominal muscles with full relaxation at the end of the contraction (as you would for any other action). Alternate phrases: 'If you find this posture difficult, you may wish to consciously engage your pelvic floor/abdominal/gluteal muscles during the posture. Try to continue breathing normally, and at the end of the posture, relax your pelvic floor/abdominal/gluteal muscles as well'. 'Some options for this posture: if you know you tend to hold a lot of tension around your back /pelvis/hips, try to relax the muscles in that area. This may help you achieve better quality or a more comfortable pose/ movement'. 'If you are weak in this region, then try pre-tensing your pelvic floor/abdominals/gluteal muscles during the posture to see if it makes it more accessible for you. Try to continue breathing normally, and at the end of the posture, relax your pelvic floor/abdominal/gluteal muscles as well'.

This table provides examples of instructions to balance facilitating postures and movements that are well controlled, while allowing flexibility for the variation of normal movements and patterns. Examples of instructions to potentially avoid are also included.

GLOSSARY

Glossary of Scientific Terms		
Term	**Definition**	**In more detail**
Action potential	Electrical nerve signal.	An electrical signal that travels along the axon, away from the cell body to the axon terminal, where it triggers the release of neurotransmitters.
Afferent	Information coming into or towards the central nervous system.	
Algesia	Relates to sensitivity to pain.	
Analgesia	Absence of pain.	Absence of pain in response to stimulation which would normally be painful.*
Hyperalgesia	Increased pain sensitivity.	Increased pain in response to a stimulus that normally provokes pain.*
Hypoalgesia	Reduced pain sensitivity.	Diminished pain in response to a stimulus that normally provokes pain.*
Allostasis	How our bodies adjust to maintain physiological balance in response to stressors.	The process by which we maintain physiological stability (homeostasis) in response to actual or perceived physical, environmental or psychological stressors. This is achieved through activation of neural, endocrine and neuroendocrine-immune mechanisms. Allostatic load refers to the price of this: the wear and tear that adapting to stress and activation of different systems entails.
Autonomic nervous system	A branch of the nervous system that regulates involuntary physiologic processes including stress responses, heart rate, respiration, digestion and sexual arousal. It comprises the sympathetic nervous system and the parasympathetic nervous system.	
Sympathetic nervous system	A branch of the autonomic nervous system associated with elevated activity and attention: governs our fight, flight or freeze responses.	
Parasympathetic nervous system	A branch of the autonomic nervous system associated with reduced excitability: governs our rest and digest responses.	

continued

Glossary

Glossary of Scientific Terms *continued*		
Term	**Definition**	**In more detail**
Cortical	Relating to the cerebral cortex (see Glossary of Brain Areas).	
Disinhibition (within nervous system)	Loss of normal inhibition within the nervous system. Results in an over-excited (sensitized) state.	
Efferent	Information traveling away from or out of the central nervous system (towards the periphery).	
Endocrine system	System of glands and groups of cells that secrete hormones to control internal body states.	
Exteroceptive senses	Sensory inputs from outside the body including tactile inputs (e.g. touch, textures on the skin), visual, auditory, olfactory (smell) and gustatory (taste) inputs.	
Homeostasis	Self-regulating process by which a system remains stable by adjusting to changing conditions.	
Homunculus	Translates as 'Little Man'. Describes neurological maps in the brain dedicated to representations of the body.	
Motor homunculus	A map of brain areas dedicated to motor processing for different parts of the body.	
Sensory homunculus	A map of brain areas dedicated to sensory processing for different parts of the body.	
Hypothalamic–pituitary–adrenal (HPA) axis	Part of our central stress response system connecting the nervous system with the hormonal system. Represents a pathway of communication between the hypothalamus, pituitary gland and adrenal glands.	
Inhibition (within nervous system)	Inhibition of target nerve cells. Calms down signaling. Effected by the release of inhibitory neurotransmitters, e.g. GABA.	
Insomnia	Persistent difficulty with getting to sleep and staying asleep or sleep quality.	"A complaint of persistent difficulty with sleep initiation, duration, consolidation, or quality, that occurs despite adequate opportunity and circumstances for sleep, and results in some form of daytime impairment".[1]
Interoception	The sense of the internal workings of the body, e.g. systems of the body, cardiovascular, gastrointestinal, etc.	

continued

Term	Definition	In more detail
Kinesthetic awareness	Awareness of the body's position and movement in relation to the surrounding environment.	
Limbic system	Areas of the brain involved in emotional processing (see Glossary of Brain Areas).	
Mechanoreceptor	Sensory receptor that responds to mechanical pressure or distortion.	
Nerve		
Axon	Long projection of a nerve cell or neuron that conducts electrical signals – the transmission line of the nerve.	
Ion channel	Opening in neuron that allows ions to pass through, which in turn change the resting potential of the neuron to allow electrical signals (action potentials) to be sent.	A protein that acts as a pore or hole through the plasma membrane. When the ion channel is open, ions move between the inside and outside of the cell.
Nerve terminal	The end region of an axon; usually a site of synaptic contact with another cell.	
Synapse	The place where one neuron connects to another; a junction between neurons.	Junction between neurons. The synapse includes the nerve terminal of the first neuron, the place on the second neuron with receptors, and the space between them. The electrical signal in the axon of the first neuron triggers a chemical signal to be released into the gap that is picked up by receptors in the second neuron.
Nervous system	A vast network of cells that carry information to and from all parts of the body. It is comprised of the brain, the spinal cord and all the nerves in the body.	
Central nervous system	The brain and spinal cord.	
Peripheral nervous system	Nerves in the body (beyond the brain and spinal cord).	
Neuromatrix	A theory that our awareness of self results from, and is influenced by, activation of multiple brain areas in a coordinated way, and further that this awareness drives various responses when we're injured, unwell or under stress. This may be extrapolated into other experiences.	"A conceptual model that proposes that the body-self neuromatrix (a conscious awareness of the self, that is influenced by integrated brain activity) activates perceptual, homeostatic and behavioral responses following injury, pathology or chronic stress".[2]
Pain neuromatrix	Brain areas typically activated during pain experiences, which influence the pain experience and drive various physiological and behavioral responses.	

continued

Glossary

Glossary of Scientific Terms *continued*

Term	Definition	In more detail
Neuron	Nerve cell: basic functional unit of the nervous system.	
Neural circuit/ neural pathway	A set of neurons that are connected in sequence to produce a sensation, behavior or function; neural network.	
Neuron, dorsal root ganglion neurons	The cell bodies of sensory neurons that are grouped together (ganglions) and located just outside the spinal cord.	
Neuron, sensory	A neuron that picks up information from the body's sensory receptors (in the skin, muscle, joints, tongue, ear, nose and eyes) and carries it toward the central nervous system.	Sensory neurons detect environmental information necessary for the body to survive, e.g. touch, nociception, temperature, light, sound, taste, smell, balance, and information about muscles and joints.
Interneuron	A neuron that carries information between neurons. There are different types: projection neuron, inhibitory interneuron and excitation interneuron.	
Neuron, excitatory (interneuron)	A neuron (interneuron) that causes another neuron to fire a signal – excites the next neuron.	
Neuron, inhibitory (interneuron)	A neuron (interneuron) whose neurotransmitter produces inhibition in target cells, making it harder for the target cell to reach threshold.	
Neuron, projection (interneuron)	Neurons (interneurons) in the spinal cord that receive information from the sensory neurons and carry them to the brain.	
Neuroplasticity	How the nervous system adapts and changes in response to the demands that are placed on it.	
Neurotransmitters	Chemical messengers that communicate between neurons at junctions called synapses.	Chemicals released by nerve terminals at a synapse that crosses the synapse carrying information from the nerve terminal (pre-synaptic cell) to the dendrite (post-synaptic cell). Neurotransmitters relay information across the space between one neuron's nerve terminal and another neuron's dendrites. Examples: acetylcholine, glutamate, serotonin, GABA, endorphins, endocannabinoids, dopamine, adrenaline (epinephrine), noradrenaline (norepinephrine).

continued

Glossary of Scientific Terms *continued*

Term	Definition	In more detail
Nociception	The process of detecting a noxious stimulus – danger detection. Nociception does not necessarily mean pain occurs.	The neural process of encoding noxious stimuli.* *Note:* Consequences of encoding may be autonomic (e.g. elevated blood pressure) or behavioral (motor withdrawal reflex or more complex nocifensive behavior). Pain sensation is not necessarily implied.
Descending modulation of nociception	The 'brain's pharmacy': the brain and brain stem's ability to turn up or turn down the dial on nociceptive signaling. It does this by controlling release of various neurotransmitters.	
Modulation (of nociceptive pathways)	Adjustment of the excitability of nociceptive pathways and/or nociception.	
Nociceptive neuron	Neuron capable of detecting and transmitting a warning signal. Can be within either the peripheral or the central nervous system.	A central or peripheral neuron of the somatosensory nervous system that is capable of encoding noxious stimuli.*
Nociceptive stimulus	A stimulus that can indicate actual or potential tissue damage.	An actually or potentially tissue-damaging event transduced and encoded by nociceptors.*
Nociceptor	A receptor that responds when there is danger – danger detector.	A high-threshold sensory receptor of the peripheral somatosensory nervous system that is capable of transducing and encoding noxious stimuli.*
Anti-nociception/ anti-nociceptive state	A state within the nervous system where nociceptive signaling is reduced. Warning signals are turned down.	
Pro-nociception/ pro-nociceptive state	A state within the nervous system where nociceptive signaling is enhanced. Warning signals are turned up.	
Nocifensive	Describes a response to pain or discomfort.	
Noxious stimulus	An intense stimulus that is more likely to provoke pain	A stimulus that is damaging or threatens damage to normal tissues.*
Proprioception	Awareness of the body's position in relation to our environment based on the sensations generated by its own actions.	
Proprioceptors	Sensory receptors in the joints, muscles and ligaments which detect position and movement and relay this information to the brain.	

continued

Glossary of Scientific Terms *continued*		
Term	**Definition**	**In more detail**
Receptors	Molecules on nerve endings that detect stimuli and/or chemical messengers (neurotransmitters).	Special molecules on a nerve that detect, and may be activated by, neurotransmitters; neurotransmitter and receptor are specific to one another and must fit together like a lock and key.
Sensitization (nervous system)	Increased excitability of neurons in the nervous system, making it easier for them to fire.	Increased responsiveness of nociceptive neurons to their normal input, and/or recruitment of a response to normally subthreshold inputs.*
Central sensitization	Increased excitability of neurons in the *central* nervous system, making it easier for them to fire.	Increased responsiveness of nociceptive neurons in the central nervous system to their normal or subthreshold afferent input.*
Peripheral sensitization	Increased excitability of neurons in the *peripheral* nervous system, making it easier for them to fire.	Increased responsiveness and reduced threshold of nociceptive neurons in the periphery to the stimulation of their receptive fields.*

*Formal definition from the International Association for the Study of Pain.[3,4]

References

1. World Health Organisation. International Classification of Diseases, 11th Revision (ICD-11). 2018; Available from: https://icd.who.int/en.

2. Melzack, R. From the Gate to the Neuromatrix. Pain, 1999. Suppl 6: S121-6.

3. International Task Force on Taxonomy. Part III: Pain Terms, A Current List with Definitions and Notes on Usage, in: Classification of Chronic Pain, H. Merskey and N. Bogduk, Editors. 1994, Seattle: IASP Press. pp. 209–14.

4. International Association for the Study of Pain. IASP Terminology. 2019; Available from: http://www.iasp-pain.org.

Glossary of Brain Areas and Spinal Cord

Area	Main function
Amygdala	Part of the cerebral cortex involved in processing emotions, particularly fear; processes the memory of emotional reactions and adds emotional context to nociceptive information.
Anterior cingulate cortex (ACC)	Area of the cerebral cortex that forms part of the limbic system, which is involved with emotion formation and processing, learning and memory. Also involved in processing interoceptive inputs.
Brain stem	Part of the central nervous system connecting the brain to the spinal cord and cranial nerves. Involved in motor and sensory function.
	Functions to regulate cardiac and respiratory function as well as having an important role in modulating nociception. The periaqueductal gray (PAG) and rostral ventral medulla (RVM) are important parts of the brain's pharmacy that are housed in the brain stem.
Cerebellum	Part of the brain above the brain stem that primarily helps control movement, balance and muscle coordination.
Cerebral cortex	The main part of the brain. Consists of two hemispheres and 52 different component areas. Responsible for all forms of conscious experience, including perception, emotion, thought and planning.
Dorsal horn (of spinal cord)	Dorsal (back) part of the spinal cord gray matter where axons from sensory neurons enter and make their first synapses or connections with projection neurons that relay information to the brain.
Frontal cortex/frontal lobe	Any part of the frontal lobe of the cerebral cortex; responsible for attention, decision making, abstract thinking, problem solving, emotion, intellect, smell and personality; also includes the motor cortex so involved with movement.
Hippocampus	Part of the cerebral cortex responsible for spatial localization, formation of declarative memory, and transfer of short-term to long-term memories.
Hypothalamus	A small part of the cerebral cortex that lies below the thalamus, near the pituitary gland. It has important roles in regulating homeostatic and autonomic nervous system functions, e.g. releasing hormones, regulating body temperature, appetite, thirst, etc. It provides a key link between the nervous system and the endocrine (hormonal) system.
Insula	Part of the cerebral cortex involved in multisensory, emotional and cognitive processing. Sensorimotor processing involves processes of sensory information including interoception, and plays an important role in autonomic control. Thought to be involved in present-moment awareness, attention and salience processing.
Motor cortex	Part of the cerebral cortex involved in the planning, control and execution of voluntary movements.
Orbitofrontal cortex (OFC)	Part of the pre-frontal cortex involved in decision making.
Parietal cortex	Part of the cerebral cortex involved in processing and integration of spatial information and guiding initial physical responses based on this information.
Periaqueductal gray (PAG)	A cell-dense region surrounding the midbrain aqueduct. Involved in modulation of nociception, as well as cardiovascular and autonomic control.

continued

221

Glossary of Brain Areas and Spinal Cord *continued*

Area	Main function
Pituitary gland	Gland at the base of the brain. Makes and releases growth, reproductive and other hormones into the bloodstream.
Prefrontal cortex (PFC)	The most anterior (frontal) part of the cortex, which controls planning and thought. Has medial and lateral aspects.
Rostral ventromedial medulla (RVM)	Located in the brain stem. Main regulator of the sympathetic nervous system (autonomic control). Has an important role in descending modulation of nociceptive signaling.
Somatosensory cortex I and II (SI/SII)	Part of the cortex that receives sensory information about the body. Has a representative map of the body, which is updated based on sensory inputs and other experiences. Provides information for other regions to drive attention, decision-making and sensory-guided action, e.g. assists movement planning.
Thalamus	Area that lies above the brain stem between the cerebral cortex and midbrain. The main function of the thalamus is to relay motor and sensory signals to, and around, the cerebral cortex. Can be considered the reception desk or relay station of the brain.

Glossary of Yoga Terms			
Term	Definition	Traditional perspective[1]	How it relates to pain
Ahimsa	An intention to be kind to yourself.	Non-violence, reducing harm (yama).	An intention to use care when we think or talk about our impairments and pain; mindfulness with participation in activities; self-compassion.
And this too	A mantra to help facilitate inclusion of all that is present.	If this exists, then that exists; if we have happiness, we also have sadness – both are true.	Pain can be included in the story of a person without taking away the person. Allows for consideration of multiple contributions to a person's pain without a focus on one aspect.
Aparigraha	An intention to ourselves that we will find gratitude for what we have, we will give back to nature and to others, and we will be careful in relationships and scenarios of not grasping or attaching or escaping.	Non-possessiveness, non-greed, non-attachment, non-grasping (yama).	Allows for a balance of acceptance of our painful scenario without grasping for a way out of it or holding on to it as a way of life.
Asana	A physical practice to facilitate the ability to be stable in our bodies.	A position that is comfortable and steady.	Facilitates moving with mindfulness and care for pain with a sense of curiosity rather than avoiding and fearing (all) movement.
Asteya	An intention to not take more than what we need, strive for a balance of giving and receiving.	Non-stealing (yama).	Encourages taking responsibility for our pain care and needs; being an active participant in our care.
Brahmacharya	An intention to maintain an outlook and participate in behaviors that feed us rather than deplete us.	Appropriate use of one's vital energy (yama).	Encourages being proactive in our thoughts and actions during times of pain and struggle, e.g. spending time doing the things we can rather than ruminating on what we can't do.
Dharana	A practice of mindfulness to aid maintaining conscious concentration while limiting distractions.	Focus, concentration.	A practice of conscious choice of focus – be it breath, an object or movement – and letting other inputs be present without allowing them to distract you.
Dhyana	Meditation/mindfulness practice where a high level of focus is maintained.	Meditation, maintaining focus.	Specific meditation practices to help develop the ability to be mindful or present. Can improve self-regulation and improve descending modulation of nociception.
Dualism	A comparative way of living and thinking, e.g. us vs. them, bad vs. good.	A separation of any domain into two distinct categories.	Viewing pain as something that is bad and is meant to be eradicated, rather than recognizing the true role of pain as a normal sensory experience meant to protect us.

continued

Glossary of Yoga Terms *continued*			
Term	**Definition**	**Traditional perspective[1]**	**How it relates to pain**
Isvarapranidha	Faith	Devotion, surrender to a higher source.	Encourages maintaining faith that healing is possible and that not all things are in our control and that is OK. Can allow for including current personal spiritual or religious practices into pain care.
Meditation	See Dhyana above.		
Mindfulness	The act of being fully aware and present each moment: moment-to-moment awareness.	Being aware.	Encourages being aware and present in our body, mind and spirit during all moments, even those that include experience of pain. Developing mindfulness can improve self-regulation, and reduce distress and pain interference.
Niyama	Intentions we set for ourselves in hopes of living a balanced life of growth with a sense of contentment and freedom.	Personal ethics, internal restraints.	Taking care of the body, mind and spirit in a balanced, productive manner while participating in pain care.
Non-dualism	The ability to see the connectiveness and unity of all things.	Advaita: 'not two' or 'no second', the true self is the same as absolute reality.	Pain is a means of protection and connection. Persistent pain may give us an opportunity to learn more about ourselves and find greater compassion for all those around us. We are all human and we all have an element of struggle.
Pranayama	A practice of mindfulness using breath regulation as a focal point.	Regulation of breath to purify and strengthen energy.	Practicing breath focus for observation and control can facilitate relaxation (reduce stress responses) and mindfulness, anchoring both in stillness and movement.
Pratyahara	Awareness of our thoughts, emotions and physical sensations, regardless of what is happening around us. The practice of turning off the outside in order to turn inward.	Internalization of senses: to draw back from the outside world.	Harnessing the ability to turn inward during a painful experience to observe what is here, separating the internal inputs from the external inputs. Encourages the ability to recognize sensations (inputs) for what they are.
Real but not true	A mantra to help remind us that there are always real feelings behind our thoughts but often the thoughts themselves are not true.		We will acknowledge and lean into the emotional feelings or fear, grief, sadness, etc. associated with our pain experiences, at the same time looking for the falsities of our thoughts and emotions that may be driving unhelpful patterns and responses.

continued

Glossary of Yoga Terms *continued*			
Term	**Definition**	**Traditional perspective[1]**	**How it relates to pain**
Samadhi	A sense of blissfulness and inner joy. The culmination of the practice that remains, regardless of our life's situations and scenarios.	Complete absorption.	The culmination of moving beyond the person who is suffering with pain to a person who has pain AND a sense of inner joy and connection.
Santosha	An intention to acknowledge that contentment comes from within and not from the outside world of material gains or recognition – can be part of a practice of gratitude for what we have.	Contentment.	Encourages knowing that we are struggling with pain but we are also OK, both can exist and we can find gratitude in the midst of our hardships.
Satya	An intention to see a scenario for what it is, recognizing all that is present without placing blame or taking credit.	Truth (yama).	Encourages being honest with ourselves and others, fully recognizing our current abilities and struggles, and avoiding blaming or being a victim of our painful scenarios.
Saucha (Sauca)	An intention to start and end the day 'clean' in mind, body and emotions – letting go of experiences and expectations to allow what is to be.	Purity, cleanliness (niyamas).	An intention to clean our expectations around pain – how, when and why it is, or will be present. Holding each experience for what it is in the moment that it is there.
Self	The consistent center of 'you'.	The witness or conscious observer.	Acknowledging that the inner self is maintained during the pain experience.
Spirit	The way in which our inner self connects with the outside world.	The non-physical aspect of you that anchors emotions and character.	The way in which our inner self is present and expressed during pain care.
Svadhyaya	An intention to study ourselves from the inside rather than the exterior, with a sense of care and kindness, and attempting to avoid judgment and comparisons.	Self-study/observation (niyama).	Encourages self-study and learning about our pain from the scientific biological side as well as observing the internal behaviors, kindly identifying areas where we are not helping ourselves and maximizing areas where we are helping or can help ourselves.
Tapas	An intention to participate in the actions and behaviors that help to take us in the direction we want to go.	Self-will, practice causing change (niyama) – can be said to have an element of heat.	Taking an active, disciplined and potentially difficult role in our pain care; choosing to find our own resilience.

continued

Glossary

Glossary of Yoga Terms *continued*			
Term	**Definition**	**Traditional perspective**[1]	**How it relates to pain**
Yama	Ethics or intentions that promote co-existence in a peaceful community.	Social ethics, restraints (five subcategories).	Intentions to promote a cooperative nature to pain care – acknowledging and taking personal responsibilities in the process.
Yoga	The study of self through a practice or discipline that brings together the mind, body and spirit through physical postures, meditation and mindfulness during daily life.	To yoke the mind, body and soul (emotions) together in study with a goal to live with awareness.	An inclusive practice or 'container' to hold the many dimensions of ourselves, our pain experiences and our ability to move beyond a life controlled by pain. Can be used as a vehicle for self-study with pain experiences and includes tools that can facilitate moving beyond pain.

References

1. Bachman, N. (2005). Language of Yoga: Complete A To Y Guide to Asana Names, Sanskrit Terms and Chants. 2005, Boulder, CO: Sounds True, Inc.

INDEX

Index continued